Trigeminal Neuralgia

Kwan Park • Kyung Rae Cho
Editors

Trigeminal Neuralgia

A Comprehensive Guide

Springer

Editors
Kwan Park
Department of Neurosurgery
Konkuk University Medical Center
Seoul, Korea (Republic of)

Kyung Rae Cho
Department of Neurosurgery
Konkuk University Medical Center
Seoul, Korea (Republic of)

ISBN 978-981-19-9170-7 ISBN 978-981-19-9171-4 (eBook)
https://doi.org/10.1007/978-981-19-9171-4

This Springer imprint is published by the registered company Springer Nature Singapore Pte Ltd.
The registered company address is: 152 Beach Road, #21-01/04 Gateway East, Singapore 189721, Singapore

Preface

This book provides a comprehensive guide from A to Z of trigeminal neuralgia. This book is composed of three parts: basics of trigeminal neuralgia, microvascular decompression, and ablative treatment and related issues.

In the first part, we introduce recent advances of pathophysiology, clinical diagnosis, differential diagnosis, and concerns about electrophysiological diagnosis. Moreover, radiological evaluation of trigeminal neuralgia is discussed with recent advances of magnetic resolution imaging techniques. Finally, medical treatments used in neuralgic patients are discussed in this part.

The second part is the key part in this book. Dr. Park, the Chief Editor of this book, has over 5000 cases of microvascular decompression for hemifacial spasm and trigeminal neuralgia. In this chapter, we have included everything that you need to know about microvascular decompression surgery for trigeminal neuralgia. From anesthesia, intraoperative neuromonitoring, key surgical technique with interposition and transposition techniques, surgical pearls and pitfalls in MVD, how to prevent CSF leak, possible complications, prognosis and concerns about re-do surgery. We have tried to include every knowledge about MVD for TN in this part.

The last part is about ablative therapies. From percutaneous procedures and stereotactic radiosurgery, balloon and glycerol rhizotomy and neuromodulatory treatments are not yet clear in the field. Finally, we have included related issues about secondary TN, glossopharyngeal neuralgia, and otalgia. We should differentiate that with classic TN.

This book would be helpful for medical school students, residents, and physicians of neurology, pain, and anesthesiology, especially neurosurgery. We hope this book can help anyone who is taking care of those suffering from this devastating pain syndrome.

Seoul, Republic of Korea — Kwan Park
Seoul, Republic of Korea — Kyung Rae Cho

Contents

Part I

Basics of Trigeminal Neuralgia

Overview of Trigeminal Neuralgia

Jae Sung Park and Kwan Park

1 Definition of Trigeminal Neuralgia

Trigeminal neuralgia (TN) is a manifestation of orofacial neuropathic pain that is recurrent, abrupt in onset and termination, triggered by innocuous stimuli, and typically compared to an electric shock or described as shooting or stabbing; the pain is typically restricted to one or more divisions of the fifth cranial nerve (CN V) [1]. Since the term TN may encompass several disease entities that are related to one another, yet not exactly identical, a number of classification systems have been suggested and used: classical vs. secondary, typical vs. atypical, type I vs. II, idiopathic vs. iatrogenic, related to multiple sclerosis (MS) or herpes zoster, etc. [2]. To minimize confusion, this chapter will use the classification according to The International Classification of Headache Disorders, third edition (ICHD-3) [3]. Diagnosis of TN must be based on the clinical history and physical examination, although subcategorization and differential diagnosis often require other imaging assessment such as magnetic resonance imaging (MRI) or computed tomography (CT).

J. S. Park
Department of Neurosurgery, Konyang University Hospital, Konyang University College of Medicine, Daejeon, Republic of Korea

K. Park (✉)
Department of Neurosurgery, Konkuk University Medical Center, Konkuk University School of Medicine, Seoul, Republic of Korea
e-mail: kwanpark@skku.edu

2 History

Prior to the current official term that is TN, the neuropathic pain syndrome in the face used to be referred as Fothergill's disease since John Fothergill presented arguably the first and accurate description of symptoms of TN in 1773 [4]. He regarded TN as a "cancerous acrimony" because of its persistence and incurability and stated that it can be triggered by light touch. A few years earlier, in 1756, a French surgeon Nicolas Andre reported three patients' symptom that was quite consistent with TN which he then named "Tic douloureux," and he treated them with neurectomy [5]. If we go back further in time, the famous Ibn Sina, also known as Avicenna (980–1037), mentioned a condition equivalent to TN in his book "Cannon of Medicine": pain over the facial skeleton, numbness and involuntary facial tics [6]. His understanding that the nerves conducted pain was later shared by a near contemporary scholar, Esmail Jorjani (1042–1137), a Persian physician. Jorjani described syndromes that were probably consistent with trigeminal neuralgia, hemifacial spasm, and Bell's palsy in his book "Treasure of the Khawarazm Shah" where he concurred with Avicenna in that pain was conducted via nerves, yet he also implicated

K. Park, K. R. Cho (eds.), *Trigeminal Neuralgia*, https://doi.org/10.1007/978-981-19-9171-4_1

an artery-nerve conflict as an etiology of trigeminal neuralgia [6]. In the 1820s, Charles bell attributed this pain syndrome of the face to the trigeminal nerve; accordingly, the disease gained a new term, TN. TN however was interchangeably used with Fothergill's disease and tic douloureux, during the nineteenth century and up until the early twentieth century. TN in the twentieth century entered into a new phase, especially since the use of antiepileptic drugs and introduction of microvascular decompression. Starting from difenylhydantoin in 1942, other antiepileptics were introduced, among which, Carbabazepine has become the drug of choice [7, 8]. Surgical treatment for TN includes open neurectomy, percutaneous ablative techniques, radiosurgery, and microvascular decompression(MVD). MVD was first introduced by Dandy in 1925, then adopted and practiced by Taarnhøj and Gardener in 1950s [9–11]. Jannetta's application of microscope-assisted MVD in 1972 certainly initiated a new era in the treatment of not only TN but also HFS and glossopharyngeal neuralgia [12]. MVD is currently accepted worldwide, and it deserves a special place among all treatment options, given that it can provide a cure despite its nondestructive nature.

3 Epidemiology

The reported annual incidence rate of TN varies, e.g., 2 per 100,000/year (PY) in 1966 or 8/100,000 PY in 2000 [13, 14]. A meta-analysis performed in 2014 concluded that it was estimated as 12.6–28.9/100,000 PY [15, 16]. The overall prevalence of TN was reported around 0.7/1000 persons, but it tends to be higher in more advanced age groups since the initial onset of the symptoms most frequently starts at the age of 50–60 years [14, 17]. The female to male ratio in the incidence of TN is about 3:2 [18]. In terms of ethnic differences, Jannetta stated that among cranial nerve dysfunction syndromes, HFS is more prevalent in Asians than in Caucasians, whereas TN is more common in Caucasians, although no cohort study is available for this observation [19].

4 Etiology and Pathophysiology

Neurovascular compression is now the generally accepted etiology of TN [20]. Classical TN refers to TN where an actual neurovascular compression, not just a contact, is identified in MRI or during the surgery [1]. Secondary TN is defined as the trigeminal neuropathy caused by underlying diseases mainly by either demyelinating conditions (e.g., multiple sclerosis) or space-occupying lesions (e.g., cerebellopontine angle tumor). Those with proper TN symptoms, yet met with criteria of neither classical nor secondary TN, are classified as idiopathic TN.

Three known causes of TN, i.e., neurovascular compression, space-occupying lesions, and multiple sclerosis, share one microscopic feature—the demyelination process found in the root entry zone (REZ). The REZ which belongs to central nervous system (CNS) tissues rather than peripheral nervous system (PNS) is known to harbor the transition of peripheral Schwann cell myelination to central oligodendroglial myelination [21]. According to Jannetta and numerous other authors, vascular compression on the REZ or its close vicinity is responsible for TN in up to 90% of entire cases [22, 23]. Microscopic and neurophysiological pathophysiology of TN when the REZ is compressed by a vessel has not reached a unanimous conclusion; abnormal impulses of gasserian ganglion, demyelinated nerve root, or the trigeminal nucleus in the brain stem have been detected and attributed to the cause of TN. Ectopic generations of sensory impulses alongside ephaptic transmission, or cross-talk, between demyelinated fibers seem to be acknowledged by the majority of researchers [24, 25]. A central role in the brain stem was also suggested, given that some neuralgic attacks could be triggered by a stimulation that is not on the trigeminal branch with symptoms, such as bright lights or loud noises [26]. However, the fact that the majority of patients with TN experience symptomatic relief immediately after MVD might preclude the involvement of the trigeminal nucleus as the main pathogenesis [27].

5 Diagnosis

Diagnosis of TN is mainly based on clinical features, but it is neither simple nor straightforward. Several diagnostic criteria and classifications have been suggested, which indicates still ongoing controversy about them. The first condition in the diagnosis of TN is, of course, its location—distribution of the trigeminal nerve. Most individuals suffer pain in the areas where maxillary and mandibular branches innervate, while only 4% of TN cases involve the ophthalmic division only [28]. When the pain is located in the tongue base, a sharp differentiation from glossopharyngeal neuralgia (GPN) is imperative, for it is where the trigeminal and glossopharyngeal nerves may overlap. Further inquiries must be made if the pain also involves deep throat or ear, which may lead to the diagnosis of GPN. One must remember that diagnosis of TN does not automatically rule out GPN, and vice versa. Concurrent TN and GPN can be possible and very challenging in diagnosis, and consequently successful treatment. Other frequent differential diagnosis includes neuropathic trigeminal pain, pulpitis, temporomandibular disorder, paroxysmal hemicrania, short unilateral neuralgiform pain with autonomic symptoms, etc. [29].

The second condition of diagnosis is the characteristics—severe in intensity, electric shock-like, shooting, stabbing and sharp in quality, and periodicity of paroxysmal occurrences, each lasting less than 2 min with definite refractory periods. Unlike other neuropathic pains, up to 63% of TN patients can enjoy complete, yet temporary remission that can be as long as years [30]. In terms of frequency of attacks, it can vary from 1 to over 50 a day, and it may or may not increase during the course of the disease [31].

The third condition is that it can be triggered by innocuous stimuli such as chewing, talking, cold wind, or brushing teeth. Spontaneous attacks are not impossible, but a thorough investigation into patients' history would probably reveal the triggering factors in the past. These innocuous stimuli can be similar to those of GPN, and whether or not an individual identifies these triggering factors cannot be a differentiation criterion. The diagnosis of TN can be made when the aforementioned three conditions are met and there are no better-accounted diseases according to ICHD-3 classifications [3].

After a clinical observation and thorough history taking yields the diagnosis of TN, CT or MRI is recommended for further classification and differential diagnosis. Classical, secondary, or idiopathic TN can be identified via MRI with or without gadolinium enhancement. When MRI is unavailable, neurophysiologic recordings including trigeminal evoked potentials and trigeminal reflexes might be helpful for differentiation [32].

6 Treatment

6.1 Nonsurgical Treatment

Pharmaceutical treatment for TN should start with carbamazepine in primary care [33]. Carbamazepine, the treatment of choice, is reported to yield 100% pain relief in 70% of patients during the initial application, though its side effects including memory and cognition impairment oftentimes cannot be overlooked [34]. Aside from carbamazepine (300–1000 mg), 4 other drugs recommended by randomized clinical trials(RCTs) can also be considered: oxcarbazepine (300–1200 mg), baclofen (50–80 mg), lamotrigine (200–400 mg), and gabapentin (1800–3600 mg) with 4 mg injection of ropivacaine [35–37]. Pregabalin (150–600 mg) also has been used yielding a substantial improvement of the pain, although yet to be proven by RCTs. Intravenous fosphenytoin can be administered for acute pain management, as well as topical injections of lidocaine. In spite of the excellent initial response to the aforementioned medications for TN in its early stage, the improvement of pain appears to decline to 50% over time. It is estimated that about 44–50% of TN patients no longer benefit from the medication only, due to either intolerable side effects or loss of therapeutic effects [38]. For these medically intractable subjects, surgical options should be offered.

Onabotulinumtoxin A (BTX-A), when 20–50 IU of it injected into the trigger zone, might be helpful in decreasing the pain intensity of TN in the long term [39]. BTX-A for TN patients showed a superior result to a placebo in a meta-analysis, although it was not recommended to replace the pharmacological treatment [40].

6.2 Surgical Treatment

Surgical procedures for TN can be divided into destructive and nondestructive techniques. Destructive techniques include percutaneous rhizotomy and gamma knife radiosurgery (RS); the percutaneous rhizotomy again can be divided into thermal (radiofrequency), mechanical (balloon compression of the Gasserian ganglion), and chemical (glycerol injection) rhizotomy. Regardless of the type of the source (thermal, mechanical, or chemical), percutaneous rhizotomy overall can yield pain improvement in up to 90% population at their initial procedure. The recurrence rate however was reported as 25–50% in 3–5 years [41, 42]. Moreover, permanent complications such as loss of sensation, dysesthesia, and anesthesia dolorosa often cannot be tolerated by patients [43]. Unlike percutaneous approaches, RS is performed noninvasively other than application of the Leksell frame. Under MR imaging guidance, a single isocenter of 4 mm size with a maximum dose of 80Gy radiation is most frequently used. According to a meta-analysis concerning RS vs. MVD in 2017, the success rate of RS was highest in the second year (77.8%) and it declined to 63.8% after 5 years, whereas that of MVD was 91.4% in 2 years and 84% in 5 years [44]. Dysesthesia was more frequent in RS group compared to MVD one (28.1 vs. 2.3%), whereas the incidence of hearing loss was lower in the former (0.7% vs. 1.5%).

MVD is the only nondestructive and the most frequently performed surgical option for TN, though it is most invasive in that it requires a retro-sigmoid craniotomy under general anesthesia. The basic technique of MVD is well described in the literature, but the detailed maneuver varies depending on surgeons. Once a lateral retrosigmoid suboccipital craniectomy or craniotomy is performed under general anesthesia, the dura is incised to reveal the cerebellar cortex. With or without traction of the cerebellum, the root entry zone (REZ) of the trigeminal nerve is observed. Upon the identification of the compressing vessels, or the offending arteries, which is most frequently superior cerebellar artery (SCA), they are separated from the fifth nerve, which then can be perpetuated by insertion of Teflon pieces. A few more additional techniques, including transposition of the vessels, snare technique, vascular sling, etc., have been proposed.

The estimated overall success rate (pain-free) of MVD for TN varies. According to the previously mentioned meta-analysis in 2017 with 12,450 TN patients, it was estimated as 84% in 5 years, whereas another meta-analysis in 2020 with 3897 subjects reported that it was 75.8% (mean follow-up duration of 1.7 ± 1.3 year) [44, 45]. Factors that affect the favorable outcome following MVD for TN include shorter disease duration (4.6 vs. 6.4 years), identifiable artery compression during MVD, preoperatively noted compression by MRI, classical TN, and involvement of SCA [45]. Major complications after MVD are hearing loss, CSF leak, meningitis, or facial palsy, while minor complications would include dysesthesia, vertigo, wound infection, etc.

Other possible treatment options for TN, yet to be acknowledged as a standard treatment, would be neuromodulation via motor cortex stimulation, deep brain stimulation in the posterior hypothalamus, and peripheral stimulation/magnetic stimulation, etc. [46]

References

1. Scholz J, Finnerup NB, Attal N, et al. The IASP classification of chronic pain for ICD-11: chronic neuropathic pain. Pain. 2019;160:53.
2. Eller JL, Raslan AM, Burchiel KJ. Trigeminal neuralgia: definition and classification. Neurosurg Focus. 2005;18:1–3.
3. Arnold M. Headache classification committee of the international headache society (IHS) the international classification of headache disorders. Cephalalgia. 2018;38:1–211.

4. Stookey A, Ransohoff J. Trigeminal neuralgia: its history and treatment. Oxford; 1959.
5. Brown JA, Coursaget C, Preul MC, Sangvai D. Mercury water and cauterizing stones: Nicolas Andre and tic douloureux. J Neurosurg. 1999;90:977–81.
6. Shoja MM, Tubbs RS, Khalili M, Khodadoost K, Loukas M, Cohen-Gadol AA. Esmail Jorjani (1042–1137) and his descriptions of trigeminal neuralgia, hemifacial spasm, and Bell's palsy. Neurosurgery. 2010;67:431–4.
7. Bergouignan M. Cures heureuses de nevralgies faciales essentielles par le diphenylhydantoinate de soude. Rev Laryngol Otol Rhinol. 1942;63:34–41.
8. Liu JK, Apfelbaum RI. Treatment of trigeminal neuralgia. Neurosurgery Clinics. 2004;15:319–34.
9. Dandy WE. Section of the sensory root of the trigeminal nerve at the pons: preliminary report of the operative procedure. Baltimore: Johns Hopkins Hospital; 1925.
10. Taarnhøj P. Decompression of the trigeminal root and the posterior part of the ganglion as treatment in trigeminal neuralgia: preliminary communication. J Neurosurg. 1952;9:288–90.
11. Gardner WJ, Pinto JP. The tarrnhoj operation; relief of trigeminal neuralgia without numbness. Cleve Clin Q. 1953;20:364–7.
12. Barker FG, Jannetta PJ, Bissonette DJ, Larkins MV, Jho HD. The long-term outcome of microvascular decompression for trigeminal neuralgia. N Engl J Med. 1996;334:1077–84.
13. Brewis M, Poskanzer DC, Rolland C, Miller H. Neurological disease in an English city. Acta Neurol Scand. 1966;42:1–89.
14. MacDonald B, Cockerell O, Sander J, Shorvon S. The incidence and lifetime prevalence of neurological disorders in a prospective community-based study in the UK. Brain. 2000;123:665–76.
15. Kurtzke JF. Neuroepidemiology. Ann Neurol. 1984;16:265–77.
16. Van Hecke O, Austin SK, Khan RA, Smith B, Torrance N. Neuropathic pain in the general population: a systematic review of epidemiological studies. Pain. 2014;155:654–62.
17. Katusic S, Beard CM, Bergstralth E, Kurland LT. Incidence and clinical features of trigeminal neuralgia, Rochester, Minnesota, 1945–1984. Ann Neurol. 1990;27:89–95.
18. Khan M, Nishi SE, Hassan SN, Islam M, Gan SH. Neuralgia, Glossopharyngeal neuralgia, and myofascial pain dysfunction syndrome: an update. Pain Res Manag. 2017;2017:7438326.
19. Jannetta PJ. Observations on the etiology of trigeminal neuralgia, hemifacial spasm, acoustic nerve dysfunction and glossopharyngeal neuralgia. Definitive microsurgical treatment and results in 117 patients. Neurochirurgia. 1977;20:145–54.
20. Maarbjerg S, Di Stefano G, Bendtsen L, Cruccu G. Trigeminal neuralgia–diagnosis and treatment. Cephalalgia. 2017;37:648–57.
21. Peker S, Kurtkaya Ö, Üzün I, Pamir MN. Microanatomy of the central myelin-peripheral myelin transition zone of the trigeminal nerve. Neurosurgery. 2006;59:354–9.
22. Jannetta PJ. Neurovascular compression in cranial nerve and systemic disease. Ann Surg. 1980;192:518.
23. McLaughlin MR, Jannetta PJ, Clyde BL, Subach BR, Comey CH, Resnick DK. Microvascular decompression of cranial nerves: lessons learned after 4400 operations. J Neurosurg. 1999;90:1–8.
24. Magerl W, Treede R-D. Secondary tactile hypoesthesia: a novel type of pain-induced somatosensory plasticity in human subjects. Neurosci Lett. 2004;361:136–9.
25. Love S, Coakham HB. Trigeminal neuralgia: pathology and pathogenesis. Brain. 2001;124:2347–60.
26. Bowsher D. Trigeminal neuralgia: an anatomically oriented review. Clin Anat. 1997;10:409–15.
27. Leandri M, Eldridge P, Miles J. Recovery of nerve conduction following microvascular decompression for trigeminal neuralgia. Neurology. 1998;51:1641–6.
28. Rozen TD. Trigeminal neuralgia and glossopharyngeal neuralgia. Neurol Clin. 2004;22:185–206.
29. Zakrzewska JM, McMillan R. Trigeminal neuralgia: the diagnosis and management of this excruciating and poorly understood facial pain. Postgrad Med J. 2011;87:410–6.
30. Maarbjerg S, Gozalov A, Olesen J, Bendtsen L. Trigeminal neuralgia–a prospective systematic study of clinical characteristics in 158 patients. Headache. 2014;54:1574–82.
31. Di Stefano G, La Cesa S, Truini A, Cruccu G. Natural history and outcome of 200 outpatients with classical trigeminal neuralgia treated with carbamazepine or oxcarbazepine in a tertiary centre for neuropathic pain. J Headache Pain. 2014;15:1–5.
32. Cruccu G, Finnerup NB, Jensen TS, et al. Trigeminal neuralgia: new classification and diagnostic grading for practice and research. Neurology. 2016;87:220–8.
33. Zakrzewska JM, Linskey ME. Trigeminal neuralgia. BMJ. 2014;348:g474.
34. Wiffen PJ, Derry S, Moore RA, McQuay HJ. Carbamazepine for acute and chronic pain in adults. Cochrane Database Syst Rev. 2011;(1):CD005451.
35. Wiffen PJ, Derry S, Moore RA, Kalso EA. Carbamazepine for chronic neuropathic pain and fibromyalgia in adults. Cochrane Database Syst Rev. 2014;4:CD005451.
36. Zakrzewska JM, Linskey ME. Trigeminal neuralgia. BMJ. 2009;2009:1207.
37. Longson D. Neuropathic pain–pharmacological management: the pharmacological management of neuropathic pain in adults in non-specialist settings. NICE. 2013:173.
38. Taylor J, Brauer S, Espir M. Long-term treatment of trigeminal neuralgia with carbamazepine. Postgrad Med J. 1981;57:16–8.
39. Hu Y, Guan X, Fan L, et al. Therapeutic efficacy and safety of botulinum toxin type a in trigeminal

neuralgia: a systematic review. J Headache Pain. 2013;14:1–8.
40. Morra ME, Elgebaly A, Elmaraezy A, et al. Therapeutic efficacy and safety of botulinum toxin a therapy in trigeminal neuralgia: a systematic review and meta-analysis of randomized controlled trials. J Headache Pain. 2016;17:1–9.
41. Baabor MG, Perez-Limonte L. Percutaneous balloon compression of the gasserian ganglion for the treatment of trigeminal neuralgia: personal experience of 206 patients. Acta Neurochir Suppl. 2011;108:251–4.
42. Kondziolka D, Lunsford LD. Percutaneous retrogasserian glycerol rhizotomy for trigeminal neuralgia: technique and expectations. Neurosurg Focus. 2005;18:1–4.
43. Gronseth G, Cruccu G, Alksne J, et al. Practice parameter: the diagnostic evaluation and treatment of trigeminal neuralgia (an evidence-based review): report of the quality standards Subcommittee of the American Academy of neurology and the European Federation of Neurological Societies. Neurology. 2008;71:1183–90.
44. Gubian A, Rosahl SK. Meta-analysis on safety and efficacy of microsurgical and radiosurgical treatment of trigeminal neuralgia. World Neurosurg. 2017;103:757–67.
45. Holste K, Chan AY, Rolston JD, Englot DJ. Pain outcomes following microvascular decompression for drug-resistant trigeminal neuralgia: a systematic review and meta-analysis. Neurosurgery. 2020;86:182–90.
46. Jones MR, Urits I, Ehrhardt KP, et al. A comprehensive review of trigeminal neuralgia. Curr Pain Headache Rep. 2019;23:1–7.

Pathogenesis of Trigeminal Neuralgia

Soonwook Kwon and Ju-Hong Min

1 Basic Anatomy

Trigeminal nerve is the largest cranial nerve and the sensory nerve of the face and innervates to the mastication muscles [1]. This one-pair nerve divides into two pure sensory nerves, ophthalmic and maxillary nerves, and one mixed nerve, mandibular nerve. The ophthalmic nerve is responsible for sensory in the upper part of the eyebrow of the head, meninx, and cornea through the superior ophthalmic fissure, the maxillary nerve for sensory in the upper lip, maxillary teeth, and mucosa through the foramen rotundum, and the mandibular nerve for the sensory of the mandible, lower lip, mucosa, and mandibular teeth through the foramen ovale crossing the Gasserian ganglion to the pons [2]. Motor component of the trigeminal nerve leaves the pons, passes beneath the Gasserian ganglion, and then merges with the sensory nerve to make the mandibular nerve [3].

The sensory afferents that transmit ipsilateral discriminative sensation, light touch proprioception of the jaw, make synapses in the principal sensory nucleus of the trigeminal nerve in the dorsal pons. The second-order neurons from the ventrolateral nucleus have synapses in the contralateral ventral posteromedial (VPM) nucleus of the thalamus along the trigeminothalamic tract. Fibers from the dorsomedial principal sensory nucleus make synapses in the ipsilateral VPM of the thalamus [4].

The sensory afferents that transmit the sense of pain and temperature make synapses in the ipsilateral spinal nucleus of the trigeminal nerve, which is distributed from the lateral medulla to the third or fourth segments of the cervical spinal cord. The spinal nucleus of the trigeminal nerve is divided into pars oralis, pars interpolaris, and pars caudalis, according to the area responsible for the facial sense with the onion-skin pattern. Second-order neurons cross the medulla and synapse in the contralateral VPM of the thalamus along the ventral trigeminothalamic tract. The third neurons from the thalamus project to the primary and secondary somatosensory cortex and limbic system which include insula, and anterior cingulate gyrus [5].

S. Kwon
Department of Neurology, Inha University School of Medicine, Incheon, Republic of Korea

J.-H. Min (✉)
Department of Neurology, Samsung Medical Center, Sungkyunkwan University School of Medicine, Seoul, Republic of Korea

Department of Neurology, Neuroscience Center, Samsung Medical Center, Seoul, Republic of Korea

Department of Health Sciences and Technology, SAIHST, Sungkyunkwan University, Seoul, Republic of Korea

K. Park, K. R. Cho (eds.), *Trigeminal Neuralgia*, https://doi.org/10.1007/978-981-19-9171-4_2

2 Pain Transmission

The pain and temperature stimuli are transmitted by Aδ and C. Innocuous and proprioceptive stimuli are transmitted by myelinated Aα and Aβ fibers to the mesencephalic trigeminal nucleus. The thinly myelinated Aδ fiber and unmyelinated C-fiber are widely distributed in the head and neck regions and transmit the signal from the thermal or mechanical nociceptors of free nerve ending [6, 7]. Nociceptors of Aδ fibers are mechanothermal nociceptors which are responsive to high-threshold mechanical or thermal stimuli. Nociceptors in free nerve ending of C-fibers are called C multimodal nociceptors because they respond to various sources of stimuli, such as heat, mechanical stimuli, or chemical stimuli [6]. Aδ mechanoreceptors are sensitive to repeated stimuli and C multimodal nociceptors have a wider range than Aδ mechanoreceptors. The conduction velocity (CV) of Aδ fibers is about 5–40 m/s and the CV of C-fiber is slower than Aδ fibers, about 0.5–2.0 m/s due to the unmyelination of the axon, which may explain different pain responses to noxious stimuli in these two fibers. When a noxious stimulus occurs, immediate and temporary sharp pain is caused by the Aδ fibers, followed by burning pain by the C-fibers [8, 9]. Signals from Aδ and C-fibers are transmitted to the spinal nucleus of the trigeminal nerve, mostly [10].

Various molecules are involved in pain transmission. At the site of injured peripheral nerves, inflammatory mediators such as prostaglandin E2 (PGE2), TNFα, IL-1β, IL-6, and brain-derived neurotrophic factor (BDNF) are increased, stimulate the nociceptor fibers of Aδ and C-fibers and increase neuronal excitability [11, 12]. Expression of transient receptor potential vanilloid 1 (TRPV1) receptors which are polymodal receptors and transient receptor potential cation channel subfamily A, member (TRPA1) receptors which transmit signals for pain, cold, and itch are increased and have a lower threshold for activation after nerve injury [13–16]. The level of substance P and CGRP which are pronociceptive neuropeptide in trigeminal nerve and Gasserian ganglion are increased [17].

3 Pain Modulation in Central Nervous System

Pain modulation is controlled by the descending pathway of the central nervous system (CNS) [18]. Activation of periaqueductal gray matter (PAG) decreases pain, which is thought to be due to an opioid-mediated response [19]. PAG is connected with nucleus raphe magnus (NRM) and rostral ventromedial medulla (RVM) [20]. They affect the spinal dorsal horn, suppressing or enhancing the pain in the pain modulation. On-cell in RVM promotes the transmission of noxious stimuli and morphine or mu-agonists inhibit the activation of these cells. Off cells in RVM inhibit the transmission of noxious stimuli and opioid agonists activate the activation of these cells [21].

4 Pathophysiology of Trigeminal Neuralgia

4.1 Nerve Vascular Compression and Focal Demyelination

Classic trigeminal neuralgia (TN) is known to result from neurovascular compression (NVD) [22]. The trigeminal nerve is the site of pain, and nerve damage and dysfunction occur as it is compressed by the artery in the dorsal root entry zone by repeated microtrauma from the pulsating vessel. Dorsal root zone (DRZ, Redlich-obersteiner's zone) is the transition area between CNS and peripheral nerve system, where myelin produced by Schwann cell changes myelin produced by oligodendrocyte. The transition area has a length of about 1.0–2.5 mm [23]. Demyelination occurs when the DRZ is pressed for a long time by artery, mainly the superior cerebellar artery followed by anterior inferior cerebellar artery, posterior inferior cerebellar artery, and vertebral artery [24, 25]. Atrophy or hypertrophy of the trigeminal nerves was observed, and axonal loss, damaged Schwann cells, demyelination, and dysmyelination were confirmed in pathology [26]. In particular, the Aδ fiber is vulnerable to nociceptive stimuli which cause spontaneous activity (ectopic action potential) and ephaptic conduction to the surrounding fibers, causing pain. (Ignition hypothesis) Pain relief after microvascular decompression surgery which separates the trigeminal nerve and blood vessels that compress the nerve is considered as the evidence of mechanism [27, 28].

4.2 Sodium Channel and Potassium Channel in Trigeminal Neuralgia

Dandy et al. reported that 40% of patients with TN did not have a gross lesion including NVD [29]. Using high-resolution MRI, the occurrence of TN without NVD was about 27% and the age of onset was younger than those of TN patients with NVD [30, 31]. Rarely, TN patients without NVD have an autosomal dominant inheritance family history [32]. Although the molecular basis is not yet clear, dysregulation in ion channels is thought to be an important mechanism. Dysregulation of the voltage-gated sodium channel is important to induce ectopic activity and neuronal excitability in TN [33]. In a previous study, downregulation of Nav1.7 and upregulation of Nav 1.3 which had rapid activation and inactivation, and a three times faster recovery after hyperpolarization than Nav1.7 was confirmed in the TN animal model [34]. At the trigeminal nuclei system, dysregulation of voltage-gated sodium channels is involved in secondary hyperalgesia and central sensitization [35]. In addition, a gain-of-function mutation of the *SCN8A* gene, a gene of Nav1.6, was reported to cause infantile epileptic encephalopathy [33]. The mutation of Nav1.6 reduces the threshold for action potential and enhances significant hyperexcitability of trigeminal ganglia and neuron. Dysregulation of voltage-gated potassium channel Kv7.2 has also been confirmed, which is associated with allodynia and hyperalgesia caused by cold stimulation. The increase in Kv7.2 appears to be due to a compensatory mechanism of decreased neuronal excitability after nerve injury [36, 37].

References

1. Williams LS, Schmalfuss IM, Sistrom CL, et al. MR imaging of the trigeminal ganglion, nerve, and the perineural vascular plexus: normal appearance and variants with correlation to cadaver specimens. AJNR Am J Neuroradiol. 2003;24:1317–23.
2. Baumel JJ. Trigeminal-facial nerve communications. Their function in facial muscle innervation and reinnervation. Arch Otolaryngol. 1974;99:34–44.
3. Kamel HA, Toland J. Trigeminal nerve anatomy: illustrated using examples of abnormalities. AJR Am J Roentgenol. 2001;176:247–51.
4. Nash PG, Macefield VG, Klineberg IJ, et al. Bilateral activation of the trigeminothalamic tract by acute orofacial cutaneous and muscle pain in humans. Pain. 2010;151:384–93.
5. Corkin S, Milner B, Rasmussen T. Somatosensory thresholds–contrasting effects of postcentral-gyrus and posterior parietal-lobe excisions. Arch Neurol. 1970;23:41–58.
6. Hall JE, Guyton AC. Guyton and hall textbook of medical physiology. Philadelphia, PA: Elsevier; 2011.
7. Van der Cruyssen F, Politis C. Neurophysiological aspects of the trigeminal sensory system: an update. Rev Neurosci. 2018;29:115–23.
8. Campbell JN, LaMotte RH. Latency to detection of first pain. Brain Res. 1983;266:203–8.
9. Lewis TPE. The double pain response of the human skin to a single stimulus. Clin Sci. 1937;3:67–76.
10. Luccarini P, Cadet R, Duale C, et al. Effects of lesions in the trigeminal oralis and caudalis subnuclei on different orofacial nociceptive responses in the rat. Brain Res. 1998;803:79–85.
11. Takeda M, Takahashi M, Kitagawa J, et al. Brain-derived neurotrophic factor enhances the excitability of small-diameter trigeminal ganglion neurons projecting to the trigeminal nucleus interpolaris/caudalis transition zone following masseter muscle inflammation. Mol Pain. 2013;9:49.
12. Bista P, Imlach WL. Pathological mechanisms and therapeutic targets for trigeminal neuropathic pain. Medicines. 2019;6:91.
13. Demartini C, Greco R, Zanaboni AM, et al. Antagonism of transient receptor potential Ankyrin Type-1 channels as a potential target for the treatment of trigeminal neuropathic pain: study in an animal model. Int J Mol Sci. 2018;19:3320.
14. Park CK, Kim MS, Fang Z, et al. Functional expression of thermo-transient receptor potential channels in dental primary afferent neurons: implication for tooth pain. J Biol Chem. 2006;281:17304–11.
15. Mickle AD, Shepherd AJ, Mohapatra DP. Nociceptive TRP channels: sensory detectors and transducers in multiple pain pathologies. Pharmaceuticals (Basel). 2016;9:72.
16. Kim HY, Park CK, Cho IH, et al. Differential changes in TRPV1 expression after trigeminal sensory nerve injury. J Pain. 2008;9:280–8.

17. Goto T, Iwai H, Kuramoto E, et al. Neuropeptides and ATP signaling in the trigeminal ganglion. Jpn Dent Sci Rev. 2017;53:117–24.
18. Loyd DR, Murphy AZ. The role of the periaqueductal gray in the modulation of pain in males and females: are the anatomy and physiology really that different? Neural Plast. 2009;2009:462879.
19. Basbaum AI, Fields HL. Endogenous pain control mechanisms: review and hypothesis. Ann Neurol. 1978;4:451–62.
20. Dostrovsky JO, Shah Y, Gray BG. Descending inhibitory influences from periaqueductal gray, nucleus raphe magnus, and adjacent reticular formation. II. Effects on medullary dorsal horn nociceptive and nonnociceptive neurons. J Neurophysiol. 1983;49:948–60.
21. Fields HL, Malick A, Burstein R. Dorsal horn projection targets of ON and OFF cells in the rostral ventromedial medulla. J Neurophysiol. 1995;74:1742–59.
22. Cruccu G, Bonamico LH, Zakrzewska JM. Cranial neuralgias. Handb Clin Neurol. 2010;97:663–78.
23. Prasad S, Galetta S. Trigeminal neuralgia: historical notes and current concepts. Neurologist. 2009;15:87–94.
24. Hardy DG, Rhoton AL Jr. Microsurgical relationships of the superior cerebellar artery and the trigeminal nerve. J Neurosurg. 1978;49:669–78.
25. Yoshino N, Akimoto H, Yamada I, et al. Trigeminal neuralgia: evaluation of neuralgic manifestation and site of neurovascular compression with 3D CISS MR imaging and MR angiography. Radiology. 2003;228:539–45.
26. Devor M, Govrin-Lippmann R, Rappaport ZH. Mechanism of trigeminal neuralgia: an ultrastructural analysis of trigeminal root specimens obtained during microvascular decompression surgery. J Neurosurg. 2002;96:532–43.
27. Rappaport HZ, Devor M. Trigeminal neuralgia: the role of self-sustaining discharge in the trigeminal ganglion. Pain. 1994;56:127–38.
28. Devor M, Amir R, Rappaport ZH. Pathophysiology of trigeminal neuralgia: the ignition hypothesis. Clin J Pain. 2002;18:4–13.
29. Dandy WE. Concerning the cause of trigeminal neuralgia. Am J Surg. 1934;24:447–55.
30. Lee A, McCartney S, Burbidge C, et al. Trigeminal neuralgia occurs and recurs in the absence of neurovascular compression. J Neurosurg. 2014;120:1048–54.
31. Ko AL, Lee A, Raslan AM, et al. Trigeminal neuralgia without neurovascular compression presents earlier than trigeminal neuralgia with neurovascular compression. J Neurosurg. 2015;123:1519–27.
32. Savica R, Lagana A, Siracusano R, et al. Idiopathic familial trigeminal neuralgia: a case report. Neurol Sci. 2007;28:196–8.
33. Tanaka BS, Zhao P, Dib-Hajj FB, et al. A gain-of-function mutation in Nav1.6 in a case of trigeminal neuralgia. Mol Med. 2016;22:338–48.
34. Siqueira SR, Alves B, Malpartida HM, et al. Abnormal expression of voltage-gated sodium channels Nav1.7, Nav1.3 and Nav1.8 in trigeminal neuralgia. Neuroscience. 2009;164:573–7.
35. Sandkuhler J. Understanding LTP in pain pathways. Mol Pain. 2007;3:9.
36. Abd-Elsayed AA, Ikeda R, Jia Z, et al. KCNQ channels in nociceptive cold-sensing trigeminal ganglion neurons as therapeutic targets for treating orofacial cold hyperalgesia. Mol Pain. 2015;11:45.
37. Tatulian L, Delmas P, Abogadie FC, et al. Activation of expressed KCNQ potassium currents and native neuronal M-type potassium currents by the anti-convulsant drug retigabine. J Neurosci. 2001;21:5535–45.

Clinical Diagnosis of Trigeminal Neuralgia

Kyung Rae Cho and Kwan Park

1 Introduction

"It is very common that patients experiencing neuralgia of the second or third branch of the trigeminal nerve, at the beginning of their suffering, will have extracted all teeth of the affected region. Generally, on a thorough examination, it will be easily recognized, whether the pain originates from the teeth or not."

—Fedor Krause (1857–1937), [1].

Trigeminal neuralgia(TN) is a devastating neuropathic pain that affects basic human psychological, physical, and social needs and activities, such as touching the face, talking, eating, and drinking [2]. TN can be frequently misdiagnosed as dental problems and patients take nerve treatments or even extraction of normal teeth. Those misdiagnoses can result in unnecessary treatments and even delays in accessing specialist care and proper treatment [3]. Many advances in symptomatology, etiology, pathophysiology, classification, and treatment were made and now we know neurovascular contact with morphological changes of the trigeminal nerve is highly associated with the symptomatic side of trigeminal neuralgia [4, 5]. Although many advances in imaging help to diagnose this symptom in detail, diagnosis of TN is still based on clinical symptoms.

2 Clinical Diagnosis of TN

The diagnosis of trigeminal neuralgia is based on the following three criteria [6]

1. Pain should be restricted to the territory of one or more divisions of the trigeminal nerve
2. Paroxysms of pain that are sudden, intense, and very short (usually a few seconds) and are described as a "shock" or an "electric sensation"
3. Pain triggered by innoculus stimuli on the face or intraoral trigeminal territory.

Triggered paroxysmal pain is a pathognomic feature of TN [7]. The most frequently affected distribution of trigeminal nerve is maxillary or mandibular division, or both [8]. Thus, a most common symptom of TN is triggered by talking (59%), washing the face (43%), and chewing (41%) which is affected by the maxillary or mandibular branch of trigeminal nerve [6].

Though TN is one of the neuropathic pain syndrome, it follows the common mechanism of neuropathic pain. That is hyperalgesia, an increased response to a painful stimulus, and allodynia, a painful response to a normally non-painful stimulus, which is caused by damage to nociceptors or peripheral nerves.TN also is

K. R. Cho (✉) · K. Park
Department of Neurosurgery, Konkuk University Medical Center, Konkuk University School of Medicine, Seoul, Republic of Korea
e-mail: kwanpark@skku.edu

K. Park, K. R. Cho (eds.), *Trigeminal Neuralgia*, https://doi.org/10.1007/978-981-19-9171-4_3

triggered by "normally nonpainful stimulus" such as washing the face or eating and exaggerated to feel like "stabbing and electric shock like." TN can be classified according to the lesion resulting in damage to the trigeminal nerve. Neurovascular contact on the nerve is the most common type of TN but other conditions that affect the nerve by mechanical compression or demyelinating pathology also affect the nerve to be sensitive and occur neuropathic pain. But regardless of the type of underlying etiology, chronic influence by lesion makes damage to the nerve and results in demyelination to develop the symptoms.

3 Classifications of TN

Internal headache society (IHS) and the international association for the study of pain (IASP) published classifications for TN. Although the two classifications differ in format, the classifications are similar regarding the clinical characteristics required for diagnosis [2, 9, 10]. According to the third edition of the International Classification of Headache Disorders (ICHD-3), TN is defined by recurrent severe paroxysmal pain restricted to the trigeminal territory, lasting from a fraction of a second up to 2 min, with the pain described as electric shock-like, stabbing, or sharp, and being triggered by innocuous stimuli [2]. Trigeminal neuralgia that was derived from neurovascular conflict was termed classical neuralgia before, but is now termed either classical or idiopathic trigeminal neuralgia in both classifications, depending on whether there is a neurovascular contact with morphological changes of the trigeminal nerve on the symptomatic side. Because neurovascular contact at the trigeminal nerve entry zone is frequently observed in healthy subjects, neurovascular contact seen on MRI with evidence of morphological change (e.g., atrophy or displacement) in the nerve root is classified as classical TN, otherwise classified as idiopathic TN. Trigeminal neuralgia caused by other pathological characteristics, such as tumors, arterio-venous malformation in the cerebellopontine angle, or multiple sclerosis, is now termed secondary trigeminal neuralgia. Classical and idiopathic trigeminal neuralgia are subdivided into groups with purely paroxysmal pain or with concomitant continuous pain—i.e., with continuous or near-continuous pain between attacks in the affected trigeminal distribution [11]. ICHD-3 classification of TN is described in the Fig. 1.

Classification of TN published by IASP start from peripheral neuropathic pain in the chronic neuropathic pain category. From the definition, chronic peripheral neuropathic pain is defined as chronic pain caused by a lesion or disease of the peripheral somatosensory nervous system [7]. TN is categorized as one of chronic peripheral neuropathy along with chronic neuropathic pain after peripheral nerve injury, painful polyneuropathy, post-herpetic neuralgia, painful radiculopathy, and other specified and unspecified chronic peripheral neuropathic pain. They define TN as a manifestation of orofacial neuropathic pain restricted to one or more divisions of the trigeminal nerve. The pain is recurrent, abrupt in onset and termination, triggered by innocuous stimuli, and typically compared to an electric shock or described as shooting or stabbing. Some patients experience continuous pain between these painful paroxysms. The diagnosis comprises idiopathic trigeminal neuralgia, classical neuralgia produced by vascular compression of the trigeminal nerve, and secondary neuralgias caused by a tumor or cyst at the cerebellopontine angle, or multiple sclerosis [7, 9]. IASP classification of TN is much simpler and not sub-divided into smaller categories than that of IHS classification and described in Fig. 2.

Summary

Recently, many of the neurological disorders are diagnosed and categorized by imaging and/or laboratory examinations. However, diagnosis of TN can be solely made by clinical presentations, rather than imaging studies. Imaging or other exams may help subdivide TN to know better about its pathophysiology and alter its treatment, but not mandatory for its diagnosis. Correct clinical diagnosis may help patients suffering from this pain and be saved from unnecessary loss of their teeth.

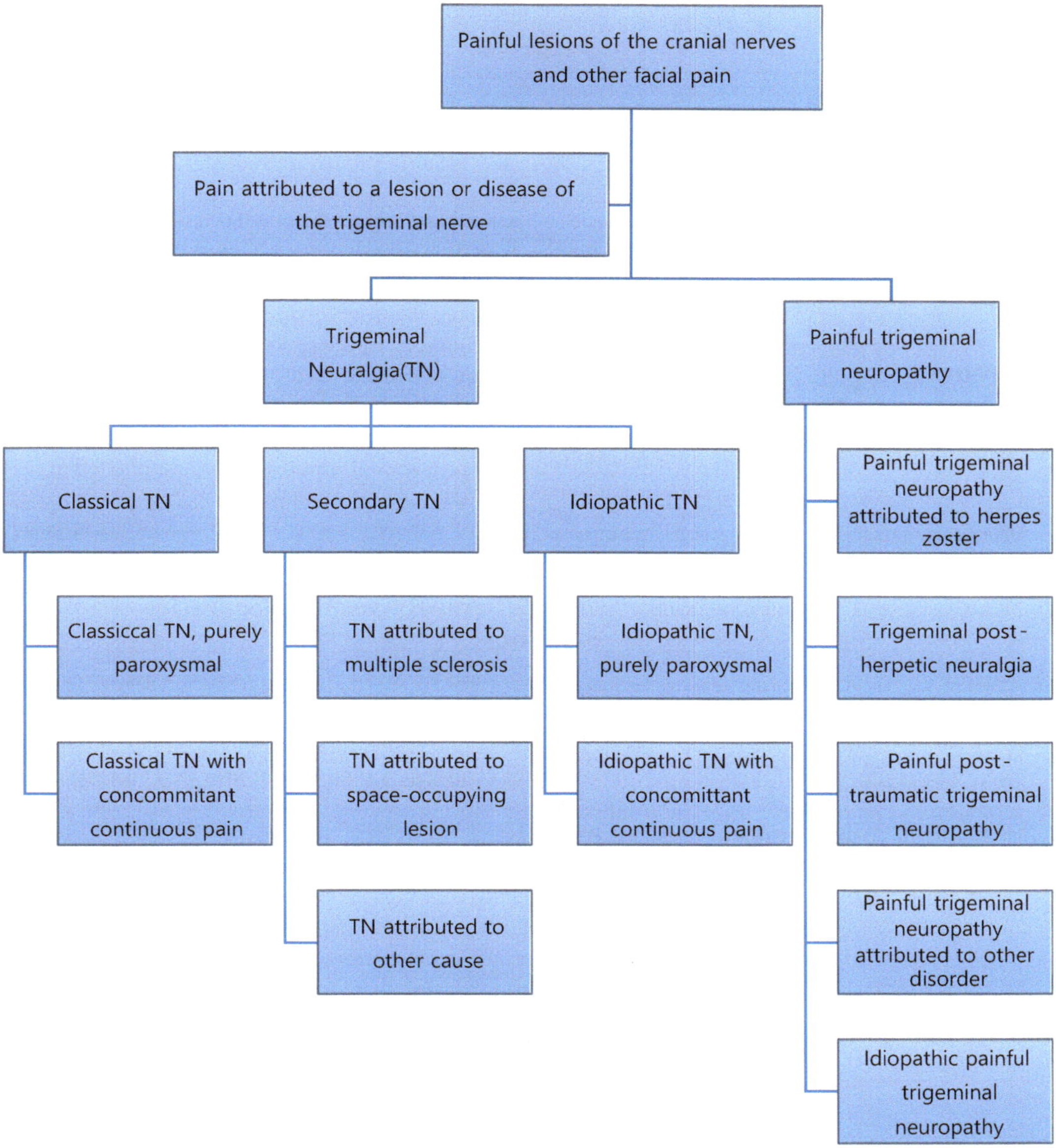

Fig. 1 The classification of Trigeminal Neuralgia and related disorders. International Headache Society (IHS) suggested classification of trigeminal neuralgia and its related disorder in International classification of headache disorders third edition (ICHD). Diagnostic criteria were defined on pain character and its underlying pathophysiology

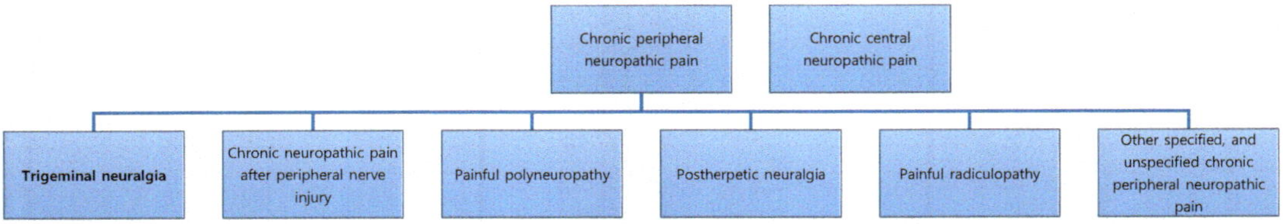

Fig. 2 IASP classification of TN. International association for the study of pain(IASP) also suggested clinical criteria for trigeminal neuralgia. IASP classification is simpler and broader than ICHD classification. However, diagnostic criteria does not differ between the two other classifications

References

1. Tripathi M, et al. Please spare my teeth! Dental procedures and trigeminal neuralgia. Surg Neurol Int. 2020;11:455.
2. Headache classification Committee of the International Headache Society (IHS). The international classification of headache disorders, 3rd edition. Cephalalgia. 2018;38(1):1–211.
3. Maarbjerg S, et al. Trigeminal neuralgia–a prospective systematic study of clinical characteristics in 158 patients. Headache. 2014;54(10):1574–82.
4. Antonini G, et al. Magnetic resonance imaging contribution for diagnosing symptomatic neurovascular contact in classical trigeminal neuralgia: a blinded case-control study and meta-analysis. Pain. 2014;155(8):1464–71.
5. Maarbjerg S, et al. Significance of neurovascular contact in classical trigeminal neuralgia. Brain. 2015;138(Pt 2):311–9.
6. Cruccu G, Di Stefano G, Truini A. Trigeminal neuralgia. N Engl J Med. 2020;383(8):754–62.
7. Scholz J, et al. The IASP classification of chronic pain for ICD-11: chronic neuropathic pain. Pain. 2019;160(1):53–9.
8. Park SH, Chang JW. Gamma knife radiosurgery on the trigeminal root entry zone for idiopathic trigeminal neuralgia: results and a review of the literature. Yonsei Med J. 2020;61(2):111–9.
9. Cruccu G, et al. Trigeminal neuralgia: new classification and diagnostic grading for practice and research. Neurology. 2016;87(2):220–8.
10. Benoliel R, et al. The IASP classification of chronic pain for ICD-11: chronic secondary headache or orofacial pain. Pain. 2019;160(1):60–8.
11. Bendtsen L, et al. Advances in diagnosis, classification, pathophysiology, and management of trigeminal neuralgia. Lancet Neurol. 2020;19(9):784–96.

Differential Diagnosis of Trigeminal Neuralgia

Mi Ji Lee

The diagnosis of trigeminal neuralgia is made primarily by clinical symptoms. Although neuroimaging findings of neurovascular contact can be helpful to diagnose "classical" trigeminal neuralgia, trigeminal neuralgia may develop without apparent evidence of neurovascular contact ("idiopathic" trigeminal neuralgia) or be caused by other disorders ("secondary" trigeminal neuralgia). Differential diagnosis starts with the recognition of clinical features that support trigeminal neuralgia or suggest the possibility of other disorders.

The International Classification of Orofacial Pain (ICOP), 1st edition, has been recently developed and published by the International Headache Society [1]. According to the ICOP, pain within the trigeminal nerve territory is classified into trigeminal neuralgia and trigeminal neuropathic pain (Table 1). Trigeminal neuropathic pain is an important differential diagnosis of trigeminal neuralgia, as the two entities are closely related but a nerve damage is present in trigeminal neuropathic pain. Thus, the prognosis is unfavorable and the decompression surgery would not benefit patients with trigeminal neuropathic pain. In addition to trigeminal neuropathic pain, primary headaches such as trigeminal autonomic cephalalgias (TACs) should be differentiated. Lastly, idiopathic pain conditions such as persistent idio-

Table 1 ICOP classification for pain within the territory of the trigeminal nerve

4. Orofacial pain attributed to lesion or disease of the cranial nerves
4.1 Pain attributed to lesion or disease of the trigeminal nerve
4.1.1 Trigeminal neuralgia
4.1.1.1 Classical trigeminal neuralgia
4.1.1.1.1 Classical trigeminal neuralgia, purely paroxysmal
4.1.1.1.2 Classical trigeminal neuralgia with concomitant continuous pain
4.1.1.2 Secondary trigeminal neuralgia
4.1.1.2.1 Trigeminal neuralgia attributed to multiple sclerosis
4.1.1.2.2 Trigeminal neuralgia attributed to space-occupying lesion
4.1.1.2.3 Trigeminal neuralgia attributed to other cause
4.1.1.3 Idiopathic trigeminal neuralgia
4.1.1.3.1 Idiopathic trigeminal neuralgia, purely paroxysmal
4.1.1.3.2 Idiopathic trigeminal neuralgia with concomitant continuous pain
4.1.2 Other trigeminal neuropathic pain
4.1.2.1 Trigeminal neuropathic pain attributed to herpes zoster
4.1.2.2 Trigeminal postherpetic neuralgia
4.1.2.3 Post-traumatic trigeminal neuropathic pain
4.1.2.3.1 Probable post-traumatic trigeminal neuropathic pain
4.1.2.4 Trigeminal neuropathic pain attributed to other disorder
4.1.2.4.1 Probable trigeminal neuropathic pain attributed to other disorder
4.1.2.5 Idiopathic trigeminal neuropathic pain

ICOP International Classification of Orofacial Pain

M. J. Lee (✉)
Department of Neurology, Seoul National University Hospital, Seoul National University College of Medicine, Seoul, Republic of Korea

K. Park, K. R. Cho (eds.), *Trigeminal Neuralgia*, https://doi.org/10.1007/978-981-19-9171-4_4

pathic facial pain (PIFP) and constant unilateral facial pain with additional attacks (CUFPA) can be considered in atypical cases. This section will follow the terminology defined by the ICOP.

1 Trigeminal Neuropathic Pain

The principle of facial pain/headache classification is to classify the clinical symptom into neuralgia and neuropathy, of which the latter indicates the apparent symptoms and/or signs of the lesion exist within the affected nerve territory, and then add the adjective "idiopathic" or "secondary" after appropriate investigations for secondary causes. Trigeminal neuropathic pain indicates pain originating from disorders causing neural damage of one or more branches of the trigeminal nerve. The feature most distinguishing trigeminal neuropathic pain from trigeminal neuralgia is that the pain is primarily continuous or near continuous. The superimposed brief pain paroxysms can accompany the continuous pain but are not predominant, whereas trigeminal neuralgia is characterized by extremely severe painful paroxysms with no or mild background pain. Signs of neural damage are present in trigeminal neuropathic pain and include hypesthesia, numbness, hyperesthesia, mechanical allodynia, and cold hyperalgesia/allodynia. Characteristics of neuropathic pain are usually sharp and described as burning, stabbing, shooting, aching, tingling, electrical shock-like, or of pins-and-needles nature.

Common causes of trigeminal neuropathic pain are herpes zoster and trauma. When these two causes do not exist, high-resolution neuroimaging and systemic work-ups should be performed to reveal the secondary cause, as tumorous conditions, demyelinating diseases, and systemic disorders can result in trigeminal neuropathic pain.

1.1 Herpes Zoster/Postherpetic Pain

In patients with herpes zoster affecting the trigeminal ganglion, V1 division is most commonly affected ("herpes zoster ophthalamicus"). Trigeminal neuropathic pain develops over a few days. Pain is usually severe and burning and accompanied by cutaneous allodynia. Herpes zoster ophthalmicus may present with ocular involvement such as conjunctivitis, keratitis, iritis, and uveitis [2]. Vesicular rash within the affected territory is the most characteristic and diagnostic finding for herpes zoster. However, some individuals may not show skin rash (*Zoster sine herpete*). In such cases, PCR detection of varicella zoster virus in the cerebrospinal fluid is required to confirm the diagnosis.

When pain within the affected nerve territory persists for more than 3 months after the onset of herpes zoster, postherpetic neuralgia can be diagnosed. Pain is typically described as burning and itching. The degree of allodynia and sensory loss varies among individuals.

1.2 Trauma

Traumatic injury to the branches of trigeminal nerve can cause trigeminal neuropathic pain. In addition to pain, negative symptoms and signs suggestive of trigeminal nerve dysfunction such as numbness and hypesthesia also exist; thus, traumatic trigeminal neuropathic pain was previously called *Anesthesia Dolorosa*. Any mechanical, thermal, radiation, or chemical injury can damage the trigeminal nerve. Sources of traumatic injury can be external trauma, dental treatments including extraction, local anesthetic injection, root canal therapy, oral surgery, and dental implants, neuroablative procedures targeting the trigeminal ganglion or nerve root.

In addition to the clinical history showing a clear temporal relationship, it is required to confirm the lesion of affected trigeminal nerve using objective diagnostic tests to make a definite diagnosis of traumatic trigeminal neuropathy. Diagnostic tests include surgical or radiological findings of nerve compression or lesion, nerve conduction study, blink reflex, or histological confirmation of nerve damage. However, it is often challenging to apply these investigations to

Table 2 ICOP criteria for traumatic trigeminal neuropathic pain

A.	Pain, in a neuroanatomically plausible area within the distribution(s) of one or both trigeminal nerve(s), persisting or recurring for >3 months and fulfilling criteria C and D
B.	Both of the following:
	1. History of a mechanical, thermal, radiation or chemical injury to the peripheral trigeminal nerve(s)
	2. Diagnostic test confirmation of a lesion of the peripheral trigeminal nerve(s) explaining the pain
C.	Onset within 6 months after the injury
D.	Associated with somatosensory symptoms and/or signs in the same neuroanatomically plausible distribution
E.	Not better accounted for by another ICOP or ICHD-3 diagnosis

ICOP international classification of orofacial pain, *ICHD-3* international classification of headache disorders, 3rd version

distal branches of the trigeminal nerve. Table 2 shows the diagnostic criteria of traumatic trigeminal neuropathic pain.

1.3 Other Secondary Causes

Tumorous conditions, demyelinating diseases, and systemic diseases can result in trigeminal neuropathic pain. Although disease conditions are much uncommon than herpes zoster and trauma, they can be a sign of significant disorders such as malignancy. Pathologies should be investigated along the trigeminal pathway including trigeminal nuclei, nerve, ganglion, courses of affected branch (V1, V2, or V3), and adjacent structures. Partial or complete sensory loss is the most important sign of trigeminal neuropathy, warranting a need for work-ups for secondary causes. Careful neurological examination including sensory examination (i.e., cheiro-oral syndrome, dissociated sensory loss), jaw jerk, and other cranial nerve function tests and neurophysiological tests such as blink reflex and electromyography can aid the localization of trigeminal neuropathy and sometimes give a clue to a central pathology.

Table 3 Causes of trigeminal neuropathy

Trauma
– Accidental, surgical, dental (especially at 3rd molar), chemical (glycerol rhizotomy), radiation
Inflammatory/autoimmune
– Undifferentiated and mixed connective tissue disease
– Progressive systemic scleroderma, Sjögren's syndrome, sarcoidosis, multiple sclerosis
Vascular
– Pontomedullary ischemia or hemorrhage (CNS mimic)
– Vascular malformation
Neoplastic
– Intra- or extracranial compression (meningioma, trigeminal or vestibular schwannoma, nasopharyngeal carcinoma)
– Perineural spread (adenoid cystic carcinoma, squamous cell carcinoma, lymphoma)
– Metastasis (breast and lung carcinoma, melanoma)
– Carcinomatous meningitis (breast and lung carcinoma, melanoma, lymphoma)
Infectious
– Leprosy, viruses (varicella zoster virus, herpes simplex virus), Lyme disease, syphilis, fungi (actinomycosis)
Degenerative
– Kennedy's disease
Toxic-metabolic
– Stilbamidine, trichloroethylene, oxaliplatin, diabetes mellitus
Congenital
– Congenital trigeminal anesthesia with or without Goldenhar-Gorlin syndrome or Möbius syndrome
– Skull base anomalies
Idiopathic trigeminal neuropathy
Other
– Amyloidosis, pseudotumor cerebri

When the localization is successful, neuroimaging should focus on the localized pathways of trigeminal nerve. However, as it is often challenging to localize, it is helpful to cover all the pathways of the trigeminal nerve from the nuclei (brainstem and upper cervical spinal cord), cavernous sinus, skull base, and the adjacent extracranial structures. Laboratory evaluations include autoantibodies (e.g., anti SS-A and SS-B autoantibodies) and serological evaluation for Lyme and syphilis in suspected cases. Table 3 lists the conditions that can cause secondary trigeminal neuropathy [3].

2 Primary Headache Disorders

As the nomenclature "headache" suggests, primary headache disorders commonly present with head pain. Among trigeminal nerve divisions, V1 is often affected in primary headaches. However, although uncommonly, primary headache can present with predominantly orofacial pain. Such clinical entities, e.g., orofacial migraine and orofacial cluster headache, have been recently suggested and defined in the ICOP. Primary headache disorders presenting orofacial pain are coded in the ICOP as 5.1 orofacial migraine, 5.2 tension-type orofacial pain, and 5.3 trigeminal autonomic orofacial pain. In this chapter, we will focus on trigeminal autonomic cephalalgias as they can be overlapped with trigeminal neuralgia in several aspects of pain characteristics.

2.1 Trigeminal Autonomic Cephalalgia (TAC)/Orofacial TAC

Trigeminal autonomic cephalalgias (TACs) include cluster headache, paroxysmal hemicrania, short-lasting unilateral neuralgiform headache attacks, and hemicrania continua (Table 4) [4]. TACs and trigeminal neuralgia share common features such as strictly unilaterality, severe intensity, and in some cases sharp quality. The differential point can be (1) duration of attack, (2) location of pain, and (3) accompanying symptoms.

Attack duration is the most important factor in the classification of TACs. Cluster headache typically lasts 15–180 min, whereas attacks of paroxysmal hemicrania lasts 2–30 min. Duration of short-lasting unilateral neuralgiform headache attacks is typically 1–600 s. As the pain paroxysm of trigeminal neuralgia can last 1 s to 2 min, although longer in rare instances, ultra-short paroxysms of neuralgic pain favor the diagnosis of trigeminal neuralgia or short-lasting unilateral neuralgiform headache attack rather than cluster headache and paroxysmal hemicrania.

Location of pain is usually within the V1 territory in TACs, while trigeminal neuralgia commonly involves V2/3 dermatomes. However, TACs can also present with orofacial pain, as stated above. Orofacial TACs have been relatively less recognized, but they can be an important differential diagnosis in patients with diagnostically challenging orofacial pain. It was

Table 4 ICHD-3 diagnostic criteria of trigeminal autonomic cephalalgias

Cluster headache
A. At least five attacks fulfilling criteria B–D
B. Severe or very severe unilateral orbital, supraorbital, and/or temporal pain lasting 15–180 min (when untreated)
C. Either or both of the following:
1. At least one of the following symptoms or signs, ipsilateral to the headache:
(a) Conjunctival injection and/or lacrimation
(b) Nasal congestion and/or rhinorrhoea
(c) Eyelid edema
(d) Forehead and facial sweating
(e) Miosis and/or ptosis
2. a sense of restlessness or agitation
D. Occurring with a frequency between one every other day and eight per day
E. Not better accounted for by another ICHD-3 diagnosis
Paroxysmal hemicranias
A. At least 20 attacks fulfilling criteria B–E
B. Severe unilateral orbital, supraorbital, and/or temporal pain lasting 2–30 min
C. Either or both of the following:
1. At least one of the following symptoms or signs, ipsilateral to the headache:
(a) Conjunctival injection and/or lacrimation
(b) Nasal congestion and/or rhinorrhoea
(c) Eyelid edema
(d) Forehead and facial sweating
(e) Miosis and/or ptosis
2. a sense of restlessness or agitation
D. Occurring with a frequency of >5 per day
E. Prevented absolutely by therapeutic doses of indomethacin
F. Not better accounted for by another ICHD-3 diagnosis
Short-lasting unilateral neuralgiform headache attacks
A. At least 20 attacks fulfilling criteria B–D
B. Moderate or severe unilateral head pain, with orbital, supraorbital, temporal, and/or other trigeminal distribution, lasting for 1–600 s and occurring as single stabs, series of stabs, or in a saw-tooth pattern
C. at least one of the following five cranial autonomic symptoms or signs, ipsilateral to the pain:
1. Conjunctival injection and/or lacrimation
2. Nasal congestion and/or rhinorrhoea
3. Eyelid edema
4. Forehead and facial sweating
5. Miosis and/or ptosis
D. Occurring with a frequency of at least one a day
E. Not better accounted for by another ICHD-3 diagnosis

Table 4 (continued)

Hemicrania continua
A. Unilateral headache fulfilling criteria B–D
B. Present for >3 months, with exacerbations of moderate or greater intensity
C. either or both of the following:
1. At least one of the following symptoms or signs, ipsilateral to the headache:
(a) Conjunctival injection and/or lacrimation
(b) Nasal congestion and/or rhinorrhoea
(c) Eyelid oedema
(d) Forehead and facial sweating
(e) Miosis and/or ptosis
2. a sense of restlessness or agitation, or aggravation of the pain by movement
D. Responds absolutely to therapeutic doses of indomethacin
E. Not better accounted for by another ICHD-3 diagnosis

ICHD-3 international classification of headache disorders, 3rd version

reported that 44% were diagnosed with suspected TACs in patients visiting a tertiary multidisciplinary orofacial pain clinic [5].

Accompanying symptoms are essential in the diagnosis of TACs as they are called trigeminal "autonomic" cephalalgias. Tearing, conjunctival injection, rhinorrhea, nasal congestion, eyelid edema, forehead and facial sweating, miosis, and ptosis are considered as autonomic symptoms of TACs, and restlessness and agitation are also supportive of cluster headache, paroxysmal hemicrania, and hemicrania continua. Tearing and conjunctival injection are essential to diagnose short-lasting unilateral neuralgiform headache attacks with conjunctival injection and tearing (SUNCT), which is a subtype of short-lasting unilateral neuralgiform headache attacks. The other subtype, short-lasting unilateral neuralgiform headache attacks with cranial autonomic symptoms (SUNA), has cranial autonomic features but no more than one conjunctival injection and tearing.

Short-lasting unilateral neuralgiform headache attack has a significant overlap with trigeminal neuralgia. Actually, there has been reported a case of trigeminal neuralgia whose pain phenotype evolved into typical SUNCT over time. One differential point is that SUNCT and SUNA can be triggered without a refractory period, whereas trigeminal neuralgia is typically triggered by innocuous stimuli but there is usually a refractory period after pain paroxysm. SUNCT and SUNA can occur as a single stab, series of stabs, or in a saw-tooth pattern.

3 Idiopathic Pain Conditions: Persistent Idiopathic Facial Pain (PIFP) and Constant Unilateral Facial Pain with Additional Attacks (CUFPA)

There are several idiopathic orofacial pain syndromes recognized so far. Among these, persistent idiopathic facial pain (PIFP) and constant unilateral facial pain with additional attacks (CUFPA) should be noted for the differential diagnosis of trigeminal neuralgia (Table 5). PIFP were previously called "atypical facial pain".

Table 5 ICOP diagnostic criteria of PIFP and CUFPA

Persistent idiopathic facial pain (PIFP)
A. Facial pain fulfilling criteria B and C
B. Recurring daily for >2 h/day for >3 months
C. Pain has both of the following characteristics:
1. Poorly localized, and not following the distribution of a peripheral nerve
2. Dull, aching, or nagging quality
D. Clinical and radiographic examinations are normal, and local causes have been excluded
E. Not better accounted for by another ICOP or ICHD-3 diagnosis
Constant unilateral facial pain with additional attacks (CUFPA)
A. Constant strictly unilateral facial pain fulfilling criterion B, with exacerbations fulfilling criterion C
B. Background pain, with both of the following characteristics:
1. Mild to moderate intensity
2. Constantly present for >3 months
C. Exacerbations occurring as distinct attacks, up to 6 times daily, with all of the following three characteristics:
1. In the same location as the background pain
2. Moderate to severe intensity
3. Lasting 10–30 min
D. Clinical and radiographic examinations are normal, and local causes have been excluded
E. Not better accounted for by another ICOP or ICHD-3 diagnosis

ICOP international classification of orofacial pain, *ICHD-3* international classification of headache disorders, 3rd version

Indeed, there is a significant difference between trigeminal neuralgia and PIFP: pain is poorly localized and not following a dermatome of the peripheral trigeminal nerve in PIFP. In addition, the pain of PIFP is usually dull, aching, or nagging. In terms of duration, patients with PIFP usually report persistent pain, but in cases where pain is not strictly persistent, pain from PIFP lasts longer than pain paroxysms of trigeminal neuralgia. CUFPA is a relatively new entity. Patients with CUFPA complain of two types of pain: constant, unremitting, dull, unilateral facial pain of mild to moderate intensity and distinct attacks of moderate to severe pain in the same location lasting 10–30 min. Not enough literature currently exists on this entity.

References

1. International classification of orofacial pain, 1st edition (ICOP). Cephalalgia. 2020;40:129–221.
2. Ting DSJ, Ghosh N, Ghosh S. Herpes zoster ophthalmicus. BMJ. 2019;364:k5234.
3. Smith JH, Cutrer FM. Numbness matters: a clinical review of trigeminal neuropathy. Cephalalgia. 2011;31:1131–44.
4. Headache Classification Committee of the International Headache Society (IHS). The international classification of headache disorders, 3rd edition. Cephalalgia. 2018;38:1–211.
5. Wei DY, Moreno-Ajona D, Renton T, Goadsby PJ. Trigeminal autonomic cephalalgias presenting in a multidisciplinary tertiary orofacial pain clinic. J Headache Pain. 2019;20:69.

Electrophysiological Diagnosis "Now and Future" for Trigeminal Neuralgia

Byung-Euk Joo

1 Introduction

Trigeminal neuralgia is a chronic neuropathic pain disorder characterized by spontaneous and elicited paroxysms of electric shock-like or stabbing pain in a region of the face. The diagnosis of trigeminal neuralgia is clinical features and is based on the three main criteria: pain restricted to the territory of one or more divisions of the trigeminal nerve; paroxysms of pain that are sudden, intense, and very short (<1 s–2 min, but usually a few seconds) and are described as a shock or an electrical sensation; and pain triggered by innocuous stimuli on the face or intraoral trigeminal territory. The pain of trigeminal neuralgia most frequently affects the distribution of the second (maxillary) or third (mandibular) division of the trigeminal nerve. Three types of trigeminal neuralgia have been classified: classical, secondary, and idiopathic. The clinical features of classical and secondary trigeminal neuralgia are similar. The electrophysiological studies of the reflex activity mediated by the trigeminal nerves allow the evaluation of their integrity and their central pathways. Their clinical applications include the evaluation of cranial neuropathies, polyradiculoneuropathies, peripheral neuropathies, and brainstem lesions. So far, many studies using electrophysiological studies such as corneal reflex, blink reflex, jaw jerk, masseter inhibitory reflex, and evoked potentials have been conducted to diagnose trigeminal neuralgia and clarify the pathologic mechanism of trigeminal neuralgia. This chapter reviews the electrophysiologic studies for trigeminal neuralgia and discusses the usefulness and implications of those studies.

2 Electrophysiological Study

2.1 Corneal Reflex

The corneal reflex is designed to protect the eye and is considered purely nociceptive. The reflex afferent nerve is an Aδ fiber that passes through the eye of the long ciliary nerve and the trigeminal nerve and reaches the pons [1, 2]. The central circuit is similar to that of the R2 response of the blink reflex, but because it is purely nociceptive and therefore relayed through a few different interneurons that are more resistant to the effects of suprasegments is different. The efferent limb contains the motor fibers of the bilateral facial motor nuclei of the facial nerve ending in the orbicularis oculi muscle (OO).

2.1.1 Methodology

Corneal reflexes consist of involuntary eyelid closure (contraction of OO) on both sides in response to corneal irritation during spontaneous

B.-E. Joo (✉)
Department of Neurology, Soonchunhyang University Seoul Hospital, Soonchunhyang University College of Medicine, Seoul, Republic of Korea

K. Park, K. R. Cho (eds.), *Trigeminal Neuralgia*, https://doi.org/10.1007/978-981-19-9171-4_5

blinking. Stimulation can be mechanical or electrical. A reaction is simultaneously recorded from both sides of the OO muscle where the surface electrode or needle electrode is arranged at the same position as the blink reflex. Mechanical stimulation is induced by the application of a small metal sphere of 2 mm (mm) to the cornea [1]. When the sphere touches the cornea, it comes into contact between the cornea and the electrical trigger circuit that transmits the pulse. Electrical stimulation of the cornea is performed by a thin saline immersion cotton thread connected to the cathode of a constant current stimulator. The anode is placed on the earlobe or forearm. This stimulus is controlled by a square pulse with a duration of 1 millisecond (ms) and a strength of 0.1–3 milliamp (mA) to generate a reproducible response. It is rare for a normal subject to have a reflex threshold greater than 0.5 mA. Mechanical and electrical stimuli induce reflexes with similar delays. The absolute latency value ranges from 36 to 64 ms for mechanical stimuli and from 35 to 50 ms for electrical stimuli. Among the age groups, the range of latency is getting smaller. In measuring the latency, three sets of latency times from the stimulus artifact to the start of the electromagnetic wave (EMG) response are evaluated. In contrast to blinking reflexes, corneal reflexes do not produce an initial R1 reaction. When the cornea is stimulated (mechanically or electrically), there is a direct (ipsilateral) and a consensual (contralateral) response. When mechanical stimulation is used, the direct response latency shall not exceed the latency on the contralateral side response by more than 8 ms. The latency of direct reaction induced by the stimulation of the two corneas shall not differ by more than 10 ms. With electrical stimuli, the difference between direct and consensual reactions shall not exceed 5 ms, and the difference between direct reactions shall not exceed 8 ms.

2.1.2 Applications

Corneal reflex dysfunction can be caused by damage to any point in the pathway (i.e., the central nervous system or the peripheral nervous system). Peripheral damage causes a defect in ipsilateral reflection, and central dysfunction causes a bilateral reflexes defect. If the peripheral nerve (V) or facial nerve (VII) is damaged, the corneal blink circuit is interrupted. Doctors diagnose peripheral nerve damage by examining early and late blinking reflexes or secondary symptoms of nerve damage. Examining the stage of blinking reflexes, patients with trigeminal nerve (V) lesions often have early reflection defects on one side, and patients with facial nerve (VII) lesions exhibit one-sided defects in both early and late stages. When examining secondary symptoms of nerve damage, doctors examine motor and sensory functions. A trigeminal nerve (V1) causes numbness in the forehead. To test V1 functionality, close the patient's eyes and tell them when to feel the touch in different parts of the face. Patients with V1 injury cannot feel or identify the affected side of the forehead. Damage to the facial nerve causes lateral paralysis of the facial muscles. Consequently, the mouth is drooping and the forehead becomes flat, and wrinkles on the nose and lip sides are formed. To access facial exercise, ask the patient to smile or create a different facial expression. Patients with facial nerve damage cannot move facial muscles on the affected side. Central nervous system dysfunction causes a defect in bilateral blinking reflexes. Symptoms appear as dysfunction later in the day, not in the early stages of the blink reflex. A common lesion affecting the blink reaction is Wallenberg syndrome (i.e., lateral medullary lesion). The nucleus of the spinal trigeminal nerve is in the lateral medulla. Interruption of this region blocks the blink reflection path and results in a lack of late reflection on both sides due to corneal stimulation on the affected side. Net-like activation systems and damage to the red nucleus and cerebellum also affect corneal blink reflexes. These areas can affect facial nerve signals and affect the intensity and speed of late blinking reactions.

2.2 Blink Reflex

Blink reflexes detect lesions associated with the first division of the trigeminal nerve (V1), the facial nerve, or the central pathway of their pons and medulla. Kugelberg studied electromyography of blink reflexes caused by electrical stimulation of the supraorbital nerve in 1952 [3]. Blink reflex is a surface EMG recorded from the OO muscle of the reflex caused by mechanical or electrical stimulation of the supraorbital nerve. The afferent limb is mediated by the supraorbital branch of V1 and the afferent limb moves through the facial nerve. An R1 is an oligosynaptic circuit response, which is conducted through a large myelinated fiber through the pons, to the main sensory nucleus of the trigeminal nerve, before the whole circuit in the pons reaches the facial nucleus. R2 is multisynaptic and is transmitted to the facial motor neuron through the dorsal pons and medulla before reaching the most caudal part of the spinal trigeminal nerve. From there, before connecting to the facial nucleus, impulses are transmitted to the side and opposite sides of the stimulated face via a multisynaptic medullary pathway. The decussations take place in the caudal medulla.

2.2.1 Methodology

If electrical stimulation is applied to the supraorbital nerve, the surface electrode transmits a single stimulation two to three times the intensity of the perception threshold. A surface recording electrode is arranged on the lower parts OO of both sides. Electrical stimulation of the supraorbital nerve induces two reactions: a relatively constant, well-synchronized, unilateral, ipsilateral with a short EMG reaction (considered an exclusive receptor) with the latency of approximately 10–13 ms in OO. The second or slow response (R2) is considered non-infringing, variable, long-term, bidirectional, and insufficient synchronization with approximately 30 ms latency. Amplitude measurements are not usually useful for localization because they can vary by 40% in normal subjects. R1 is a relatively stable response and is used to evaluate the afferents from the superior orbit and the pons region and is not affected by supraorbital dysfunction and consciousness and cognitive impairment (except the acute phase of insult). Extending the absolute or side-to-side R1 delay is considered abnormal. The R2 reaction is related to eyelid closure and has the same latency as the corneal reflex. It is polysynaptic, more variable than R1, and is affected by the supratentorial process, but is important for the diagnosis of medullary lesions. The R2 reaction is attenuated during sleep and by sedative drugs. R2 reactions tend to become habitual when repeatedly stimulated. Simultaneous recording of both R2 responses is useful for distinguishing afferent (trigeminal nerve) patterns and efferent (facial nerve) patterns of lesions. Blinking reflexes can also be induced by stimulation of the peripheral nerve's non-trigeminal nerve input (somatosensory, acoustic, or photic) [4]. These reflections include central mechanisms, and responses exhibit greater variability in latency, more dispersion in time, vary with lengthy repetition of stimuli, and show other distinctive differences.

2.2.2 Applications

In the lesion of the trigeminal nerve, the reaction of ipsilateral R1 and bilateral R2 may be delayed or absent depending on the severity of the lesion, but the reaction of ipsilateral R1 and bilateral R2 is normal due to the stimulus of the unaffected side [5]. This pattern is usually seen in proximal or distal trigeminal neuropathy. R1 only, or both R1 and R2 abnormalities can be seen in isolated trigeminal neuropathy. In post-herpes neuralgia, significant abnormalities are frequently observed in the R1 blink reflex reaction of the affected side compared to the normal side. However, in most patients with idiopathic trigeminal neuralgia, all blinking reflexes are normal and abnormalities may suggest structural lesions.

2.3 Jaw Jerk (Masseter Reflex)

The jaw jerk is the only monosynaptic reflex that can be used for electrophysiological examinations of cranial muscles. It is pulled out by mechanically hitting the lower jaw with a tendon reflection hammer. It is difficult to evaluate jaw jerk only by examination. It is impossible to distinguish whether patients with lip reactions have abnormalities on only one side or no reflexes. EMG monitoring of masseter or temporal muscle responses is of paramount importance in evaluating suspected brainstem lesions. If you hit the jaw, the masseter-jaw-closing muscles will contract. Afferent neurons are centrally located, unlike all other stretch reflexes (the dorsal root ganglion) in the mesencephalic nucleus of the midbrain. The efferent motor neurons are located in the pons trigeminal motor nucleus and activate only ipsilateral masseter muscles. A centripetal impulse from the masseter muscle spindle moves through the motor root of V3 to the mesencephalic nucleus and activates the motor nucleus in a monosynaptic manner. The lower limb of the reflected arc contracts the ipsilateral masseter muscle. Whether afferent fibers migrate at the trigeminal nerve root or at the trigeminal nerve root remains controversial [6]. It is also different from deep tendon reflexes in the extremities because the masseter reflexes are strengthened rather than suppressed by vibration.

2.3.1 Methodology

In electrophysiological evaluation of jaw joint reflexes, the reflection hammer is fitted with a microswitch that triggers an oscilloscope sweep when the examiner's finger placed on the subject's chin is tapped [7]. An electromyogram response is simultaneously recorded in both directions by either surface electrodes arranged at a distance of 2/3 between the joint and the lower edge of the mandible or by small concentric needle electrodes inserted into each masseter (older or obese). The reference electrode is placed directly below the mandibular angle or on the cheekbones. Because it is not common in older adults, there is no clear clinical significance in situations that can occur in healthy subjects if they are absent in both directions. The normal range of latencies is from 5 to 10 ms [8]. Amplitude changes widely and measurements are not considered clinically useful. Because the latency of responses may vary depending on successive trials, the comparison of the latency of the recorded contralateral responses simultaneously is more meaningful than analyzing the absolute value. A difference of more than 0.8 ms or a consistent unilateral absence of the reflex is considered abnormal. The masseter reflexes are technically not as accurate as blinking reflexes. Technical issues can include standardization of mechanical taps and variations in the tone of the masseter muscle (interpersonal and intrapersonal variations), so four consecutive responses are used to show consistency. If the jaw is not relaxed enough, background muscle activity can obscure the response. This reflex is strongly affected by dental occlusion and may be asymmetric or absent in some patients with jaw joint problems.

2.3.2 Applications

This reflection evaluates the function of mandibular division of the trigeminal nerve (V3). The most common anomality is not the extended latency, but the absence of responses. Unilateral delay or lack of response suggests either a trigeminal nerve or a lesion in the brainstem. Using jaw reflexes in conjunction with needle examination of masseter muscles, peripheral lesions can be recorded if evidence of degeneration exists. Since the afferent nerve cell body is located in the nucleus of the brainstem patients with primarily sensory symptoms and hyporeflexia who have a normal masseter response would more likely be diagnosed with ganglionopathy rather than sensory neuropathy. This is also a reason why the response is typically normal in patients with Friedrich Ataxia [9]. Observation of lack of reflex response in the aspect of normal massage device EMG study is observed in ipsilateral midbrain lesions. However, both EMG and jaw jerk may be abnormal in pons lesions due to cell body involvement [10]. A multisynaptic brainstem reflex, such as a blinking reflex R2 reaction, shows an increase in latencies and a decrease in amplitude, especially in the lower part of the rear center. Because the machine reflection is monosynaptic, it is not similarly affected, so it is a reliable measure of the direct involvement of the reflection arch. Due to hypersegmental and cerebellar effects, no masseter reflex latency and amplitude movement beyond the normal range is observed. By utilizing both the masseter device and the blink reflex of the internuclear ptosis patient due to multiple sclerosis or lacunar brainstem infarction, the lesion can be localized to the midbrain or pons. If the abnormality is limited to the masseter reflex, this suggests a midbrain lesion, but the abnormal blink reflex R1 delay means that anastomotic pons is involved.

2.4 Masseter Inhibitory Reflex (MIR)

A jaw reflex elicited during voluntary clenching gives rise to a brief pause in the electromyographic activity of the masseter muscles. This inactivity, called as masseteric silent period, lasts about 30 ms in normal subjects. This silent period for the jaw tap starts at approximately 10–12 ms and lasts 20–40 ms [11]. This was thought to be due to the unloading of the spindle and the activation of the Golgi tendon organ, as electrical stimulation evokes double silence. Electrical stimulation of the upper and lower jaw trifurcated ganglia can cause reflex suppression in the jaw-closing muscles. This phenomenon can be caused by electrical or mechanical stimulation of infraorbital or mentalis nerves during spontaneous contraction of the masseter muscle, which induces reflex suppression and EMG silence of the jaw closure muscle (masseter, temporal muscle) and temporary relative or absolute reduction of EMG activity evoked in the midst of an otherwise sustained contraction [12]. The reflex is believed to play a major role in preventing powerful jaw closures when chewing or biting. After stimulating the mental or infraorbital nerve, the pulse reaches the pons through the sensory mandible or maxillary root of the trigeminal nerve. Response during the silence period 1 (SP1) is mediated by an inhibitory interneuron located probably near the ipsilateral trigeminal nerve nucleus. Inhibitory interneurons are projected bidirectionally on motor neurons that close the jaw. The entire circuit is in the mid-pons. The afferent point of silence period 2 (SP2) descends in the spinal trifecta and is connected via a multisynaptic chain of excitatory interneurons at the level of the cranial medullary junction, probably located in lateral reticulation.

2.4.1 Methodology

The recording electrode is placed on the masseter muscle bilaterally. Subjects are instructed to clench their teeth as hard as possible for approximately 2–3 s. The reflex can be measured properly only if the patient is able to clench the teeth and produce a full EMG interference pattern. Single electric shocks are delivered to the mental or infraorbital nerves through surface electrodes placed over the appropriate foramina. A stimulus intensity of approximately two to three times the reflex threshold (usually 20–50 mA) yields the best results. It is always necessary to perform several trials. Some authors measure the latency at the last EMG peak crossing of the isoelectric line, whereas others record the beginning of the electrical silence. Each of these methods is clinically satisfactory, provided the normal value determination is maintained and intraindividual measurement differences (between right- and left-sided stimuli) are avoided. With an electrical stimulus, two electrical silent periods occur interrupting the voluntary EMG activity in the ipsilateral and contralateral masseter muscles. The first (SP1) corresponds to the SP after a mechanical tap and the second one (SP2) begins 30–60 ms after the stimulus. Prolongation of either absolute latencies, ipsilateral-contralateral latency difference, or side-to-side latency difference when recorded from one muscle is considered abnormal. Perhaps because electrical stimuli yield mixed nociceptive and non-nociceptive inputs, whether the SP1, SP2, or both components are nociceptive reflexes remains controversial.

2.4.2 Applications

The silent period may be absent in patients with trigeminal sensory neuropathies that result in significant impairment of the reflex mechanism involved in chewing [13]. It is also sometimes absent in tetanus and may be unilaterally absent in patients with hemimasticatory spasm. The latency of SP1 is often delayed in patients with demyelinating neuropathies [14]. MIR is especially useful to confirm conduction delay secondary to demyelination in severe neuropathies with absent sensory and muscle action potentials as well as blink reflex, as it can still be measured. MIR remains normal in axonopathies. An afferent abnormality (absent or delayed direct and crossed responses to unilateral stimulation) indicates a lesion along the afferent path (intra- or extra-axial before the site of crossing of the impulse volley). SP1 is more susceptible than SP2 to extra-axial lesions, such as trigeminal neuropathy. Brainstem lesions may show an afferent delay or block to unilateral stimulation and abnormal crossed responses to contralateral stimulation, or abnormal crossed responses to stimulation of either side. The lesion involves the dorsal pontine tegmentum at the level of the mid-pons if both SP1 and SP2 are affected, and the lower pons or the pontomedullary junction if SP2 alone is affected. A unilateral efferent abnormality (absent or delayed responses confined to the muscle on one side, irrespective of the side of stimulation) is extremely rare except in cases of unilateral masticatory spasm [15].

2.5 Trigeminal Somatosensory-Evoked Potentials

Different approaches have been used to study the trigeminal system by the evoked potential techniques. As these techniques are not frequently used, clinically their practical application and utility remain poorly defined. The main problems associated with somatosensory-evoked potentials (SEPs) from the trigeminal territory are stimulus artifact (with electrical stimulation), unwanted stimulus spread to facial muscles innervated by the facial nerve, and direct or reflex muscle activities (with mechanical stimulation), which contaminate scalp recordings. In addition to the limitations related to puff stimulation that appeared to activate receptors with differing thresholds. The suggested solution was the use of invasive techniques such as the use of electrical pulses to the tooth pulp or gums and needle electrode stimulation at the mental foramen [16]. Despite the last method's reliability, its invasiveness limited its use. Another consideration was the use of short versus long latency potentials [17]. Very short latency-evoked potentials were recorded by Leandri et al. who described an invasive technique to stimulate the mental nerve without simultaneous activation of the surrounding muscles, with a technique similar to that used to stimulate the infraorbital and supraorbital nerves. Inferior alveolar nerve (IAN) SEPs have been used to evaluate the sensory function of the mandibular branch through the mental nerve, and a separate technique was reported with stimulation of the mental nerve at the mandibular foramen, with recording early evoked potentials over the scalp. With IAN SEPs, it became possible to evaluate nerve function and its central connections noninvasively. The use of near-nerve electrode over the mentalis nerve causes localized stimulation without triggering the movement of the jaw and muscle artifact. Hand stimulation of the IAN endings with surface electrodes has been successfully demonstrated and normative data have been published [18–20]. Arcuri et al. described a reliable technique of a regular pattern of peak events that were stable and not contaminated by muscle artifact [21]. In a study by Rossini et al. IAN SEPs were recorded in a noninvasive technique and represented a noninvasive objective method to evaluate sensory nerve function in the maxillofacial region with very similar results [22]. Latencies obtained by this method were more stable than amplitudes, and mean latency values were similar to those reported by Arcuri et al. 2006.

2.6 Laser-Evoked Potentials and Contact Heat-Evoked Potentials

Owing to the growing interest in the evaluation of neuropathic pain and somatosensory pain pathways, the assessment of nociceptive cerebral-evoked potentials using laser-evoked potentials (LEPs) has been extensively studied and proven to be a very reliable method. It is considered the gold standard objective test that is highly specific for small fiber/spinothalamic tract function evaluation. Because of the short conduction distance and high receptor density, the trigeminal LEPs are of higher amplitude and recorded easier than with limb stimulation [23]. Due to the radiant heat delivered through laser beams and the risk of eye damage and skin burns, another method of stimulating the skin with contact heat conveyed through thermofoil thermodes with brain electrical source analysis was developed and became of practical application in recent years. Both methods LEPs and contact heat-evoked potentials (CHEPs) stimulate the same type of nociceptors in cutaneous Aδ and C fibers. The main difference in stimulation for LEPs versus CHEPs during the thermode skin application of stimulus is a slope of the temperature rise which is 70 °C/s (centigrade/second) for CHEPs that is considerably less than that for LEPs, which is about 1000 °C/s [24, 25]. A large multicenter international study by Granowsky et al. provided a previously lacking data set of normative values that facilitated the clinical use of CHEPs 26]. The data are valid only for the equipment, setup, and stimulation parameters used in the study. Normative values at different body parts (face, upper and lower limbs, cervical and lumbar spine) were analyzed for both males and females, compared between both sides of the body, and correlated their amplitudes and latencies with age and sex. Contact heat-evoked potentials latencies and amplitudes were similar on both sides of the body hence were both reliable and sufficient for normative data with unilateral assessment. Prolonged latencies and reduced amplitudes were associated with aging and correlated with age-related changes in thermal pain perception. Females responded with higher amplitudes and shorter latencies compared with males, but both genders reported similar pain scores.

3 Conclusion

The described electrophysiological studies of the trigeminal nerves and their application in the right clinical contexts provide useful diagnostic tools to localize the lesion to the peripheral or central nervous systems and sometimes assist in prognostication. Moreover, the addition of these tests to the routine diagnostic armamentarium (nerve conduction studies, EMG, SEP, MRI, etc.) in combination with the neurological examination and disease phenotype increases the yield of identifying and/or classifying the peripheral nerve process, and ultimately guiding further disease-targeted evaluation and therapy.

References

1. Aramideh M, de Visser BWO. Brainstem reflexes: electrodiagnostic techniques, physiology, normative data, and clinical applications. Muscle Nerve. 2002;26:14–30.
2. Cruccu G, Inghilleri M, Fraioli B, Guidetti B, Manfredi M. Neurophysiologic assessment of trigeminal function after surgery for trigeminal neuralgia. Neurology. 1987;37:631.
3. Kugelberg E. Facial reflexes. Brain 1952;75:385–96.
4. Kimura J, Power JM, Van Allen MW. Reflex reponse of the obicularis oculi muslce to supraobrital nerve stimulation: study in normal subjects and in peripheral facial paresis. Trans Am Neurol Assoc. 1969;94:288–90.
5. Kimura J, Rodnitzky RL, Van Allen MW. Electrodiagnostic study of trigeminal nerve. Orbicularis oculi reflex and masseter reflex in trigeminal neuralgia, paratrigeminal syndrome, and other lesions of the trigeminal nerve. Neurology. 1970;20:574–83.
6. de Visser BWO. Afferent limb of the human jaw reflex: electrophysiologic and anatomic study. Neurology. 1982;32:563–6.
7. de Visser BWO, Goor C. Jaw reflexes and masseter electromyograms in mesencephalic and pontine lesions: an electrodiagnostic study. J Neurol Neurosurg Psychiatry. 1976;39:90–2.
8. Cruccu G, de Visser BWO. The jaw reflexes. The international federation of clinical neurophysiology. Electroencephalogr Clin Neurophysiol Suppl. 1999;52:243–7.
9. Auger RG. Preservation of the masseter reflex in Friedreich's ataxia. Neurology. 1999;42:875–8.
10. Goodwiil CJ, O'Tuama L. Electromyographic recording of the jaw reflex in multiple sclerosis. J Neurol Neurosurg Psychiatry. 1969;32:6–10.
11. Valls-Sole J. Neurophysiological assessment of trigeminal nerve reflexes in disorders of central and peripheral nervous system. Clin Neurophysiol. 2005;116:2255–65.
12. Godaux E, Desmedt JE. Exteroceptive suppression and motor control of the masseter and temporalis muscles in normal man. Brain Res. 1975;85:447–58.
13. Auger RG, McManis PG. Trigeminal sensory neuropathy associated with decreased oral sensation and impairment of the masseter inhibitory reflex. Neurology. 1990;40:759–63.
14. Cruccu G, Agostino R, Inghilleri M, Innocenti P, Romaniello A, Manfredi M. Mandibular nerve involvement in diabetic polyneuropathy and chronic inflammatory demyelinating polyneuropathy. Muscle Nerve. 1998;21:1673–9.

15. Cruccu G, Pauletti G, Agostino R, Berardelli A, Manfredi M. Masseter inhibitory reflex in movement disorders. Huntington's chorea, Parkinson's disease, dystonia, and unilateral masticatory spasm. Electroencephalogr Clin Neurophysiol. 1991;81:24–30.
16. Singh N, Sachdev KK, Brisman R. Trigeminal nerve stimulation: short latency somatosensory evoked potentials. Neurology. 1982;32:97–101.
17. Soustiel JF, Feinsod M, Hafner H. Short latency trigeminal evoked potentials: normative data and clinical correlations. Electroencephalogr Clin Neurophysiol. 1991;80:119–25.
18. Bennett MH, Jannetta PJ. Trigeminal evoked potentials in humans. Electroencephalogr Clin Neurophysiol. 1980;48:517–26.
19. Pogrel MA, Mouhabaty D, Dodson T, Rampil I, Grecco M. Trigeminal somatosensory evoked potentials: a normal value study. J Dent. 1992;20:298–301.
20. Barker GR, Bennett AJ, Wastell DG. Normative studies of the TSEP. The basis of an objective sensory testing procedure in oral and maxillofacial surgery. Int J Oral Maxillofac Surg. 1987;16:586–92.
21. Arcuri C, Muzzi F, Docimo R, Fusco E, Pauri F, Rossini PM. Somatosensory evoked potentials of inferior alveolar nerve. J Oral Maxillofac Surg. 2006;64:594–9.
22. Rossini, C, Luigetti M, Romanello R, Gnoni V, Virdis D, Cordaro M, Rossini P.M. Somatosensory Evoked Potentials of Inferior Alveolar Nerve: confirmation of a possible non-invasive neurophysiological approach. Clin. Ter. 2016;167:25–8.
23. Bromm B, Chen AC. Brain electrical source analysis of laser evoked potentials in response to painful trigeminal nerve stimulation. Electroencephalogr Clin Neurophysiol. 1995;95:14–26.
24. Cruccu G, Romaniello A, Amantini A, Lombardi M, Innocenti P, Manfredi M. Assessment of trigeminal small-fiber function: brain and reflex responses evoked by CO2-laser stimulation. Muscle Nerve. 1999;22:508–16.
25. Kakigi R, Shibasaki H, Tanaka K, et al. CO2 laser-induced painrelated somatosensory evoked potentials in peripheral neuropathies: correlation between electrophysiological and histopathological findings. Muscle Nerve. 1991;14:441–50.
26. Granovsky Y, Anand P, Nakae A, et al. Normative data for Adelta contact heat evoked potentials in adult population: a multicenter study. Pain 2016;157:1156–63.

Magnetic Resonance Imaging Evaluation of Trigeminal Neuralgia

Hyung-Jin Kim, Yi Kyung Kim, and Minjung Seong

Trigeminal neuralgia (TN) is probably the most well-known type of facial pain under the category of chronic peripheral neuropathic pain disorders [1, 2]. It is the most common disease entity in the spectrum of neurovascular compression syndrome (NVCS) of the intracranial cavity, defined as a direct contact with mechanical irritation of the cranial nerves by the blood vessels [3–6]. Although a wide variety of diseases are categorized as NVCS according to the affected CNs and the resulting symptoms, the evidence-based firm cause-and-effect relationship was generally recognized in only three conditions, including TN for the trigeminal nerve, hemifacial spasm (HFS) for the facial nerve, and vago-glossopharyngeal neuralgia for the vagus and glossopharyngeal nerves [5, 7].

According to the revised classification system adopted by the International Headache Society (IHS) and the International Association for the Study of Pain (IASP) to align classification and to standardize terminology between the two groups, TN is now classified as classical, secondary (symptomatic), and idiopathic types [1, 8–13]. In this classification, the classical type refers to TN that is associated with vascular compression with the radiological or surgical evidence of morphologic changes of the root of the trigeminal nerve, while the secondary type accounting for approximately 15% of cases, refers to TN attributable to an underlying disease such as multiple sclerosis or tumor in the cerebellopontine angle (CPA). When there is no cause of neural disturbance identified on the diagnostic tests, it is classified as idiopathic TN and accounts for approximately 10% of cases [1, 10–13]. Primary TN encompasses both classical and idiopathic TNs [14]. Although paroxysmal facial pain is the hallmark of TN, 14–50% of patients also have a concomitant continuous pain between paroxysmal attacks in the same area as the paroxysmal pain. This type of TN was previously known as Type 2 or atypical TN [15] and is now simply referred to TN with concomitant continuous pain [12, 13].

As in the other categories of NVCS, recent technical advances have firmly established magnetic resonance imaging (MRI) as the gold standard for imaging evaluation of patients with classical TN. With the aid of magnetic resonance angiography (MRA), MRI provides valuable information on the detailed neurovascular relationship that might be responsible for the clinical symptoms [6, 7, 16–20].

In this chapter, we will discuss the role of MRI in patients with TN—how to image and what to look. The current MRI techniques used for TN and the MRI features of classical and secondary TN are described. Compression of the trigeminal nerve by the blood vessels in asymptomatic

H.-J. Kim (✉) · Y. K. Kim · M. Seong
Department of Radiology, Samsung Medical Center, Sungkyunkwan University School of Medicine, Seoul, Republic of Korea
e-mail: hyungkim@skku.edu; yk2009.kim@samsung.com; m.seong@samsung.com

K. Park, K. R. Cho (eds.), *Trigeminal Neuralgia*, https://doi.org/10.1007/978-981-19-9171-4_6

subjects and the imaging issues on failed microvascular decompression (MVD) will be addressed as well. For the sake of simplicity, we will focus on the cisternal segment of the trigeminal nerve, where neurovascular compression (NVC) on the root entry zone (REZ) is believed to cause classical TN.

1 MR Imaging Techniques Used for Trigeminal Neuralgia

High-resolution three-dimensional (3D) MRI has proved useful and highly accurate in the preoperative evaluation of all of the different types of TN. Recent advances in hardware and software of MRI enabled us to obtain images of high quality in a reasonably short time. Transversely oriented axial images obtained with a 3D heavily T2-weighted fast imaging sequence, so-called magnetic resonance cisternography (MRC), is well suited for evaluation of the complex relationship between the trigeminal nerve and adjacent blood vessels. In these images, the low signal intensity of the nerves and vessels contrasts with the bright signal intensity of the background cerebrospinal fluid (CSF) (Fig. 1a) [16, 19, 21]. Based on the isotropic images obtained with the 3D technique, the images can be displayed in any plane by multiplanar reformation (MPR) to improve the precision of evaluation [16–18]. In particular, the coronal reformatted MR images can provide additional valuable information on the site and severity of NVC, which might be underestimated if we depend on the axial images alone (Fig. 1b, c).

Various 3D steady-state fast gradient-echo (FGE) and 3D fast spin-echo (FSE) sequences have been used among the different vendors, with the former including FIESTA-C, CISS, and bTFE and the latter including CUBE, SPACE, and VISTA [6, 7, 20].

3D time-of-flight (TOF) MRA is another useful MRI technique to visualize the offending arteries (Fig. 1d) [6, 17, 22, 23]. Image fusion that combines MRC and 3D TOF MRA has been reported to display the neurovascular relationship more vividly in patients with TN [21, 24–26].

3D contrast-enhanced T1-weighted imaging sequence is useful in the evaluation of TN, especially for the evaluation of secondary TN caused by tumor, inflammation, and demyelinating disease (Fig. 1e) [6, 20]. Venous compression that may cause TN can be demonstrated much better with this technique [21, 27]. Recently, 3D contrast-enhanced CISS imaging has also been reported to be useful for the evaluation of patients with unilateral TN by improving both characterization of higher-grade NVC in the affected side and performance in predicting favorable outcomes after MVD [28].

Fluid-attenuated inversion recovery (FLAIR) sequence is useful to evaluate patients with secondary TN, as seen in patients with demyelinating diseases, such as multiple sclerosis. By using an inversion recovery pulse, the signal intensity of CSF is nulled and the lesion other than fluid is demonstrated as high signal intensity on the images (Fig. 1f) [20]. The value of the fusion images generated by 3D FLAIR and MRC has also been reported in patients with TN [29].

Diffusion-weighted imaging (DWI) is also helpful in the evaluation of patients with TN. The lesions showing restricted diffusion are seen as an area of high signal intensity on DWI and are best exemplified by the diseases causing secondary TN such as brainstem infarction and epidermoid cyst in the CPA (Fig. 2) [20]. Diffusion tensor imaging with tractography can provide important information on the microstructural alterations within the trigeminal nerve in patients with TN by demonstrating decreased fractional anisotropy (FA) due to tissue damage associated with demyelination on the affected side [6, 7, 30]. These microstructural alterations are evident in the affected trigeminal nerve in patients with both classical and idiopathic TN with or without appreciable atrophic changes of the nerve [6]. Diffusivity abnormalities are reported to be different between primary TN and TN secondary to multiple sclerosis. While abnormal diffusivity is

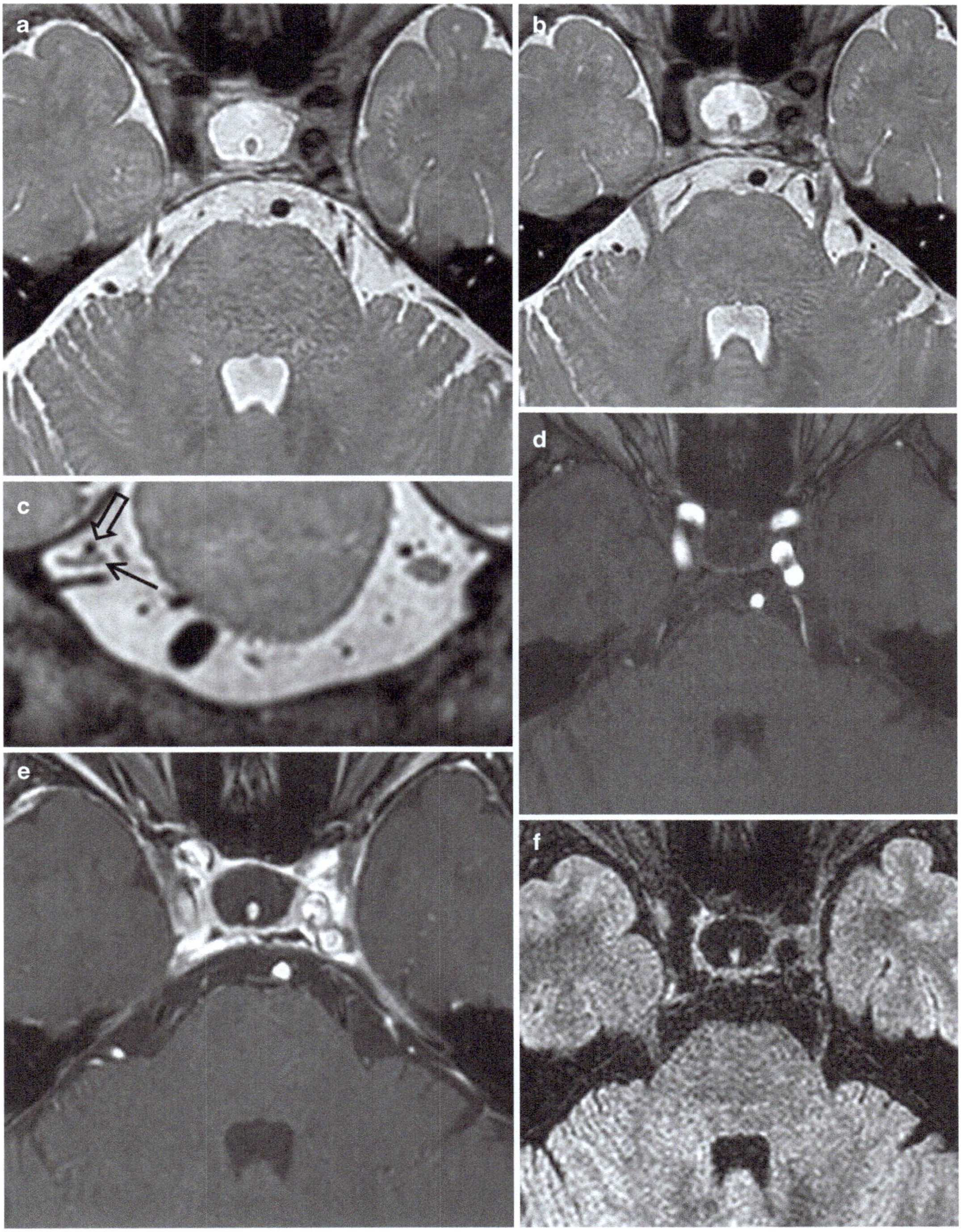

Fig. 1 Various 3D MRI sequences used for evaluation of hemifacial spasm. (**a**) MR cisternography (MRC) using 3D volumetric isotropic turbo spin echo acquisition (T2 VISTA). (**b**) and (**c**) Axial MRC (**b**) shows no significant abnormality at the cisternal segment of the right trigeminal nerve (arrow). However, MRC in coronal plane (**c**) nicely demonstrates the atrophic cisternal segment of the right trigeminal nerve which is compressed by the superior cerebellar artery (open arrow) in this patient with trigeminal neuralgia in the right side. (**d**) MR angiography (MRA) using 3D time-of-flight (TOF). (**e**) Contrast-enhanced T1-weighted imaging using 3D balanced turbo field echo (bTFE). (**f**) Fluid-attenuated inversion recovery (FLAIR) image using 3D FLAIR-VISTA

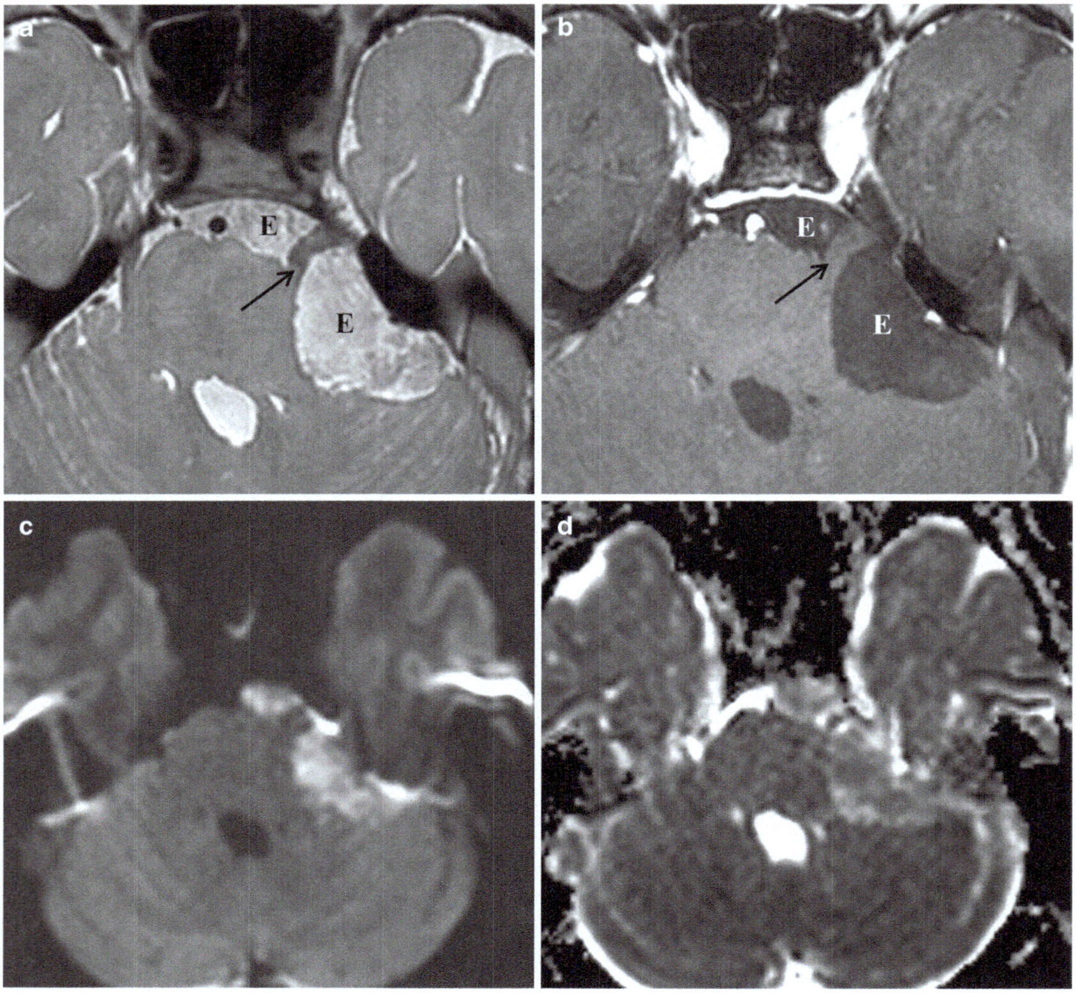

Fig. 2 Trigeminal neuralgia associated with an epidermoid cyst. (**a**) and (**b**) MRC (**a**) and 3D contrast-enhanced T1-weighted image (**b**) show a large infiltrative mass (E) in the left cerebellopontine angle, which causes encasement and displacement of the ipsilateral trigeminal nerve (arrow). The mass shows heterogeneous hyperintensity on MRC (**a**) and does not enhance after contrast injection (**b**), which represents the cystic nature of the lesion. (**c**) and (**d**) Diffusion weighted image (DWI) obtained with $b = 1000$ (**c**) and apparent diffusion coefficient (ADC) map image (**d**) demonstrate the high signal intensity and the low signal intensity within the mass, respectively, which is related to restricted diffusion, characteristic of the epidermoid cyst

typically seen in the cisternal segment of the trigeminal nerve in patients with primary TN, it mostly involves the intrapontine fibers of the trigeminal nerve in patients with multiple sclerosis [6, 13]. This observation can provide useful information preoperatively to triage patients who are likely to fail MVD [13]. Reversibility of an abnormal diffusivity has also been reported after successful MVD [7].

2 Anatomy of the Cisternal Segment of the Trigeminal Nerve

The cisternal segment of the trigeminal nerve refers to the portion of the nerve within the prepontine cistern, composed of the sensory and motor roots. After leaving the brain stem, it courses anterosuperiorly, passing over the tip of the petrous apex, and enters the Meckel's cave through the porus trigeminus, which contains the trigeminal (gasserian) ganglion (Fig. 3) [31]. The smaller motor roots, typically 1–3 in number, arise separately from the brain stem, superomedial to the larger sensory root (Fig. 3) [7, 32].

The most appealing theory as to the pathogenesis of NVCS is that NVC initiates demyelination of the nerve at the REZ, which causes ephaptic transmission of neural impulse [4, 33, 34]. In general, the sensory nerves are known to have a longer REZ than the motor nerves [33]. Anatomically, the REZ includes not only the transition zone (TZ) but also the central myelin portion of the nerve root and subpial portion of the nerve fascicles within the brain stem [5, 6, 18]. The TZ is a cone-shaped organization where a transition occurs between the oligodendrocyte-derived central myelin and the Schwann cell-derived peripheral myelin and is believed

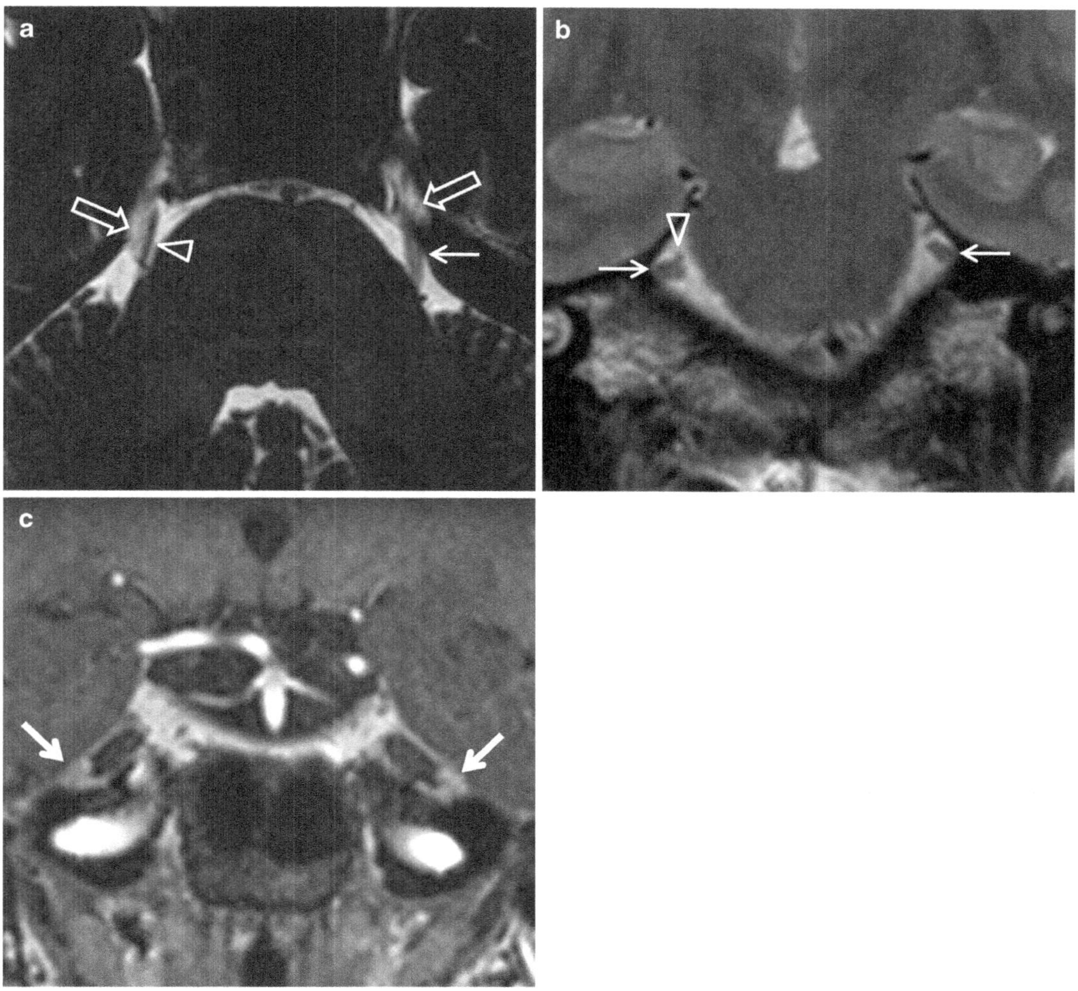

Fig. 3 Anatomy of the trigeminal nerve. (**a**) and (**b**) MRCs in axial (**a**) and coronal (**b**) planes demonstrate the cisternal segment of the trigeminal nerve within the prepontine cistern (arrows). It consists of the sensory (arrows) and motor (arrowhead) roots with the latter usually being located superomedial to the former. The nerve enters the CSF-filled Meckel's cave through the porus trigeminus (open arrows in **a**). (**c**) Within the Meckel's cave, the trigeminal ganglion normally enhances well on 3D contrast-enhanced T1-weighted image (thick arrows) because of the lack of blood-brain-barrier

particularly prone to the mechanical irritation caused by NVC [5, 6, 33]. Compared to the central myelin segment, the peripheral myelin segment of the CNs is more resistant to NVC because of the different morphological properties including the undulating nerve fibers, organized layers of supporting tissue such as endoneurium, perineurium, and epineurium, and well-organized myelination [33]. Each cranial nerve has a different length and size of the REZ. In a cadaveric study, the average length of the trigeminal nerve from the pons to Meckel's cave was reported to be 13.11 ± 1.12 mm (range, 11.9–15.2 mm). The most distal part of the TZ of the trigeminal nerve was at 4.19 ± 0.81 mm (range, 3.24–5.65 mm) from the brain stem and the volume of central myelin portion measured about 24.54 ± 9.82 mm^3 (range, 10.11–38.82 mm^3) [5]. The length of central myelin is shorter on the medial side (mean, 1.13 mm; range, 0.1–2.5 mm) than on its lateral side (mean, 2.47 mm; range, 0.17–6.75 mm) [35]. For the motor roots, central myelin is much closer to the brain stem with the average length being reported as 0.3 mm (range, 0–1.0 mm) [32].

3 MRI Evaluation of Trigeminal Neuralgia

3.1 MRI Evaluation of Classical TN

The first step of MRI interpretation in patients with TN is to exclude secondary causes, such as multiple sclerosis, CPA tumors, ischemic changes, and other vascular lesions. If those lesions are not found on MRI, one should carefully focus on the course of the trigeminal nerve within the prepontine cistern if there is evidence of vascular compression that may be responsible for the clinical symptoms. As mentioned before, in the revised classification, classical TN should satisfy NVC that is accompanied by the radiological or surgical evidence of morphologic changes of the trigeminal nerve root, such as distortion, displacement, flattening, or atrophy (Fig. 4a, b). Simple contact between the nerve and the vascular structures is considered insufficient to explain the patient's symptoms and should be classified as idiopathic TN (Fig. 4c, d) [12, 13]. To characterize the NVC in patients with classical TN, the following items should be included in the radiologic report on MRI—the type of the offending (culprit) vessels and the site and severity of NVC.

The offending vessels are usually arterial with the superior cerebellar artery being the most common artery in 57–88%, followed by the anterior inferior cerebellar artery in 7–39% [6, 7, 36]. Less often, the trigeminal nerve is compressed by the posterior inferior cerebellar, basilar, and vertebral arteries (Fig. 5a–d). Type 1 TN is significantly more likely associated with arterial compression [36]. The venous cause is less common, reported in 8–10%, with the tributaries of the superior petrosal vein accounting for the majority of cases (Fig. 5e, f) [6, 36, 37]. In contrast to Type 1 TN, Type 2 TN is reported to be associated with venous compression nearly as often as arterial compression [9]. The association of venous compression with TN isolated to the facial territory supplied by the maxillary division of the trigeminal nerve has been reported as well [36]. Not infrequently, TN is associated with multiple vascular compression in various combinations (Fig. 6) [6, 36].

The site of NVC should be addressed whether it involves the REZ or a more distal portion of the trigeminal nerve. The incidence of NVC at the REZ in classical TN is reported as 80–90% (Figs. 4a, 5a, b) [34]. As expected, the more the proximal site of NVC, the greater the likelihood that the vessel is a real offender. According to an MRI study by Suzuki et al. [38], the rate of TN was much higher in proximal (≤ 3 mm) than in distal (>3 mm) NVC (83.1% vs 19.6%). The practical cutoff of 3 mm from the brain stem may be a reasonable compromise for localizing the TZ of the trigeminal nerve on MRI [7]. In contrast to arterial compression, venous compression is reported to more commonly affect the distal cisternal segment of the trigeminal nerve (Fig. 5e, f) [6, 37].

The severity of NVC can be classified as simple contact, displacement, and atrophy as the severity increases, with the latter two being

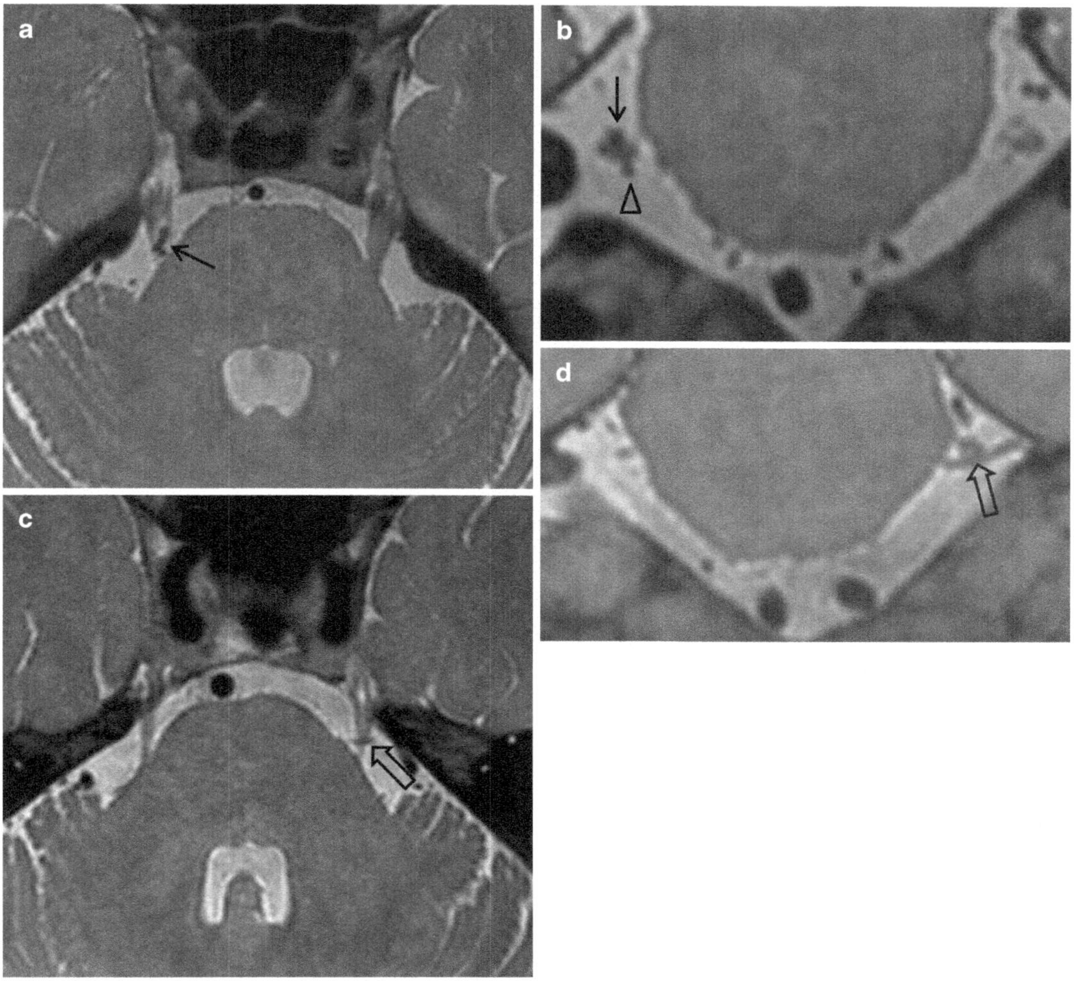

Fig. 4 (**a**) and (**b**) Classical trigeminal neuralgia. MRCs in axial (**a**) and coronal (**b**) planes demonstrate the right superior cerebellar artery that causes a severe compression on the superior aspect of the transition zone of the ipsilateral trigeminal nerve (arrows), which is most typical in patients with classical trigeminal neuralgia. Also noted is a small vein inferior to the right trigeminal nerve with no mass effect on the nerve (arrowhead in **b**). (**c**) and (**d**) Idiopathic trigeminal neuralgia. MRCs in axial (**c**) and coronal (**d**) planes in the patient with left-sided trigeminal neuralgia demonstrate a small tributary of the left superior petrosal vein that is simply in contact with the inferior margin of the transition zone of the ipsilateral trigeminal nerve (open arrows) with no evidence of morphologic changes of the nerve. This kind of a simple contact between the trigeminal nerve and the vascular structures is now believed insufficient for the cause of the clinical symptoms, and is hence classified as idiopathic trigeminal neuralgia

categorized into severe contact (Figs. 1c, 4a, 5c, 6) [39]. To reiterate the revised classification of TN, simple neurovascular contact alone without morphologic changes of the nerve is now classified as idiopathic TN (Fig. 4c, d). Severe NVC has been reported to be highly prevalent on the symptomatic side compared to the asymptomatic side [17, 26, 39]. When there are multiple offenders, each site of vascular compression should be reported one by one.

TN without significant vascular compression, so-called idiopathic TN, is well known and has been reported in 3–17% [40]. Its pathogenesis remains unclear and several potential

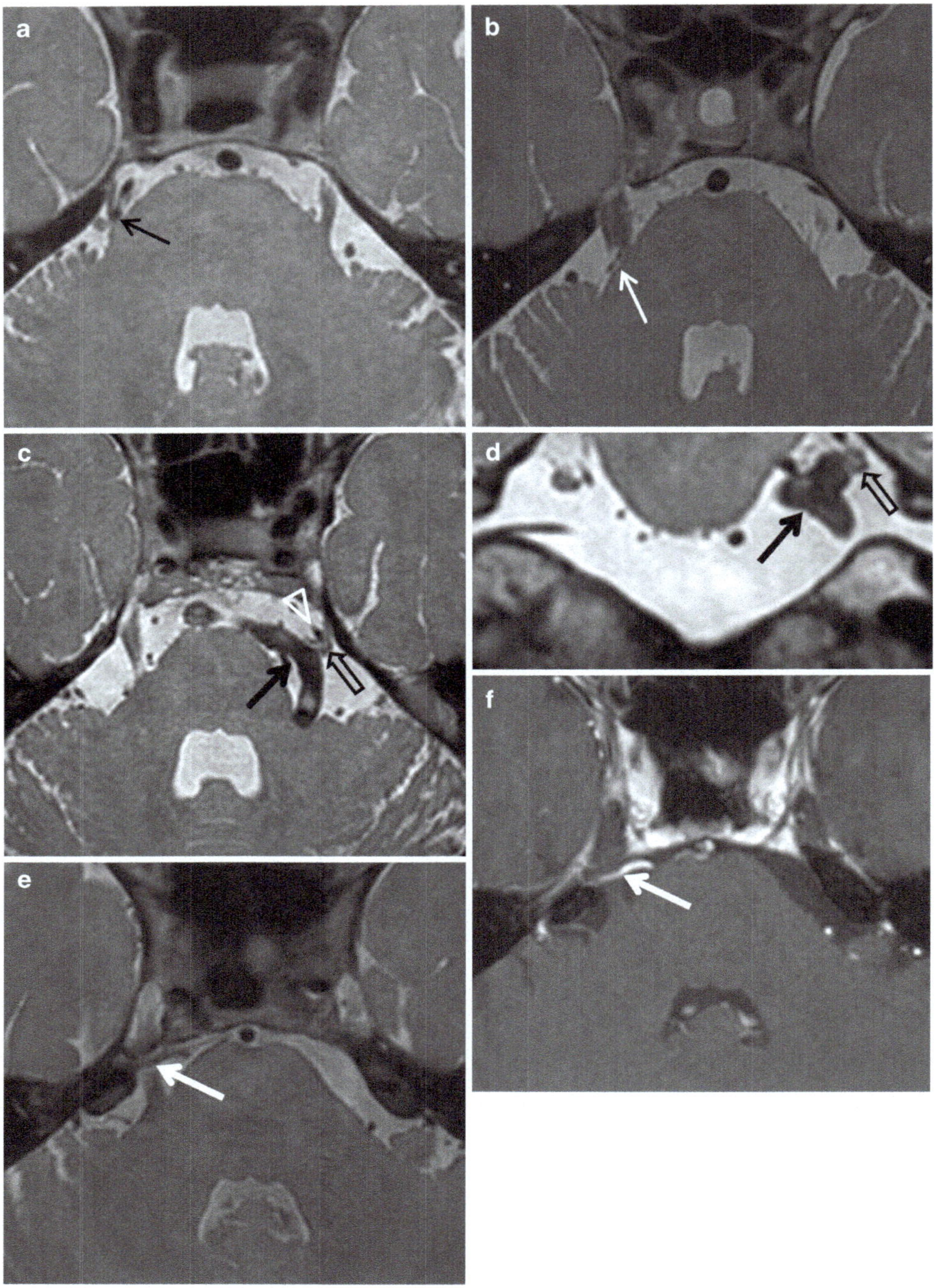

Fig. 5 Examples of various offending vessels and sites of neurovascular compression in different patients with trigeminal neuralgia. (**a**) and (**b**) MRCs in two different patients show the right superior cerebellar artery (black arrow in **a**) and the right anterior cerebellar artery (white arrow in **b**), both of which cause compression on the transition zone of each trigeminal nerve. (**c**) and (**d**) MRCs in axial (**c**) and coronal (**d**) planes in same patient demonstrate a sandwich type of neurovascular compression at the cisternal segment (open arrows) by the dolichoectatic vertebrobasilar artery (arrows) and superior cerebellar artery (arrowhead in **c**) in combination. (**e**) and (**f**) MRC (**e**) and 3D contrast-enhanced T1-weighted image (**f**) in same patient demonstrate the right superior petrosal vein that causes mild compression on the cisternal segment of the ipsilateral trigeminal nerve (arrows)

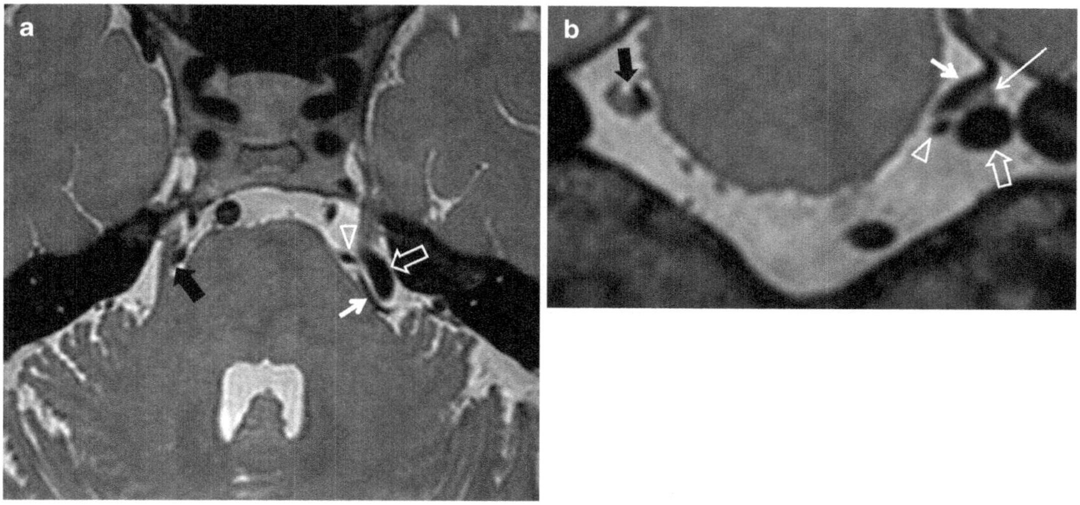

Fig. 6 Trigeminal neuralgia caused by multiple offending vessels. (**a**) and (**b**) MRCs in axial (**a**) and coronal (**b**) planes in the patient with left-sided trigeminal neuralgia demonstrate multiple offending vessels that cause a sandwich type of neurovascular compression on the transition zone of the left trigeminal nerve (long arrow in **b**), including the vertebral (open arrows), superior cerebellar (short arrows), and anterior inferior cerebellar (arrowheads) arteries. Incidentally, neurovascular compression is also noted in the asymptomatic side at the transition zone of the right trigeminal nerve by the superior cerebellar artery (thich black arrows)

explanations have been proposed. Devor et al. [4] suggested that minimal root pathology might be enough to yield significant pain in some predisposed persons and also more favorably that the primary pathology would not be in the REZ but in or near the trigeminal ganglion. Ishikawa et al. [41] proposed that tethering on the trigeminal nerve associated with arachnoid thickening or granulomatous adhesions could cause an abnormal stretching at the REZ and angulation and torsion of the root, leading to hyperexcitability. A small cerebellopontine angle cistern appears to be associated with nerve atrophy and TN [42].

It is well known that vascular contact is not infrequent on MRI in subjects with no clinical symptoms of TN and has been reported in 18–78% [29, 38, 39, 43–46]. Meta-analysis of pooled data from nine MRI studies by Antonini et al. [46] revealed that NVC was detected in 471 (88.7%) of 531 symptomatic nerves and in 244 (35.8%) of 681 asymptomatic nerves ($p < 0.0001$). Among these, NVC at the REZ was detected in 97 (76.3%) of 127 symptomatic nerves and in 34 (16.5%) of 205 asymptomatic nerves ($p < 0.0001$), while NVC distal to the REZ was detected in 12 (22.2%) of 54 symptomatic nerves and in 34 (25.7%) of 132 asymptomatic nerves ($p < 0.58$). In their study, morphologic changes of the nerves were also significantly more prevalent on the symptomatic side (152/286 [53.1%]), compared to the asymptomatic side (43/474 [9.1%]) ($p < 0.0001$). It is very likely that the site and severity of NVC are key factors to provoke the clinical symptoms. Sometimes, MRI shows the trigeminal nerve that is compressed more severely on the asymptomatic side than on the symptomatic side. To avoid such pitfalls, we need to make sure which side is symptomatic during image interpretation, because the imaging findings are valuable only when clinically relevant [6].

3.2 MRI Evaluation of Secondary TN

About 15% of patients with TN are associated with a major underlying neurologic disease such as multiple sclerosis and CPA tumors and are

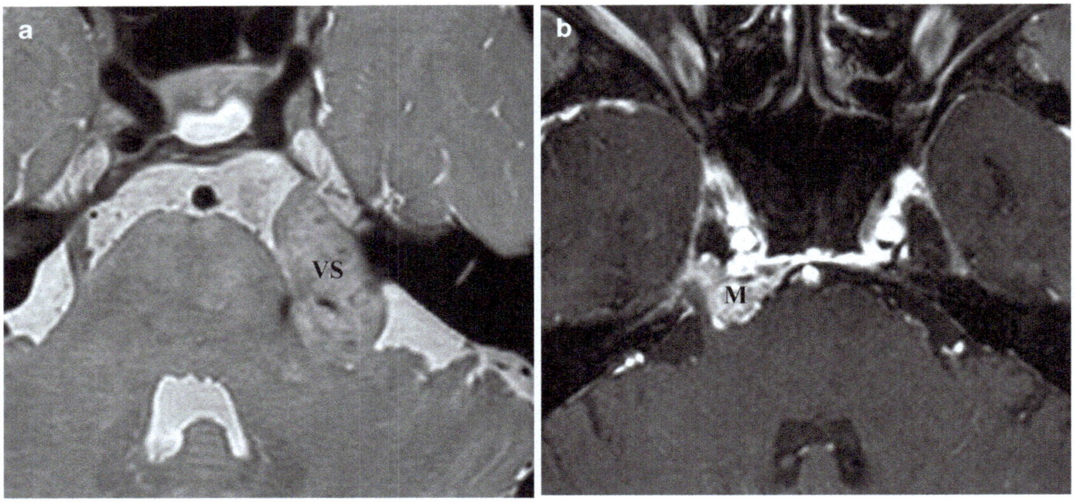

Fig. 7 Examples of secondary trigeminal neuralgia. (**a**) Vestibular schwannoma. MRC shows a large lobulated soft tissue mass (VS) in the left cerebellopontine angle, causing significant compression on the medial aspect of the ipsilateral trigeminal nerve as well as the adjacent brain stem. (**b**) Petroclival meningioma. 3D contrast-enhanced T1-weighted image shows a well-enhancing irregular dural-based soft tissue mass (M) in the right cerebellopontine angle. The mass causes significant compression on the medial aspect of the ipsilateral trigeminal nerve and infiltrates the ipsilateral Meckel's cave

classified as secondary or symptomatic TN [12, 13, 47]. TN occurs in 2–5% of patients with multiple sclerosis, sometimes bilaterally, while multiple sclerosis is present in 2–14% of patients with TN [10]. Compared with the general population, the risk of TN is increased by a factor of 20 among patients with multiple sclerosis [12]. TN related to multiple sclerosis is attributed to demyelinating plaques at the REZ or in the fascicular segment through the ventral pons [1, 12]. CPA tumors leading to TN are mostly benign and include vestibular schwannomas, meningiomas, and epidermoid cysts (Figs. 2 and 7) [10, 12]. They typically compress the REZ of the trigeminal nerve. In a study based on the meta-analysis of four studies, tumors were the cause of TN in 20 (8%) of 243 patients [47]. Interestingly, trigeminal neuromas have not been associated with TN [12]. Malignant tumors are more likely to infiltrate the nerve and cause axonal degeneration, resulting in hypoesthesia in regions of the face and persistent pain, which is different from pain in TN [10]. Other uncommon causes of secondary TN include skull base deformity, connective tissue disease, arteriovenous malformation, dural arteriovenous fistula, and genetic causes of neuropathy or nerve hyperexcitability [1]. By using the various pulse sequences, MRI plays an important role in the management of secondary TN not only for the diagnosis of the lesions but also for a precise assessment of the extent of the lesions to help clinicians determine the best treatment option for the patients. It is beyond scope of this chapter to deal with the detailed MRI findings of the various causes of secondary TN. As previously shown in Fig. 2, DWI is very useful for the diagnosis of the epidermoid cyst.

3.3 MRI Evaluation of Persistent or Recurrent TN After MVD

MVD is the first-choice surgery for patients with drug-resistant classical TN with rates of immediate postoperative pain relief being reported in 87–98% [7, 13]. However, this rate decreases to 58–68% after 8–10 years [7]. The surgical findings during repeat MVD responsible for the recurrent symptoms include the missed offending vessels, insufficient decompression, malposition and displacement of the surgical sponge, newly developed vascular compression, arachnoid

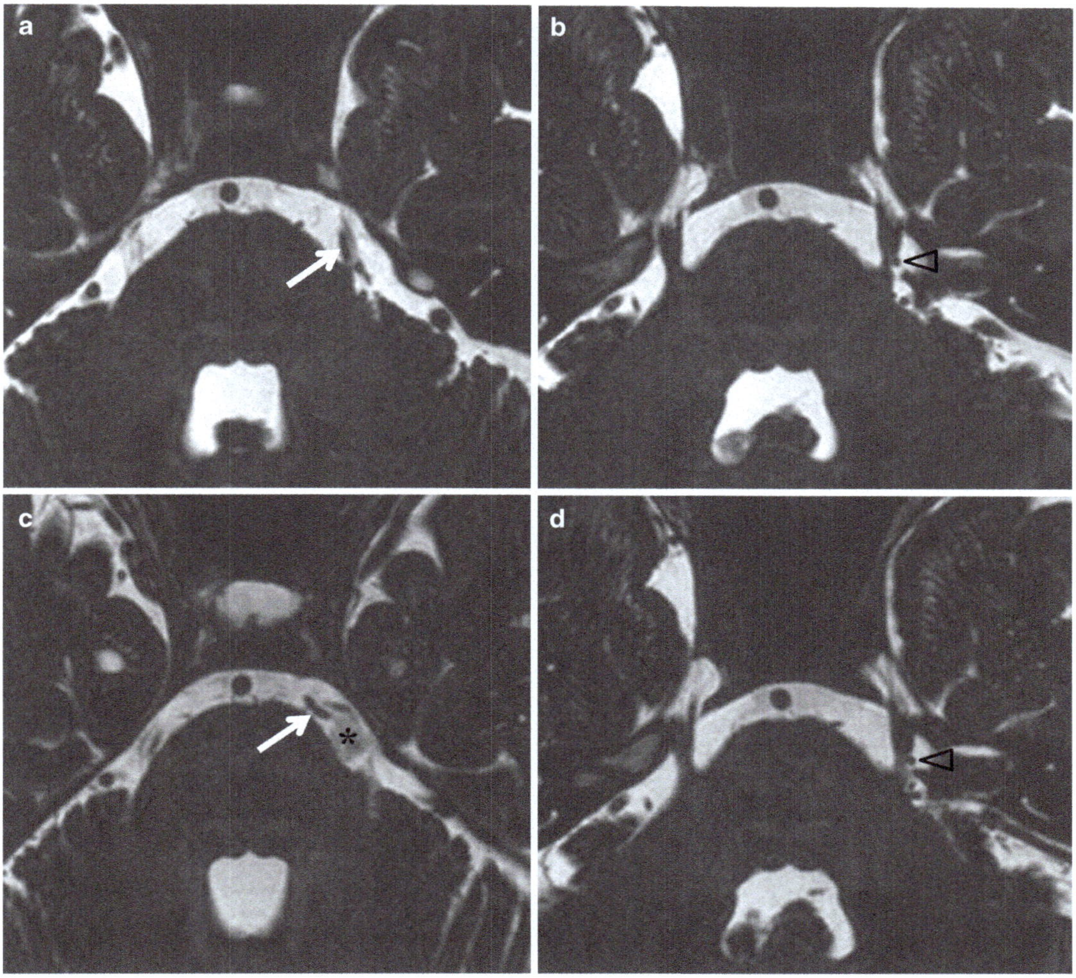

Fig. 8 Recurrent trigeminal neuralgia after microvascular decompression. (**a**) and (**b**) MRCs obtained before microvascular decompression demonstrate neurovascular compression at two different sites of the transition zone of the left trigeminal nerve by the superior cerebellar artery (arrow in **a**) and anterior inferior cerebellar artery (arrowhead in **b**), respectively. (**c**) and (**d**) MRCs obtained 1 year after microvascular decompression demonstrate well-positioned Teflon sponge (asterisk in **c**) between the left superior cerebellar artery (arrow in **c**) and trigeminal nerve. However, there is no significant change in neural compression by the anterior inferior cerebellar artery (arrowhead in **d**), which may be responsible for the recurrent symptoms of the patient

adhesion, and foreign body granuloma (Fig. 8) [14, 48–50].

Among others, due to its histocompatibility and absorption resistance, polytetrafluoroethylene (Teflon) is currently used as the material of choice in MVD for patients with NVCS. Since the early 1990s however cases of granuloma formation associated with giant cell foreign body reaction were reported in patients with TN who underwent MVD using Teflon, with an incidence ranging from 1.1 to 7.3% [50–52]. The occurrence of Teflon granuloma in patients with HFS after MVD has been reported much less commonly. As suggested by Chen et al. [50], the greater overall prevalence of Teflon granulomas in patients with TN after MVD may be attributed to the fact that owing to a longer REZ of the trigeminal nerve, there is a greater chance of Teflon to be in contact with the tentorium and dura, which provokes an inflammatory reaction.

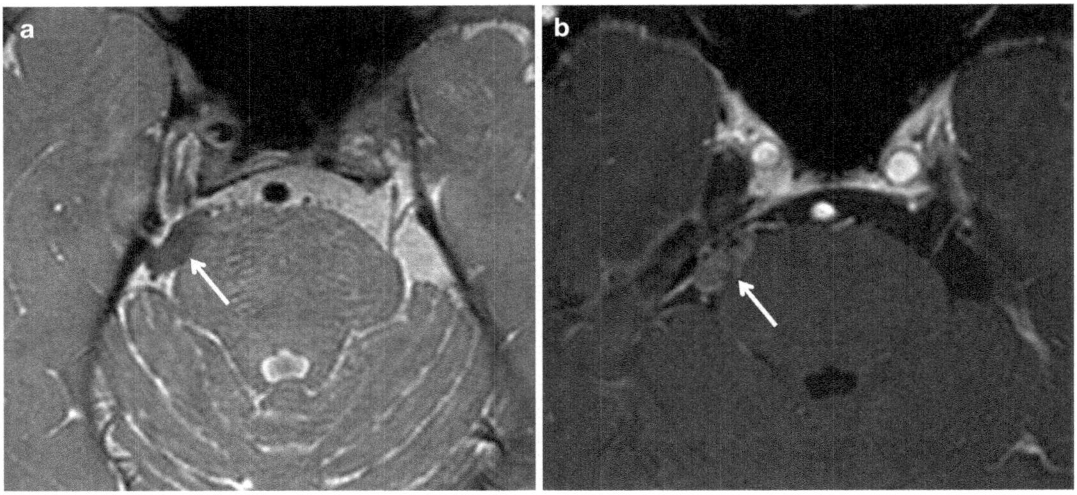

Fig. 9 Teflon granuloma causing recurrent trigeminal neuralgia after microvascular decompression. (**a**) and (**b**) MRC (**a**) and 3D contrast-enhanced T1-weighted image (**b**) obtained 11 years after microvascular decompression demonstrate a mass at the root entry zone of the right trigeminal nerve at the site of previous surgery (arrows). The lesion shows low signal intensity on T2-weighted image (**a**) and mild heterogeneous enhancement after contrast injection (**b**)

Radiologically, Teflon granuloma may present as an enhancing CPA mass on CT and MRI many years or even decades after surgery and thus can be confused with other CPA tumors (Fig. 9) [50–52]. MRI demonstrates an oval to round heterogeneous mass that is hypointense on both T1- and T2-weighted images. Early, actively growing granuloma may demonstrate avid enhancement, whereas older, quiescent granuloma shows minimal or no enhancement [51, 52]. On CT, focal calcification is often noticed. Although Teflon granuloma frequently continues to grow, associated malignant transformation has not yet been reported [52].

4 Conclusion

According to the revised classification system of TN, classical TN is the most common type and is associated with vascular compression with the radiological or surgical evidence of morphologic changes of the trigeminal nerve root, such as distortion, displacement, flattening, or atrophy, which leads to demyelination of the REZ of the trigeminal nerve. High-resolution 3D MRI such as 3D MRC and 3D TOF MRI is the imaging modality of choice for the preoperative evaluation of the complex neurovascular anatomy in terms of the type of the offending vessels and the site and severity of NVC. Because vascular contact is not infrequent in asymptomatic subjects or in the unaffected side of symptomatic patients, it is critical to refer to the clinical information to avoid mistakes during MRI interpretation. Secondary or symptomatic TN is attributed to an underlying disease such as multiple sclerosis and CPA tumors. MRI with the aid of contrast material is also useful in the management of secondary TN not only for the diagnosis but also for an accurate assessment of the lesion extent to help clinicians determine the best treatment option. Idiopathic TN refers to a condition where any cause of neural disturbance cannot be identified on diagnostic tests. Simple contact between the nerve and vessels without morphologic changes of the nerve should be categorized as idiopathic TN. High-resolution MRI is also useful in the evaluation of patients with TN who have recurrent symptoms after MVD. Teflon granuloma is a rare cause of failed MVD and may present as an enhancing CPA mass on MRI that should be differentiated from true CPA tumors.

References

1. International Headache Society. Headache classification committee of the international headache society (IHS). The international classification of headache disorders, 3rd edition. Cephalalgia. 2018;38:1–211.
2. Sholtz J, Finnerup NB, Attal N, et al. The IASP classification of chronic pain for ICD-11: chronic neuropathic pain. Pain. 2019;160:53–9.
3. Jannetta PJ. Neurovascular compression in cranial nerve and systemic disease. Ann Surg. 1980;192:518–25.
4. Devor M, Amir R, Rappaport ZH. Pathophysiology of trigeminal neuralgia: the ignition hypothesis. Clin J Pain. 2002;18:4–13.
5. Guclu B, Sindou M, Meyronet D, Streichenberger N, Simon E, Mertens P. Cranial nerve vascular compression syndromes of the trigeminal, facial and Vagoglossopharyngeal nerves: comparative anatomical study of the central myelin portion and transitional zone: correlations with incidences of corresponding hyperactive dysfunctional syndromes. Acta Neurochir. 2011;153:2365–75.
6. Donahue JH, Ornan DA, Mukherjee S. Imaging of vascular compression syndromes. Radiol Clin N Am. 2017;55:123–38.
7. Haller S, Etienne L, Kovari E, et al. Imaging of neurovascular compression syndromes: trigeminal neuralgia, hemifacial spasm, vestibular paroxysmia, and glossopharyngeal neuralgia. AJNR Am J Neuroradiol. 2016;37:1384–92.
8. Miller JP, Acar F, Hamilton BE, et al. Radiographic evaluation of trigeminal neurovascular compression in patients with and without trigeminal neuralgia. J Neurosurg. 2009a;110:627–32.
9. Miller JP, Acar F, Burchiel KJ. Classification of trigeminal neuralgia: clinical, therapeutic, and prognostic implications in a series of 144 patients undergoing microvascular decompression. J Neurosurg. 2009b;111:1231–4.
10. Cruccu G, Finnerup NB, Jensen TS, et al. Trigeminal neuralgia. New classification and diagnostic grading for practice and research. Neurology. 2016;87:220–8.
11. Bendtsen L, Zakrzewska JM, Abbott J, et al. European academy of neurology guideline on trigeminal neuralgia. Eur J Neurol. 2019;26:831–49.
12. Cruccu G, Di Stefano G, Truini A. Trigeminal neuralgia. N Engl J Med. 2020;383:754–62.
13. Bendtsen L, Zakrzewska M, Heinskou TB, et al. Advances in diagnosis, classification, pathophysiology, and management of trigeminal neuralgia. Lancet Neurol. 2020;19:784–96.
14. Huang Z, Pu B, Li F, et al. Analysis of failed microvascular decompression in patients with trigeminal neuralgia. J Neurol Surg B Skull Base. 2020;81:567–71.
15. Burchiel KJ. A new classification for facial pain. Neurosurgery. 2003;53:1164–7.
16. Yamakami I, Kobayashi E, Hirai S, et al. Preoperative assessment of trigeminal neuralgia and hemifacial spasm using constructive interference in steady state-three-dimensional Fourier transformation magnetic resonance imaging. Neurol Med Chir (Tokyo). 2000;40:545–56.
17. Fukuda H, Ishikawa M, Okumura R, et al. Demonstration of neurovascular compression in trigeminal neuralgia and hemifacial spasm with magnetic resonance imaging. Comparison with surgical findings in 60 consecutive cases. Surg Neurol. 2003;59:93–100.
18. Tanrikulu L, Scholz T, Nikoubashman O, et al. Preoperative MRI in neurovascular compression syndromes and its role for microsurgical considerations. Clin Neurol Neurosurg. 2015;129:17–20.
19. Yoshino N, Akimoto H, Yamada I, et al. Trigeminal neuralgia: evaluation of neuralgic manifestation and site of neurovascular compression with 3D CISS MR imaging and MR angiography. Radiology. 2003;228:539–45.
20. Kim H-J, Seong M. Magnetic resonance imaging evaluation of hemifacial spasm. In: Park K, Park JS, editors. Hemifacial spasm: a comprehensive guide. Singapore: Springer; 2020. p. 43–56.
21. Miller J, Acar F, Hamilton B, et al. Preoperative visualization of neurovascular anatomy in trigeminal neuralgia. J Neurosurg. 2008;108:477–82.
22. Chang JW, Chang JH, Park YG, et al. Microvascular decompression in trigeminal neuralgia: a correlation of three-dimensional time-of-flight magnetic resonance angiography and surgical findings. Stereotact Funct Neurosurg. 2000;74:167–74.
23. Patel NK, Aquilina K, Clarke Y, et al. How accurate is magnetic resonance angiography in predicting neurovascular compression in patients with trigeminal neuralgia? A prospective, single-blinded comparative study. Br J Neurosurg. 2003;17:60–4.
24. Akimoto H, Nagaoka T, Nariai T, et al. Preoperative evaluation of neurovascular compression in patients with trigeminal neuralgia by use of three-dimensional reconstruction from two types of high-resolution magnetic resonance imaging. Neurosurgery. 2002;51:956–62.
25. Satoh T, Onaoda K, Date I. Preoperative simulation for microvascular decompression in patients with idiopathic trigeminal neuralgia: visualization with three-dimensional magnetic resonance cisternogram and angiogram fusion imaging. Neurosurgery. 2007;60:104–14.
26. Satoh T, Omi M, Nabeshima M, et al. Severity analysis of neurovascular contact in patients with trigeminal neuralgia: assessment with the inner view of the 3D MR cisternogram and angiogram fusion imaging. AJNR Am J Neuroradiol. 2009;30:603–7.
27. Chun-Cheng Q, Qing-Shi Z, Ji-Qing Z, et al. A single-blinded pilot study assessing neurovascular contact by using high-resolution MR imaging in patients with trigeminal neuralgia. Eur J Radiol. 2009;69:459–63.
28. Blitz AM, Northcutt B, Shin J, et al. Neurovascular compression in trigeminal neuralgia: improved

correlation with symptoms and prediction of surgical outcomes. AJNR Am J Neuroradiol. 2018;39:1724–32.
29. Cha J, Kim ST, Kim H-J, et al. Trigeminal neuralgia: assessment with T2 VISTA and FLAIR VISTA fusion imaging. Eur Radiol. 2011;21:2633–9.
30. Lutz J, Linn J, Mehrkens JH, et al. Trigeminal neuralgia due to neurovascular compression: high-spatial-resolution diffusion-tensor imaging reveals microstructural neural changes. Radiology. 2011;258:524–30.
31. Casselman J, Mermuys K, Delanote J, et al. MRI of the cranial nerves–more than meets the eye: technical considerations and advanced anatomy. Neuroimaging Clin N Am. 2008;18:197–231.
32. Blitz AM, Macedo LL, Chonka ZD, et al. High-resolution CISS MR imaging with and without contrast for evaluation of the upper cranial nerves: segmental anatomy and selected pathologic conditions of the cisternal through extraforaminal segments. Neuroimaging Clin N Am. 2014;24:17–34.
33. De Ridder D, Møller A, Verlooy J, Cornelissen M, De Ridder L. Is the root entry/exit zone important in microvascular compression syndromes? Neurosurgery. 2002;51:427–34.
34. Prasad S, Galetta S. Trigeminal neuralgia Historical notes and current concepts. Neurologist. 2009;15:87–94.
35. Peker S, Kurtkaya O, Uzun I, et al. Microanatomy of the central myelin-peripheral myelin transition zone of the trigeminal nerve. Neurosurgery. 2006;59:354–9.
36. Thomas KL, Vilensky JA. The anatomy of vascular compression in trigeminal neuralgia. Clin Anat. 2014;27:89–93.
37. Hong W, Zheng X, Wu Z, et al. Clinical features and surgical treatment of trigeminal neuralgia caused solely by venous compression. Acta Neurochir. 2011;153:1037–42.
38. Suzuki M, Yoshino N, Shimada M, et al. Trigeminal neuralgia: differences in magnetic resonance imaging characteristics of neurovascular compression between symptomatic and asymptomatic nerves. Oral Surg Oral Med Oral Pathol Oral Radiol. 2015;119:113–8.
39. Maarbjerd S, Wolfram F, Gozalov A, et al. Significance of neurovascular contact in classical trigeminal neuralgia. Brain. 2015;138:311–9.
40. Baechil H, Gratzl O. Microvascular decompression in trigeminal neuralgia with no vascular compression. Eur Surg Res. 2007;39:51–7.
41. Ishikawa M, Nishi S, Aoki T, et al. Operative findings in cases of trigeminal neuralgia without vascular compression: proposal of a different mechanism. J Clin Neurosci. 2002;9:200–4.
42. Park SH, Hwang SK, Lee SH, et al. Nerve atrophy and a small cerebellopontine angle cistern in patients with trigeminal neuralgia. J Neurosurg. 2009;110:633–7.
43. Tanaka T, Morimoto Y, Shiiba S, et al. Utility of magnetic resonance cisternography using three-dimensional fast asymmetric spin-echo sequences with multiplanar reconstruction: the evaluation of sites of neurovascular compression of the trigeminal nerve. Oral Surg Oral Med Oral Pathol Radiol Endod. 2005;100:215–25.
44. Anderson VC, Berryhill PC, Sandquist MA, et al. High-resolution three-dimensional magnetic resonance angiography and three-dimensional spoiled gradient-recalled imaging in the evaluation of neurovascular compression in patients with trigeminal neuralgia: a double-blind pilot study. Neurosurgery. 2006;58:666–73.
45. Kakizawa Y, Seguchi T, Kodama K, et al. Anatomical study of the trigeminal and facial cranial nerves with the aid of 3.0-tesla magnetic resonance imaging. J Neurosurg. 2008;108:483–90.
46. Antonini G, Pasquale AD, Cruccu G, et al. Magnetic resonance imaging contributions for diagnosing symptomatic neurovascular contact in classical trigeminal neuralgia: a blind case-control study and meta-analysis. Pain. 2014;155:1464–71.
47. Gronseth G, Cruccu G, Alksne J, et al. Practice parameter: the diagnostic evaluation and treatment of trigeminal neuralgia (an evidence-based review). Report of the quality standards Subcommittee of the American Academy of neurology and the European Federation of Neurological Societies. Neurology. 2008;71:1183–90.
48. Gu W, Zhao W. Microvascular decompression for recurrent trigeminal neuralgia. J Clin Neurosci. 2014;21:1549–53.
49. Bakker NA, Van Dijk MC, Immenga S, et al. Repeat microvascular decompression for recurrent idiopathic trigeminal neuralgia. J Neurosurg. 2014;121:936–9.
50. Chen J-F, Lee S-T, Lui T-N, et al. Teflon granuloma after microvascular decompression for trigeminal neuralgia. Surg Neurol. 2005;53:281–7.
51. Capelle H-H, Brandis A, Tschan C, et al. Treatment of recurrent trigeminal neuralgia due to Teflon granuloma. J Headache Pain. 2010;11:339–44.
52. Deep NL, Graffeo CS, Copeland WR, et al. Teflon granulomas mimicking cerebellopontine angle tumor following microvascular decompression. Laryngoscope. 2017;127:715–9.

Recent Advances and Future Perspective in MRI Technique for the Trigeminal Neuralgia

Jin Woo Choi and Chung Hwan Kang

1 Introduction

Trigeminal neuralgia is a neurological disorder characterized by recurrent, paroxysmal, short-lasting, lancinating facial pain restricted to the unilateral trigeminal territory, and usually triggered by innoxious stimuli. Trigeminal neuralgia can be divided into classical, secondary, and idiopathic. Trigeminal neuralgia is classified as idiopathic when any diagnostic tests fail to reveal a lesion or disease that can cause trigeminal neuralgia [1]. Neurovascular compression with morphological change of the trigeminal nerve on MRI or during surgery is essential to classify trigeminal neuralgia as classical. Secondary trigeminal neuralgia is categorized when trigeminal neuralgia is caused by an underlying disease such as tumor in cerebellopontine angle/Meckel's cave or multiple sclerosis [1]. Although the diagnosis of trigeminal neuralgia is made clinically, the combination of high-resolution, 3D T2-weighted images, post-contrast 3D T1-weighted images, and TOF-MRA with 3D reconstruction have provided us reliable information about the presence and severity of neurovascular compression in classical trigeminal neuralgia [2, 3]. It also helps us to exclude other causes of trigeminal neuralgia such as infectious, inflammatory, demyelinating disease, or tumor. Moreover, recent advances in structural and functional imaging enable us to elucidate the pathomechanism of trigeminal neuralgia [4]. In this chapter, we review recent trends in the MR techniques for detecting neurovascular conflict between the trigeminal nerve and vascular structures in trigeminal neuralgia, which includes MR cisternography and post-contrast 3D T1-weighted imaging. We also provide clinical application of MR techniques such as high-resolution, T1-weighted imaging for brain morphometry, diffusion tensor imaging, and resting-state functional MRI to investigate structural and functional alteration in the central nervous system in trigeminal neuralgia. To acquire the previously mentioned, 3D, high-resolution, and various MR images within the clinically acceptable scan time, fast imaging techniques are inevitable. Fast imaging techniques such as parallel imaging, compressed sensing, or modified K-space sampling are briefly reviewed in advance. Lastly, we briefly introduce the clinical application of 7.0 T MRI in trigeminal neuralgia.

J. W. Choi (✉) · C. H. Kang
Department of Radiology, Konkuk University Medical Center, Konkuk University School of Medicine, Seoul, Republic of Korea
e-mail: cardijin@kuh.ac.kr; chkang@kuh.ac.kr

2 Fast Imaging Technique

Although modern, advanced MR machines enable us to obtain high-resolution, 3D and isotropic MR images, the important limitation for achieving these is the long acquisition time, which should be acceptable within the limits of

K. Park, K. R. Cho (eds.), *Trigeminal Neuralgia*, https://doi.org/10.1007/978-981-19-9171-4_7

the patient's cooperation, safety, and cost-effectiveness. Number of signal average, repetition time (TR), and phase-encoding steps are main components to determine the length of scan time. Reducing the number of signal average can significantly reduce signal, and therefore it is not a parameter that can be reduced further. TR affects image contrast and are limited by the type of pulse sequence and performance of the gradient system in MRI. Therefore, modern fast imaging techniques are based on the concept to reduce phase-encoding step by modulation of the K-space filling methods such as undersampling, nonlinear K-space filling, and random filling of K-space in sparse signal [5]. These commercially available fast imaging techniques can be used in combination with each advanced technique which will be described in this chapter.

K-space is a mathematical area where the frequency and phase information of the MR signal is stored. MR images are created by Fourier transformation using the digitized information in K-space. Classically, K-space has been filled sequentially, row-by-row manner in Cartesian grid using alternative use of each readout and phase-encoding gradient which is time-consuming. Novel non-Cartesian K-space sampling (spiral K-space sampling) fills K-space along the radius of the circle using simultaneous use of two gradients, and leads to oversampling of the central K-space (low-frequency area where determined image contrast) and undersampling of the peripheral K-space (high-frequency area related to resolution) (Fig. 1) [5]. Using this technique, scan time is not only reduced but also motion artifact is mitigated. In sequential data filling in Cartesian grid, motion artifact usually propagated in one direction and however it is dispersed across the entire image and reduced by applying additional motion correction using oversampled central K-space data as a reference for each step. Parallel imaging technique such as SENSE is a MR technique to reduce scan time by undersampling of K-space along the phase-encoding direction using multiple independent receiver elements with different spatial sensitivity within the phased array coils. Aliasing artifact caused by undersampling of the K-space is eliminated by using the spatial sensitivity profiles of each receiver element (Fig. 2) [6]. In compressed sensing, scan time can be reduced using random undersampling K-space data, incoherence, and iterative nonlinear reconstruction. Linear and regular undersampling of the data often results in a coherent artifact such as aliasing like parallel imaging. However, random undersampling

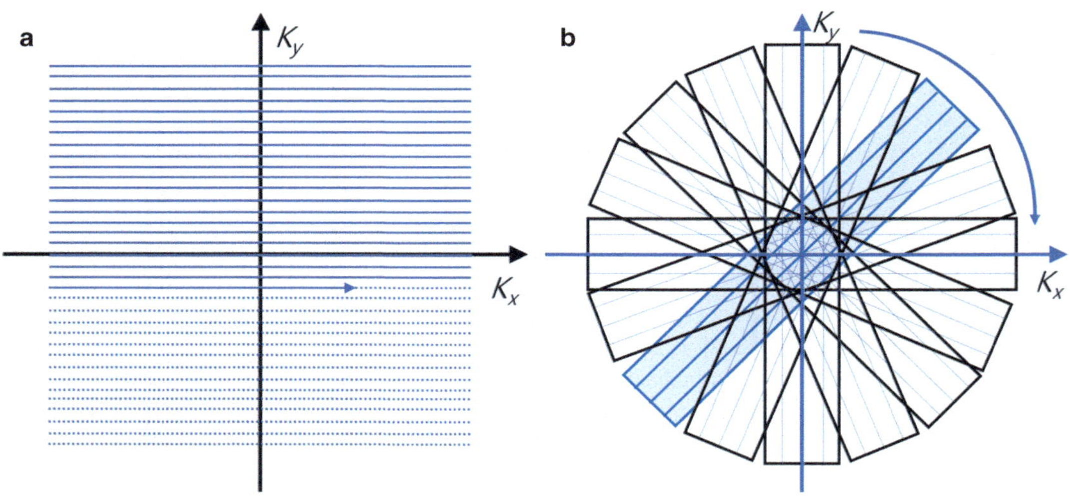

Fig. 1 Fast imaging technique—Radial K-space sampling. In a Cartesian K-space sampling (**a**), data are collected in a row-by-row manner. Each line requires separate phase-encoding step therefore it is time-consuming. In radial K-space sampling (**b**), data are filled with spoke-wheel pattern. Nowadays, multiple parallel phase-encoded lines called BLADE are rotated by a small angle until data from the entire *K*-space circle has been collected. This leads to oversampling of the central K-space and relative undersampling of the peripheral K-space

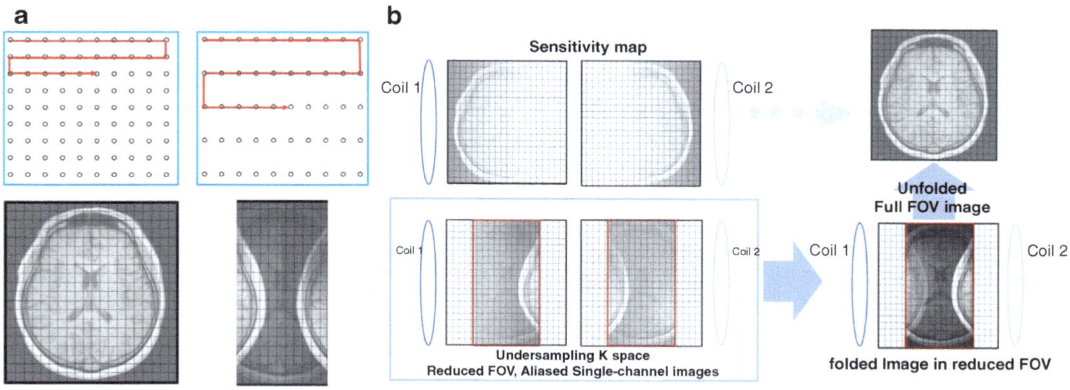

Fig. 2 Fast imaging technique—Parallel imaging. In conventional acquisition, undersampling of the K-space can reduce scan time, but cause aliased images as compared with full K-space sampling (**a**). In parallel imaging, a folded image derived from the undersampled, reduced field of view (FOV) and aliased single-channel images of each coil element is unfolded by mathematic formulation using spatial sensitivity profiles of each coil (**b**)

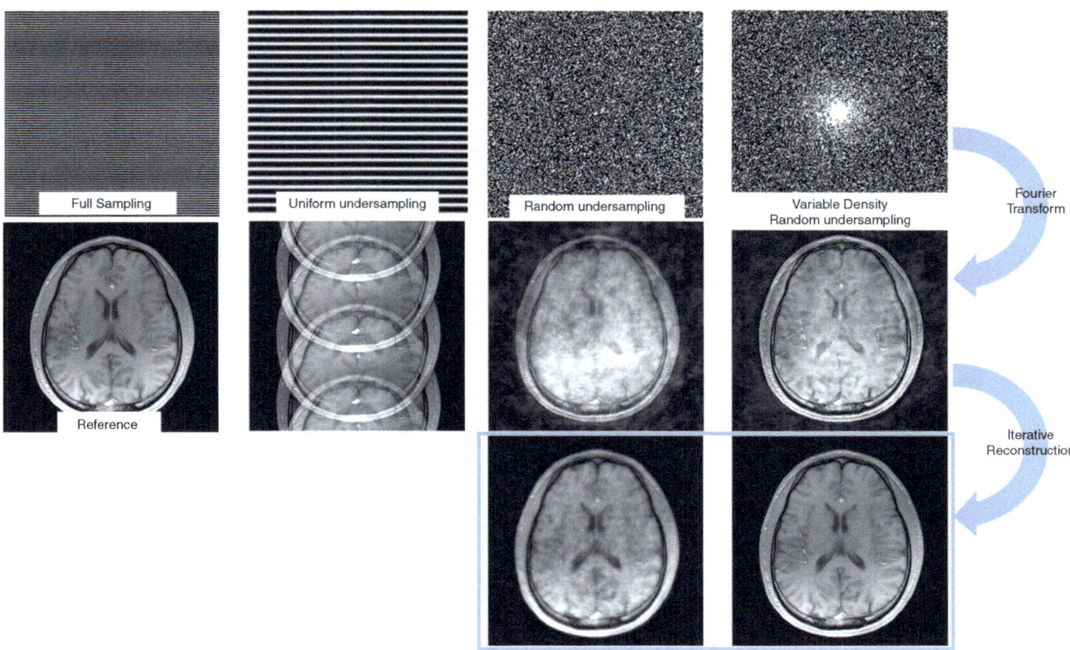

Fig. 3 Fast imaging technique—Compressed sensing. Uniform undersampling of K-space can cause structured, coherent artifact like aliasing which is difficult to eliminate by any reconstruction algorithm. Artifact caused by random undersampling is non-structured and incoherent. Variable density random undersampling results in a noise-like artifact. This noise-like artifact can be removed by an iterative nonlinear reconstruction algorithm

switched these structured artifacts into noise-like ones. These noise-like, incoherent artifacts can be removed by using nonlinear, iterative reconstruction (Fig. 3) [5]. In patients with suspected neurovascular compression, 3D T2 VISTA and CE-3D T1WI with SENSE and compressed sensing seem to provide better cerebrospinal fluid (CSF) homogeneity, less motion artifact, and shorter scan time without loss of overall image quality than those with SENSE alone (Fig. 4) [7].

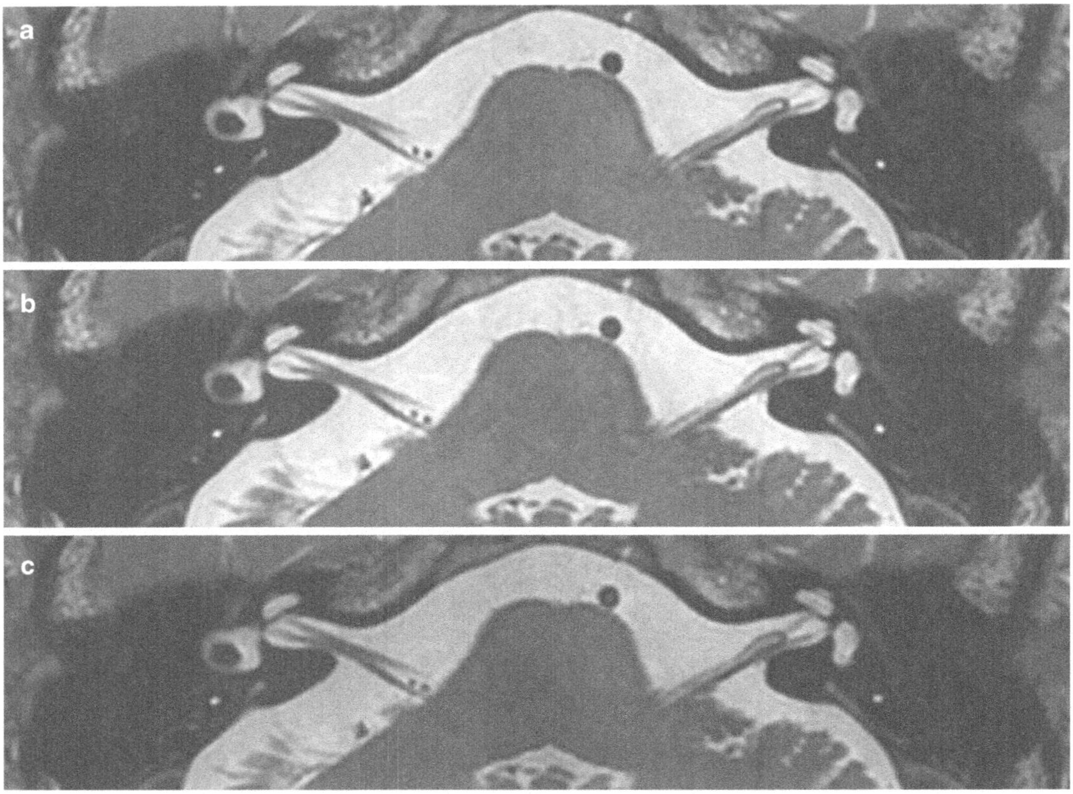

Fig. 4 Fast imaging technique—Compressed sensing. MR cisternography using parallel imaging technique and/or compressed sensing. Acquisition time for MR cisternography using parallel imaging only (**a**), parallel imaging and compressed sensing with accelerating factors of 1.25 (**b**) and 1.5 (**c**) is 6:10, 4:55, and 4:07, respectively

3 MR Cisternography (Heavily T2-Weighted/Proton Density Imaging)

3D, high-resolution, heavily T2-weighted imaging (so-called MR cisternography) is an inevitable sequence for evaluating the presence of neurovascular conflict and complex relationship between the cranial nerves and offending vessels in trigeminal neuralgia. Various T2-weighted 3D fast spin echo (FSE)- or gradient-echo (GRE)-based sequences have been developed in different MR vendors, and the basic principle of these techniques is to create high contrast between the thin cranial nerves and surrounding CSF with minimum artifact caused by CSF flow and local magnetic field inhomogeneity [8–14]. Generally, GRE-based sequences are sensitive to susceptibility artifact and inhomogeneity of the main magnetic field [8, 9, 12, 15, 16]. In spite of these disadvantages, GRE has been mainly used for acquiring a large volume of data for image reconstruction in 3D imaging due to short acquisition time [15]. In FSE, multiple 180° refocusing pulse can make the MR signal insensitive to susceptibility artifact; however, the major drawbacks of FSE-based sequences include inconsistent cisternographic effect caused by flow artifact of CSF, a relatively long-scan time and blurring of the edge between different tissue [9]. Nowadays, there are various, commercially available 3D GRE and FSE sequences which minimize the disadvantages of each sequence using advanced techniques while maintaining their innate advantages.

Balanced SSFP (Steady-State Free Precession) such as FIESTA (Fast Imaging Employing STeady-state Acquisition; GE Healthcare), true-FISP (true-Fast Imaging with Steady-state

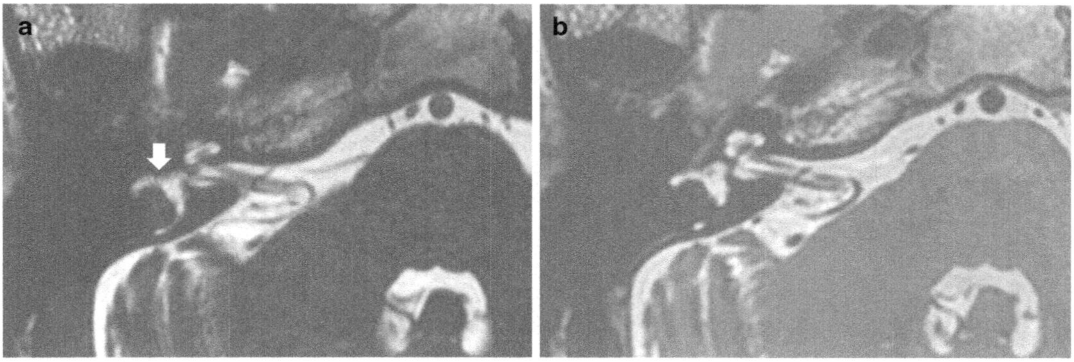

Fig. 5 3D GRE and FSE for cisternography. A banding artifact (arrow) is observed in the vestibule and anterior crus of the right lateral semicircular canal on 3D GRE (**a**, balanced SSFP; FIESTA-C) as compared with 3D TSE (**b**, CUBE). Both 3D GRE (**a**) and FSE (**b**) sequences demonstrate good definition of seventh and eighth cranial nerves in the internal acoustic canal without significant CSF artifact

Precession; Siemens) is a 3D fast GRE method to obtain high-resolution MR cisternography [15, 16]. SSFP used both longitudinal and transverse magnetization in a nonzero steady-state condition to make MR image. In SSFP, the steady state is achieved by repeating radiofrequency (RF) pulse with shorter TR than the T2 relaxation times of the tissue, and the residual transverse magnetization which is left over after each RF pulse is refocused to contribute to the steady state. In balanced SSFP, the gradients applied to all three axes (e.g., slice, readout, and phase-encoding direction) are completely balanced by opposite polarity, and therefore net dephasing of the transverse magnetization does not occur within each TR. Fully balanced gradients result in more efficient refocusing of the steady-state magnetization, and eventually increase signal-to-noise ratio and make motion insensitive. However, balanced SSFP requires complete rephase of the signal along each axis, it is extremely sensitive to off-resonance effects from nonuniform main magnetic field which cause band-like signal loss. FIESTA-C (GE Healthcare) and CISS (Constructive Interference in Steady State; SIMENS) are a modified version of the FIESTA and true-FISP to increase signal-to-noise ratio and eliminate banding artifact by canceling dephased signal using a maximum intensity projection of the two datasets created by RF pulse with opposite polarity (Fig. 5).

Recently, 3D FSE has been widely used for cranial nerve and inner ear imaging by overcoming innate weaknesses such as long-scan time, signal loss, and blurring using advanced imaging techniques such as modification of the pulse-sequence structure, K-space filling strategy, parallel imaging, and compressed sensing [12–14]. In 3D FSE, the longitudinal recovery of CSF with long T1 and T2 are partially saturated, if successive, short trains of RF pulses are applied before complete longitudinal recovery of the CSF. Partial saturation of the longitudinal relax lead to loss of the signal from the CSF. Driven equilibrium RF reset pulse can accelerate longitudinal recovery of residual transverse magnetization by applying refocusing pulse at the end of echo train length (ETL). RESTORE (Siemens), FRFSE (Fast Recovery Fast Spin Echo; GE healthcare), and DRIVE (Philips) are different trade names of 3D FSE using driven equilibrium RF reset pulse. By virtue of driven equilibrium RF reset pulse, heavily T2-weighted images can be acquired with a shorter TR, which helps reduce flow void artifact and increase brightness of the CSF in a relatively short acquisition time (Fig. 6) [10, 12, 13]. In FSE, main solution for shortening acquisition time is increased ETL and echo space as short as possible. However, increasing ETL cause imaging blurring and repeated RF pulse can increase specific absorption rate (SAR). Recent 3D FSE using short, nonspatially selective RF pulses and variable flip angles for refocusing RF pulses allow us to use an extremely long echo train for short acquisition time and to provide high-resolution volumetric images without excessive blurring or SAR [11, 14]. Using these commercially available 3D FSE sequences such as CUBE (GE Healthcare), SPACE (Sampling Perfection with Application-optimized Contrasts by using flip-angle Evolution; Siemens), and VISTA (Volume Isotropic Turbo Spin-echo Acquisition; Philips), we can obtain isotropic imaging up to 0.3 mm at 3 T and provide higher contrast-to-noise ratio (CNR) when compared with TrueFISP [17, 18]. Moreover, we cannot only get T2-weighted images, but also T1-weighted, proton density (PD), or FLAIR images by modulating imaging parameters such as flip angle, TR, and TE in these new 3D FSE sequences (Fig. 7) [14].

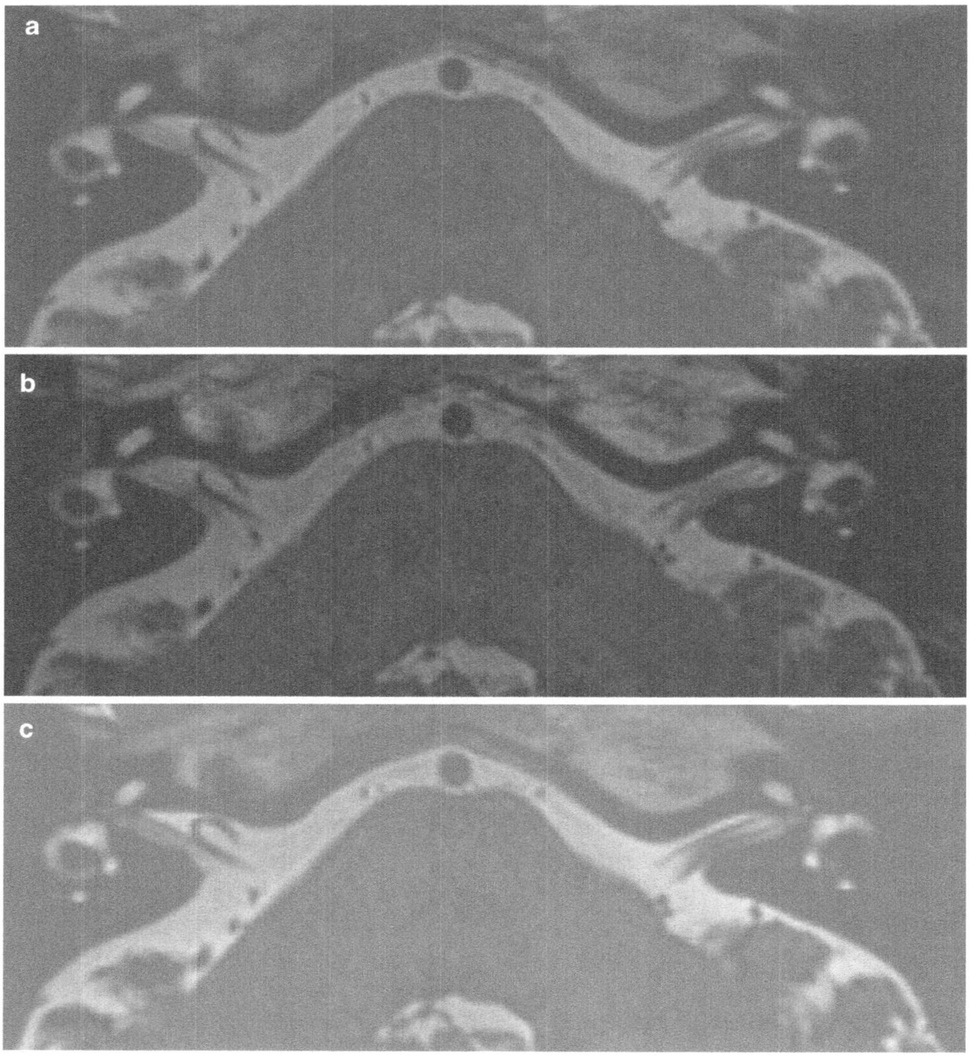

Fig. 6 3D FSE with drive equilibrium pulse. 3D TSE without driven equilibrium RF pulse with TR of 3000 ms and acquisition time of 6 min and 48 s (**a**) shows excellent contrast between the cranial nerves/vessels with low signal intensity and CSF with bright signal intensity. 3D TSE without driven equilibrium RF pulse with half the previous TR (1500 ms) and acquisition time (3 min and 24 s) (**b**) shows reduced CSF signal intensity and CSF flow artifact in the prepontine cistern. 3D TSE with driven equilibrium RF pulse with TR of 1500 ms (**c**) demonstrates excellent contrast between the cranial nerves/vessels and CSF without significant CSF flow artifact or loss of brightness of the CSF in a short acquisition time (3 min and 24 s)

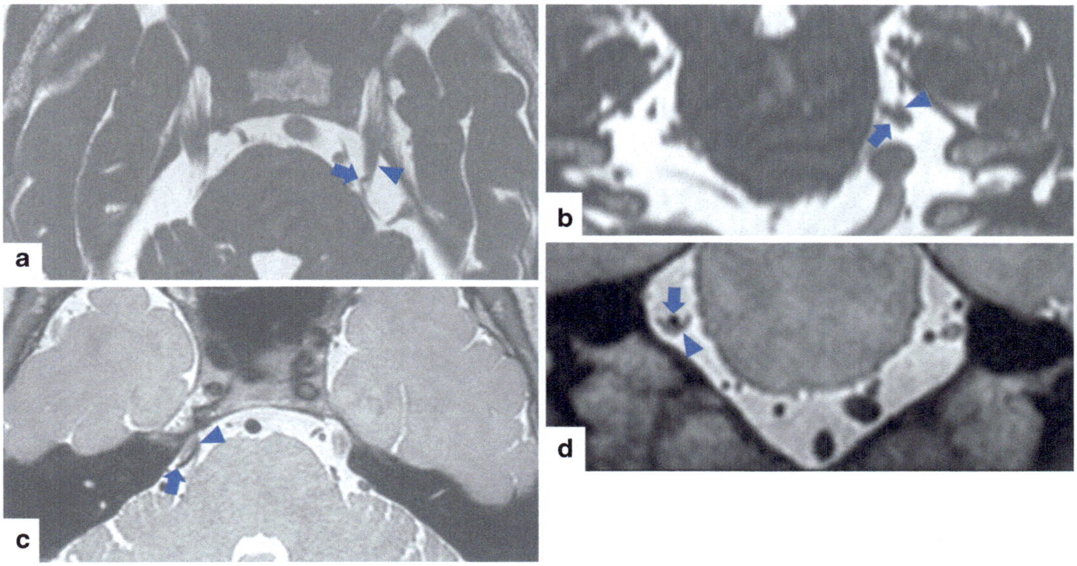

Fig. 7 Proton density MR cisternography using 3D FSE with variable flip angle. The signal intensity of the offending artery (arrows) and trigeminal nerve (arrowhead) is identical on 3D GRE images (**a** and **b**, FIESTA-C). Conversely, the signal intensity of the offending artery (arrowhead) is slightly low as compared with trigeminal nerve (arrow) on 3D FSE proton density images (**c** and **d**, 3D VISTA)

4 Post-contrast 3D T1-Weighted Images

MR cisternography in conjunction with 3D TOF-MRA can be successfully visualized by the cranial nerve and offending arteries in neurovascular conflict (NVC). However, these are not suitable for detecting contrast enhancement of cranial nerves and enhancing venous structures which cannot be ignored in trigeminal neuralgia. Moreover, volumetric analysis is increasingly being used for evaluating global or specific brain regional volume changes in trigeminal neuralgia [19–30]. For these purposes, high-resolution, 3D T1-weighted images with/without contrast enhancement are applied in patients with trigeminal neuralgia.

Since 1990, 3D MPRAGE (Magnetization-Prepared RApid Gradient-Echo) sequence has been most widely used to obtain structural T1-weighted images with high spatial resolution and excellent gray-white matter differentiation. For providing excellent tissue contrast and spatial resolution, an additional non-selective (180°) inversion pulse and a large number of K-space filling are needed in MPRAGE. This inversion pulse is modified to a null CSF signal and maximizes gray-white matter differentiation by increasing T1 weighting. However, for the purpose to detect a subtle and small contrast-enhancing lesion, MPRAGE images show less conspicuity compared with another 3D GRE image such as VIBE [31, 32]. Recently, optimal contrast conspicuity can be achieved by interpolated 3D T1-weighted GRE sequences such as VIBE (Volumetric Interpolated Breath-hold Examination, Siemens), LAVA (Liver Acquisition with Volume Acceleration; GE Healthcare), THRIVE (T1-weighted High-Resolution Isotropic Volume Examination; Philips) which are optimized for rapid acquisition and high-resolution by using asymmetric K-space sampling and interpolation; however, these sequences cannot be applied to volumetric analysis due to poor gray-white matter differentiation [17, 18]. One recent study found that VIBE sequence with compressed sensing provided more favorable image quality, better performance in the depiction of the cranial nerve enhancement than those of conventional MPRAGE [33]. The conspicuity of the contrast enhancement in the abnormal cranial nerves may be also improved in spin echo-based 3D T1-weighted images such as SPACE; however, the signal from

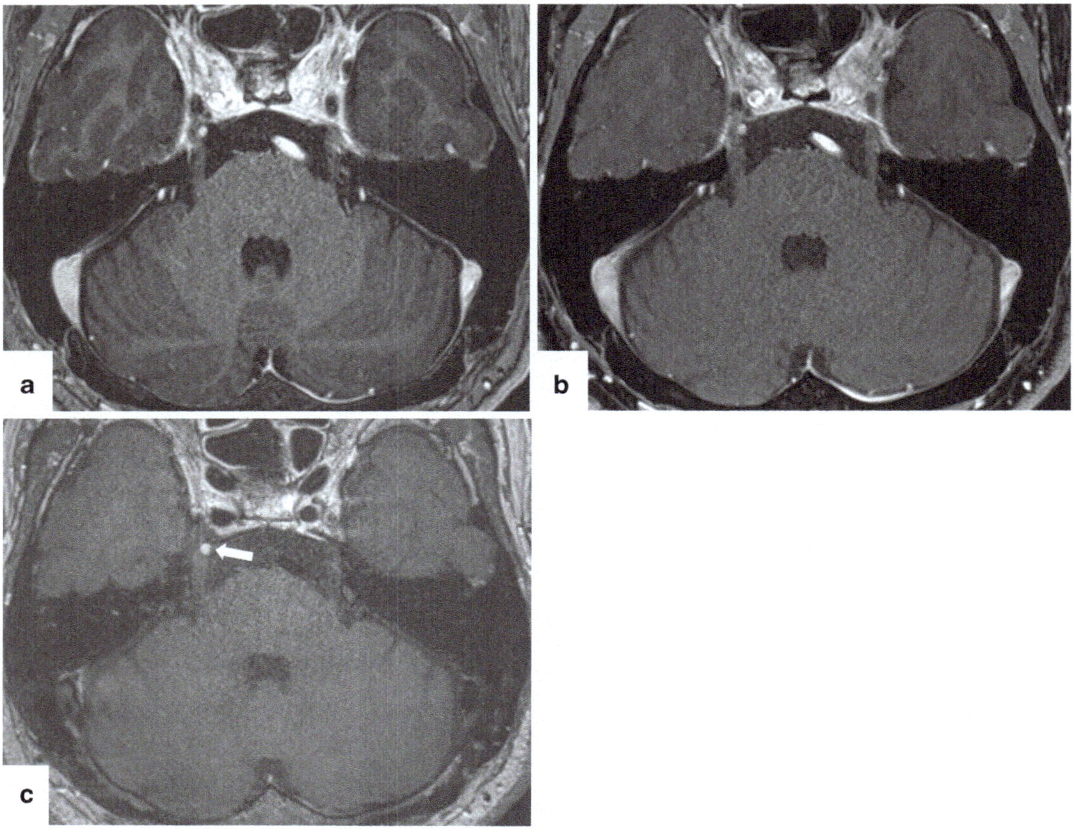

Fig. 8 Various 3D, high-resolution T1WI with contrast. Post-contrast MPRAGE (**a**) reveals excellent gray-white matter differentiation in the scanned bilateral temporal lobes and cerebellar hemispheres as compared to VIBE (**b**) and SPACE (**c**). Post-contrast MRRAGE and VIBE show good vascular enhancement. A small schwannoma in right trigeminal nerve (arrow) is easily detected on post-contrast SPACE due to vascular enhancement being canceled out

the offending vessels can be nulled. Therefore, new 3D FSE such as SPACE seems to be more sensitive to detect enhancing lesions in the brain parenchyma and cranial nerves, but it is not suitable to identify offending vessels in neurovascular compression syndrome (Fig. 8).

5 Volumetric Analysis of the Brain in Patients with Trigeminal Neuralgia

MRI-based volumetric analysis is increasingly being used for evaluating global or specific brain regional volume changes in a wide range of neurologic diseases [19–30]. Nowadays, it is nearly impossible to segment and measure the brain volume of interest by highly trained specialists manually because multiple brain regions are simultaneously evaluated in enormous amounts of image data from a large patient group. Therefore, a large number of semi-automated or automated, and free or commercially available software packages based on voxel-based, deformation-based, and surface-based morphometry have been developed for accelerating quantitative volumetric data analysis in various neurodegenerative or neuropsychiatric disease. Although these methods are known to provide high accuracy and reproducibility in clinical studies, acquisition of the high-quality volumetric MRI source images is essential. This means the MR images should have high spatial resolution, high signal homogeneity, excellent gray/white matter differentiation, and minimum MR artifact. As stated earlier, MPRAGE has been most widely used for this purpose.

It is postulated that trigeminal neuralgia can affect gray matter volume of certain brain regions which are responsible for pain and emotional modulation [4, 30, 34, 35]. The results of the gray matter volume analysis strongly suggest that the gray matter volume of several brain regions and whole brain in patients with trigeminal neuralgia are affected as compared with that of healthy controls; however, the results are inconsistent and inconclusive [24–28]. These discrepancies may be caused by study design, sample size, disease duration, severity of the pain, analysis methods, etc. One recent systemic review revealed that gray matter volume of the anterior cingulate, posterior cingulate, insula, secondary somatosensory cortex, cerebellum, caudate nucleus, fusiform gyrus, and left cuneus decreased. The change of the gray matter volume in the periaqueductal gray matter, thalamus, amygdala, putamen, primary somatosensory cortex, and primary motor cortex showed conflicting results [4]. Although some results are conflicting, it is generally accepted that the gray matter volume changes in previously stated brain regions are affected in patients with trigeminal neuralgia (Fig. 9) [22]. Another systemic review and meta-

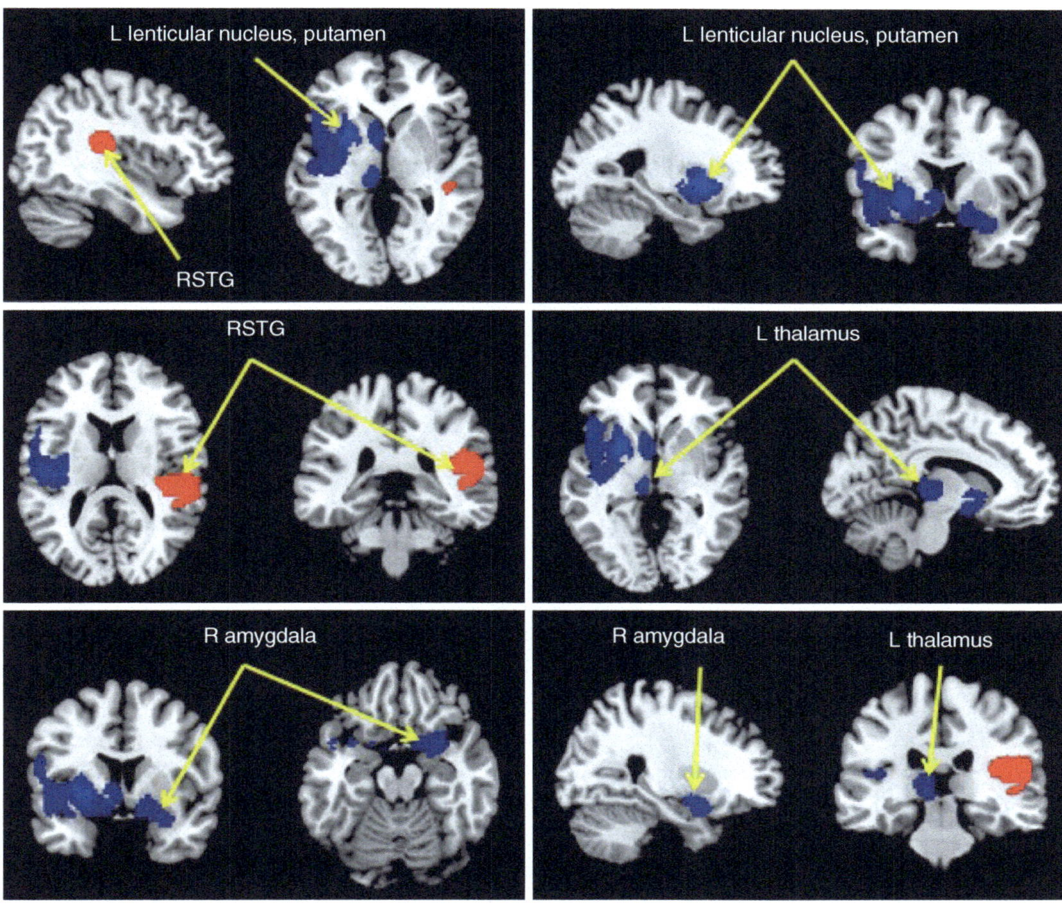

Fig. 9 Voxel-based morphometry for trigeminal neuralgia. Regions showing increased (red) and decreased (blue) GM volume in patients with TN compared to HCs. Abbreviations: *L* left; *R* right; *TN* trigeminal neuralgia; *GM* grey matter; *HCs* healthy controls; *RSTG* right superior temporal gyrus. (With permission Grey matter volume alterations in trigeminal neuralgia: A systematic review and meta-analysis of voxel-based morphometry studies. Prog Neuropsychopharmacol Biol Psychiatry. 2020 Mar 2;98:109821. doi: 10.1016/j.pnpbp.2019.109821. Epub 2019 Nov 19)

analysis showed that the gray matter volume changes are located in the basal ganglia, cingulate gyrus, thalamus, insula, and superior temporal gyrus. They also found that the left striatum and superior temporal gyrus and insula may be correlated with symptom ratings and disease duration [30]. Moreover, several studies investigated the correlation between the morphological changes in gray matter and clinical variables and found that there is a negative correlation between pain duration and cortical volume [23, 25, 28]. Some authors tried to predict postsurgical outcome after gamma knife radiosurgery or microvascular decompression (MVD) in trigeminal neuralgia. The results showed that increased thickness or volume of the frontal/temporal cortex, amygdala, and/or hippocampus are correlated with a poor response after treatment [36, 37]. Using machine learning technique, Hung et al. concluded that superior frontal gyrus and contralateral isthmus of the cingulate gyrus is most relevant brain area to predict the response after gamma knife radiosurgery [29].

6 Diffusion Tensor Imaging

Microstructural changes such as demyelination, dysmyelination, deposition of myelin debris/dense collagen materials, or even axonal loss were observed on electron-microscopic examination at the surgical specimen of the trigeminal nerve during MVD [38, 39]. High-resolution 3D T2WI can successfully demonstrate atrophy of the trigeminal nerve by measuring the mean diameter and cross-sectional area using multiplanar reconstruction in patients with trigeminal neuralgia caused by neurovascular conflicts. However, it is not capable of detecting subtle white matter tract change in trigeminal nerve or central nervous system. By virtue of diffusion tensor imaging, we have a chance to detect microstructural changes such as axonal loss or myelin injury which had occurred before gross anatomic changes were detected on conventional MR technique.

Each tissue of the organ has its innate water diffusion property influenced by various structural and physiologic factors such as size, density of the microorganelle, orientation, permeability of the cell membrane, shape, viscosity, and temperature. Innate water diffusion property of each tissue in the brain is changed in many neurologic diseases. The general concept of diffusion tensor imaging is that, by calculating water diffusion parameters measured by MRI using a diffusion-sensitizing gradient, we can infer the microstructural changes in many neurologic diseases. The motility of each water molecule in CSF is random and identical in all directions, and, therefore, probable location of each molecule will be within a complete sphere after a period (isotropic diffusion). The water molecules in white matter tract tend to move in a direction parallel to the white matter bundles, and, thus, probable location of the water molecules after a period is ellipsoid, not spherical (anisotropic diffusion). The direction and shape of the ellipsoid are characterized by three axes which are perpendicular to each other and cross at the center point of the ellipsoid. The direction of each axis is represented by eigenvector and measured lengths of three axes are eigenvalue. With diffusion-sensitized gradient pulse in at least 6 directions, we can calculate several values (FA, AD, RD, MD) derived from these eigenvalues. FA (fractional anisotropy) represents the degree of directionality of water diffusion ranges from 0 (a sphere; complete isotropic) to 1 (the ellipsoid is infinitely elongated; completely anisotropic). The degree of water diffusion is measured along the longitudinal axis (AD, axial diffusivity) and along the perpendicular plane (RD, radial diffusivity) to longitudinal axis. The mean of this orthogonal diffusivity is mean diffusivity (MD). These diffusion metrics are clinically used for evaluating microstructural changes of the white matter, but there is no specific parameter to determine the type of white matter injury. FA and MD are sensitive to detecting any alteration of the water diffusion in white matter tract, and, therefore, FA may represent the integrity of the white matter fibers. It was reported that increased RD seemed to be associated with myelin injury, while increased AD is associated with axonal loss [17]. Moreover, by assuming the largest principal diffusion direction might be related to the direction of the white matter tract, tractography can be reconstructed by connecting the directional diffusion information in each voxel using deterministic or probabilistic methods [23].

Similar to gray matter changes in trigeminal neuralgia, several studies have revealed that patients with trigeminal neuralgia not only have disruption of the white matter in their trigeminal nerves but also in those which interconnect gray matter in the pathway of modulation, attention, and psychomotor response to the pain in the central nervous system [40–46]. These pathological processes can be assumed by quantitative and qualitative analysis of the white matter bundle using tractography and diffusion metrics obtained by diffusion tensor imaging. Generally, FA value were reduced and MD, RD, and AD were increased in the root entry zone (REZ) of the trigeminal nerve [40–43, 45, 47]. These findings may be linked to neurovascular conflict-induced focal demyelination, neuroinflammation, and/or edema of the trigeminal REZ. In addition to REZ of the affected trigeminal nerve by neurovascular compression, corpus callosum, corona radiata, and/or longitudinal fasciculus showed reduced FA values and increased MD, RD, and AD values on DTI (Fig. 10) [4, 19, 26, 46, 48, 49]. Moreover, Wang et al. showed a close linkage between altered cortical gyrification and abnormalities in the underlying white matter tracts such as insular cortex and anatomically related white matter tracts such as external capsule, superior corona radiata, and posterior limb of the internal capsule [50]. Several studies demonstrated that DTI metrics can be used to predict surgical outcome in trigeminal neuralgia [51–57].

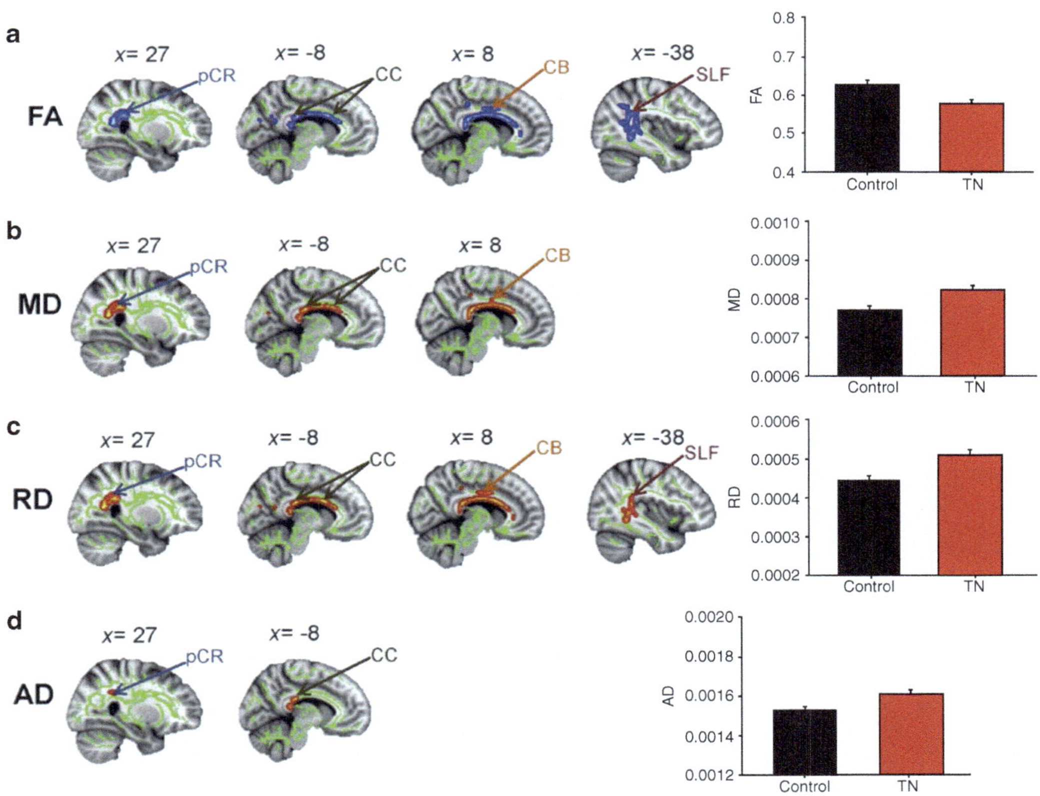

Fig. 10 Abnormal brain white matter (WM) in corpus callosum, cingulum, posterior corona radiata, and superior longitudinal fasciculus represented by FA (**a**), MD (**b**), RD (**c**) and AD (**d**). The main regions of brain WM abnormalities from the group Tract-Based Spatial Statistics results ($p < 0.05$, corrected) are highlighted for each diffusion tensor imaging (DTI) metric, with graphs of the extracted DTI-derived values ± SEM to the right: controls (black bars), patients (red bars). Blue clusters indicate patients < controls and red clusters indicate patients > controls. Abbreviations: *pCR* posterior corona radiata, *CC* corpus callosum, *CB* cingulum bundle, *SLF* superior longitudinal fasciculus, *FA* fractional anisotropy, *RD* radial diffusivity, *MD* mean diffusivity, *AD* axial diffusivity. Diffusion in mm^2/s. (With permission Pain. 2014 Jan;155(1):37–44. doi: 10.1016/j.pain.2013.08.029. Epub 2013 Aug 30. Abnormal trigeminal nerve microstructure and brain white matter in idiopathic trigeminal neuralgia)

7 Resting-State Functional MRI

In addition to structural imaging which shows subtle changes in gray matter volume and white matter tracts in the central nervous system, functional imaging can be used to obtain a deeper understanding of the brain plasticity to the trigeminal neuralgia. Functional MRI indirectly measures the neuronal activity of the brain with/without external stimuli by monitoring alterations in the brain blood-oxygen level-dependent (BOLD) signal, which reflect simultaneously the amount of local cerebral blood flow and deoxyhemoglobin. In resting-state fMRI, spontaneous neuronal activity can be investigated without external stimuli by separating weak BOLD signal from the noise. There are several analytic methods to evaluate spontaneous neuronal activity represented by BOLD signal which might be influenced by neurodegenerative, neuropsychologic disease, or chronic pain in rs-fMRI. The total power of the BOLD signal within the low-frequency range (0.01–0.1 Hz) and the synchrony of BOLD signal in a given voxel and its nearest neighbors over a time series can be represented by ALFF (Amplitude of Low-Frequency Fluctuation) and ReHo (Regional Homogeneity), respectively [58]. These analytic methods are commonly used for mapping specific brain regions with altered activity. Moreover, by calculating the degree of synchrony of the BOLD signal between different brain regions using various analytic methods such as seed-based correlation, functional connectivity density, independent component analysis, or graph analysis, functional connectivity can be assessed. A handful of studies regarding functional changes and connectivity of the brain in trigeminal neuralgia showed inconsistent results; functional change in precentral gyrus, middle and superior frontal gyri, anterior and posterior cingulate, temporal gyrus, amygdala, and cerebellum are observed, and alteration of the connectivity between insula—cingulate, hippocampus—striatum, and thalamus—precentral gyrus, etc. (Fig. 11) [4, 20, 30, 50, 59–66].

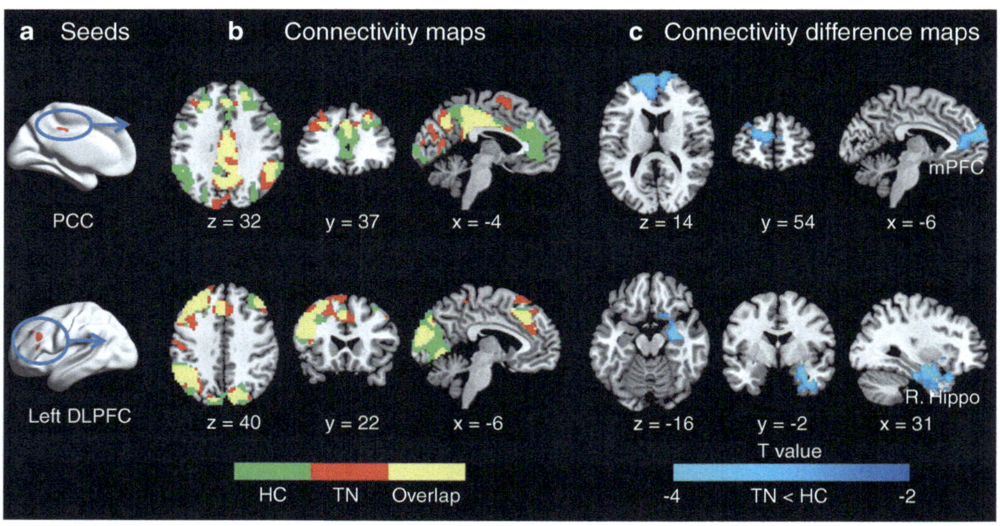

Fig. 11 ALFF/fALFF and related rsFC differences between TN patients and healthy controls. Between-group differences in rsFC analyses were only found related to the seed of PCC and left DLPFC. (**a**) Seed regions for rsFC analyses. (**b**) Functional connectivity patterns in TN patients and healthy control subjects. Green: healthy controls; red: TN patients; yellow: overlaps. (**c**) Functional connectivity differences between the two groups ($p < 0.05$, corrected). The color bar displays t-values. Abbreviations: *ALFF* amplitude of low-frequency fluctuation, *DLPFC* dorsolateral prefrontal cortex, *fALFF* fractional amplitude of low-frequency fluctuation, Hippo, hippocampus; *mPFC* medial prefrontal cortex, *PCC* posterior cingulate cortex, *rsFC* resting-state functional connectivity. (With permission Brain Imaging Behav. 2019 Dec;13(6):1497–1509. doi: 10.1007/s11682-019-00105-8. Frequency-specific alterations in cortical rhythms and functional connectivity in trigeminal neuralgia)

8 7T MRI

The main benefits of higher magnetic field strength are improvement of the signal-to-noise ratio, contrast-to-noise ratio, and increased spatial resolution. Theoretically, these advantages can be used to improve detectability of minute pathologic changes and the conspicuity between different brain tissue on DTI and high-resolution T1-weighted image. There are several studies to evaluate microstructural change in the trigeminal nerve, thalamo-somatosnsory tracts using DTI, and cingulate using volumetric analysis on ultra-high field MRI (7T) [67–71].

References

1. Bendtsen L, Zakrzewska JM, Heinskou TB, Hodaie M, Leal PRL, Nurmikko T, et al. Advances in diagnosis, classification, pathophysiology, and management of trigeminal neuralgia. The Lancet Neurology. 2020;19(9):784–96.
2. Donahue JH, Ornan DA, Mukherjee S. Imaging of vascular compression syndromes. Radiol Clin N Am. 2017;55(1):123–38.
3. Haller S, Etienne L, Kövari E, Varoquaux AD, Urbach H, Becker M. Imaging of neurovascular compression syndromes: trigeminal neuralgia, Hemifacial spasm, vestibular Paroxysmia, and glossopharyngeal neuralgia. AJNR Am J Neuroradiol. 2016;37(8):1384–92.
4. Zhang C, Hu H, Das SK, Yang MJ, Li B, Li Y, et al. Structural and functional brain abnormalities in trigeminal neuralgia: a systematic review. J Oral Facial Pain Headache. 2020;34(3):222–35.
5. Kozak BM, Jaimes C, Kirsch J, Gee MS. MRI techniques to decrease imaging times in children. Radiographics. 2020;40(2):485–502.
6. Hamilton J, Franson D, Seiberlich N. Recent advances in parallel imaging for MRI. Prog Nucl Magn Reson Spectrosc. 2017;101:71–95.
7. Cho SJ, Choi YJ, Chung SR, Lee JH, Baek JH. High-resolution MRI using compressed sensing-sensitivity encoding (CS-SENSE) for patients with suspected neurovascular compression syndrome: comparison with the conventional SENSE parallel acquisition technique. Clin Radiol. 2019;74(10):817.e9–e14.
8. Chavhan GB, Babyn PS, Jankharia BG, Cheng H-LM, Shroff MM. Steady-state MR imaging sequences: physics, classification, and clinical applications. Radiographics. 2008;28(4):1147–60.
9. Schmalbrock P. Comparison of three-dimensional fast spin echo and gradient echo sequences for high-resolution temporal bone imaging. J Magn Reson Imaging. 2000;12(6):814–25.
10. Ciftci E, Anik Y, Arslan A, Akansel G, Sarisoy T, Demirci A. Driven equilibrium (drive) MR imaging of the cranial nerves V-VIII: comparison with the T2-weighted 3D TSE sequence. Eur J Radiol. 2004;51(3):234–40.
11. Busse RF, Hariharan H, Vu A, Brittain JH. Fast spin echo sequences with very long echo trains: design of variable refocusing flip angle schedules and generation of clinical T2 contrast. Magn Reson Med. 2006;55(5):1030–7.
12. Jung NY, Moon WJ, Lee MH, Chung EC. Magnetic resonance cisternography: comparison between 3-dimensional driven equilibrium with sensitivity encoding and 3-dimensional balanced fast-field echo sequences with sensitivity encoding. J Comput Assist Tomogr. 2007;31(4):588–91.
13. Byun JS, Kim H-J, Yim YJ, Kim ST, Jeon P, Kim KH, et al. MR imaging of the internal Auditory Canal and inner ear at 3T: comparison between 3D driven equilibrium and 3D balanced fast field Echo sequences. Korean J Radiol. 2008;9(3):212–8.
14. Mugler JP 3rd. Optimized three-dimensional fast-spin-echo MRI. J Magn Reson Imaging. 2014;39(4):745–67.
15. Markl M, Leupold J. Gradient echo imaging. J Magn Reson Imaging. 2012;35(6):1274–89.
16. Bieri O, Scheffler K. Fundamentals of balanced steady state free precession MRI. J Magn Reson Imaging. 2013;38(1):2–11.
17. Avey G. Technical improvements in head and neck MR imaging: at the cutting edge. Neuroimaging Clin N Am. 2020;30(3):295–309.
18. Touska P, Connor SEJ. Recent advances in MRI of the head and neck, skull base and cranial nerves: new and evolving sequences, analyses and clinical applications. Br J Radiol. 2019;92(1104):20190513.
19. Wu M, Jiang X, Qiu J, Fu X, Niu C. Gray and white matter abnormalities in primary trigeminal neuralgia with and without neurovascular compression. J Headache Pain. 2020;21(1):136.
20. Wang Y, Cao DY, Remeniuk B, Krimmel S, Seminowicz DA, Zhang M. Altered brain structure and function associated with sensory and affective components of classic trigeminal neuralgia. Pain. 2017;158(8):1561–70.
21. Vaculik MF, Noorani A, Hung PS, Hodaie M. Selective hippocampal subfield volume reductions in classic trigeminal neuralgia. Neuroimage Clin. 2019;23:101911.
22. Tang Y, Wang M, Zheng T, Yuan F, Yang H, Han F, et al. Grey matter volume alterations in trigeminal neuralgia: a systematic review and meta-analysis of voxel-based morphometry studies. Prog Neuro-Psychopharmacol Biol Psychiatry. 2020;98:109821.
23. Shen S, Zheng H, Wang J, Guo W, Guo X, Ji H, et al. Gray matter volume reduction with different disease duration in trigeminal neuralgia. Neuroradiology. 2021:1–11.
24. Parise M, Kubo TT, Doring TM, Tukamoto G, Vincent M, Gasparetto EL. Cuneus and fusiform cor-

tices thickness is reduced in trigeminal neuralgia. J Headache Pain. 2014;15(1):17.
25. Obermann M, Rodriguez-Raecke R, Naegel S, Holle D, Mueller D, Yoon MS, et al. Gray matter volume reduction reflects chronic pain in trigeminal neuralgia. NeuroImage. 2013;74:352–8.
26. Mo J, Zhang J, Hu W, Luo F, Zhang K. Whole-brain morphological alterations associated with trigeminal neuralgia. J Headache Pain. 2021;22(1):95.
27. Li M, Yan J, Wen H, Lin J, Liang L, Li S, et al. Cortical thickness, gyrification and sulcal depth in trigeminal neuralgia. Sci Rep. 2021;11(1):16322.
28. Li M, Yan J, Li S, Wang T, Zhan W, Wen H, et al. Reduced volume of gray matter in patients with trigeminal neuralgia. Brain Imaging Behav. 2017;11(2):486–92.
29. Hung PS, Noorani A, Zhang JY, Tohyama S, Laperriere N, Davis KD, et al. Regional brain morphology predicts pain relief in trigeminal neuralgia. Neuroimage Clin. 2021;31:102706.
30. Henssen D, Dijk J, Knepflé R, Sieffers M, Winter A, Vissers K. Alterations in grey matter density and functional connectivity in trigeminal neuropathic pain and trigeminal neuralgia: a systematic review and meta-analysis. Neuroimage Clin. 2019;24:102039.
31. Danieli L, Riccitelli GC, Distefano D, Prodi E, Ventura E, Cianfoni A, et al. Brain tumor-enhancement visualization and morphometric assessment: a comparison of MPRAGE, SPACE, and VIBE MRI techniques. AJNR Am J Neuroradiol. 2019;40(7):1140–8.
32. Wetzel SG, Johnson G, Tan AG, Cha S, Knopp EA, Lee VS, et al. Three-dimensional, T1-weighted gradient-echo imaging of the brain with a volumetric interpolated examination. AJNR Am J Neuroradiol. 2002;23(6):995–1002.
33. Chung MS, Yim Y, Sung JK, Kim I, Nickel D, Chang M, et al. CS-VIBE accelerates cranial nerve MR imaging for the diagnosis of facial neuritis: comparison of the diagnostic performance of post-contrast MPRAGE and CS-VIBE. Eur Radiol. 2021;
34. Zhang Y, Mao Z, Pan L, Ling Z, Liu X, Zhang J, et al. Dysregulation of pain- and emotion-related networks in trigeminal neuralgia. Front Hum Neurosci. 2018;12:107.
35. DeSouza DD, Hodaie M, Davis KD. Structural magnetic resonance imaging can identify trigeminal system abnormalities in classical trigeminal neuralgia. Front Neuroanat. 2016;10:95.
36. Albano L, Agosta F, Basaia S, Castellano A, Messina R, Parisi V, et al. Alterations of brain structural MRI are associated with outcome of surgical treatment in trigeminal neuralgia. Eur J Neurol. 2021.
37. Danyluk H, Lee EK, Wong S, Sajida S, Broad R, Wheatley M, et al. Hippocampal and trigeminal nerve volume predict outcome of surgical treatment for trigeminal neuralgia. Cephalalgia. 2020;40(6):586–96.
38. Devor M, Govrin-Lippmann R, Rappaport ZH. Mechanism of trigeminal neuralgia: an ultrastructural analysis of trigeminal root specimens obtained during microvascular decompression surgery. J Neurosurg. 2002;96(3):532–43.
39. Rappaport ZH, Govrin-Lippmann R, Devor M. An electron-microscopic analysis of biopsy samples of the trigeminal root taken during microvascular decompressive surgery. Stereotact Funct Neurosurg. 1997;68(1–4 Pt 1):182–6.
40. Fujiwara S, Sasaki M, Wada T, Kudo K, Hirooka R, Ishigaki D, et al. High-resolution diffusion tensor imaging for the detection of diffusion abnormalities in the trigeminal nerves of patients with trigeminal neuralgia caused by neurovascular compression. J Neuroimaging. 2011;21(2):e102–8.
41. Leal PRL, Roch JA, Hermier M, Souza MAN, Cristino-Filho G, Sindou M. Structural abnormalities of the trigeminal root revealed by diffusion tensor imaging in patients with trigeminal neuralgia caused by neurovascular compression: a prospective, double-blind, controlled study. Pain. 2011;152(10):2357–64.
42. Lin W, Chen YL, Zhang QW. Vascular compression of the trigeminal nerve in asymptomatic individuals: a voxel-wise analysis of axial and radial diffusivity. Acta Neurochir. 2014;156(3):577–80.
43. Lutz J, Linn J, Mehrkens JH, Thon N, Stahl R, Seelos K, et al. Trigeminal neuralgia due to neurovascular compression: high-spatial-resolution diffusion-tensor imaging reveals microstructural neural changes. Radiology. 2011;258(2):524–30.
44. Neetu S, Sunil K, Ashish A, Jayantee K, Usha KM. Microstructural abnormalities of the trigeminal nerve by diffusion-tensor imaging in trigeminal neuralgia without neurovascular compression. Neuroradiol J. 2016;29(1):13–8.
45. Chai W, You C, Zhang W, Peng W, Tan L, Guan Y, et al. Diffusion tensor imaging of microstructural alterations in the trigeminal nerve due to neurovascular contact/compression. Acta Neurochir. 2019;161(7):1407–13.
46. Liu J, Zhu J, Yuan F, Zhang X, Zhang Q. Abnormal brain white matter in patients with right trigeminal neuralgia: a diffusion tensor imaging study. J Headache Pain. 2018;19(1):46.
47. Zhang Y, Mao Z, Cui Z, Ling Z, Pan L, Liu X, et al. Diffusion tensor imaging of axonal and myelin changes in classical trigeminal neuralgia. World Neurosurg. 2018;112:e597–607.
48. DeSouza DD, Hodaie M, Davis KD. Abnormal trigeminal nerve microstructure and brain white matter in idiopathic trigeminal neuralgia. Pain. 2014;155(1):37–44.
49. Li R, Chang N, Liu Y, Zhang Y, Luo Y, Zhang T, et al. The integrity of the substructure of the corpus callosum in patients with right classic trigeminal neuralgia. J Craniofac Surg. 2021;32(2):632–6.
50. Wang Y, Zhang Y, Zhang J, Wang J, Xu J, Li J, et al. Structural and functional abnormalities of the insular cortex in trigeminal neuralgia: a multimodal magnetic resonance imaging analysis. Pain. 2018;159(3):507–14.

51. Hung PS, Chen DQ, Davis KD, Zhong J, Hodaie M. Predicting pain relief: use of pre-surgical trigeminal nerve diffusion metrics in trigeminal neuralgia. Neuroimage Clin. 2017;15:710–8.
52. Chen ST, Yang JT, Weng HH, Wang HL, Yeh MY, Tsai YH. Diffusion tensor imaging for assessment of microstructural changes associate with treatment outcome at one-year after radiofrequency Rhizotomy in trigeminal neuralgia. BMC Neurol. 2019;19(1):62.
53. Leal PRL, Roch J, Hermier M, Berthezene Y, Sindou M. Diffusion tensor imaging abnormalities of the trigeminal nerve root in patients with classical trigeminal neuralgia: a pre- and postoperative comparative study 4 years after microvascular decompression. Acta Neurochir. 2019;161(7):1415–25.
54. Lee YL, Chen ST, Yang JT, Weng HH, Wang HL, Tsai YH. Diffusivity parameters of diffusion tensor imaging and apparent diffusion coefficient as imaging markers for predicting the treatment response of patients with trigeminal neuralgia. J Neurosurg. 2019;132(6):1993–9.
55. Pikis S, Bunevicius A, Donahue J, Lavezzo K, Patterson G, Xu Z, et al. Diffusivity metrics three months after upfront gamma knife radiosurgery for trigeminal neuralgia may be correlated with pain relief. World Neurosurg. 2021;153:e220–e5.
56. Tohyama S, Hung PS, Zhong J, Hodaie M. Early postsurgical diffusivity metrics for prognostication of long-term pain relief after gamma knife radiosurgery for trigeminal neuralgia. J Neurosurg. 2018;131(2):539–48.
57. Wu M, Qiu J, Jiang X, Li M, Wang SD, Dong Q, et al. Diffusion tensor imaging reveals microstructural alteration of the trigeminal nerve root in classical trigeminal neuralgia without neurovascular compression and correlation with outcome after internal neurolysis. Magn Reson Imaging. 2020;71:37–44.
58. Azeez AK, Biswal BB. A review of resting-state analysis methods. Neuroimaging Clin N Am. 2017;27(4):581–92.
59. Tian T, Guo L, Xu J, Zhang S, Shi J, Liu C, et al. Brain white matter plasticity and functional reorganization underlying the central pathogenesis of trigeminal neuralgia. Sci Rep. 2016;6:36030.
60. Wang Y, Xu C, Zhai L, Lu X, Wu X, Yi Y, et al. Spatial-temporal signature of resting-state BOLD signals in classic trigeminal neuralgia. J Pain Res. 2017;10:2741–50.
61. Wang Y, Zhang X, Guan Q, Wan L, Yi Y, Liu CF. Altered regional homogeneity of spontaneous brain activity in idiopathic trigeminal neuralgia. Neuropsychiatr Dis Treat. 2015;11:2659–66.
62. Xiang CQ, Liu WF, Xu QH, Su T, Yong-Qiang S, Min YL, et al. Altered spontaneous brain activity in patients with classical trigeminal neuralgia using regional homogeneity: a resting-state functional MRI study. Pain Pract. 2019;19(4):397–406.
63. Yan J, Li M, Fu S, Li G, Wang T, Yin Y, et al. Alterations of dynamic regional homogeneity in trigeminal neuralgia: a resting-state fMRI study. Front Neurol. 2019;10:1083.
64. Yuan J, Cao S, Huang Y, Zhang Y, Xie P, Zhang Y, et al. Altered spontaneous brain activity in patients with idiopathic trigeminal neuralgia: a resting-state functional MRI study. Clin J Pain. 2018;34(7):600–9.
65. Zhang Y, Mao Z, Pan L, Ling Z, Liu X, Zhang J, et al. Frequency-specific alterations in cortical rhythms and functional connectivity in trigeminal neuralgia. Brain Imaging Behav. 2019;13(6):1497–509.
66. Zhu PW, Chen Y, Gong YX, Jiang N, Liu WF, Su T, et al. Altered brain network centrality in patients with trigeminal neuralgia: a resting-state fMRI study. Acta Radiol. 2020;61(1):67–75.
67. Arrighi-Allisan AE, Delman BN, Rutland JW, Yao A, Alper J, Huang KH, et al. Neuroanatomical determinants of secondary trigeminal neuralgia: application of 7T ultra-high-field multimodal magnetic resonance imaging. World Neurosurg. 2020;137:e34–42.
68. Moon HC, You ST, Baek HM, Jeon YJ, Park CA, Cheong JJ, et al. 7.0 tesla MRI tractography in patients with trigeminal neuralgia. Magn Reson Imaging. 2018;54:265–70.
69. Moon HC, Park CA, Jeon YJ, You ST, Baek HM, Lee YJ, et al. 7 tesla magnetic resonance imaging of caudal anterior cingulate and posterior cingulate cortex atrophy in patients with trigeminal neuralgia. Magn Reson Imaging. 2018;51:144–50.
70. Rutland JW, Huang KH, Gill CM, Villavisanis DF, Alper J, Verma G, et al. First application of 7-T ultra-high field diffusion tensor imaging to detect altered microstructure of thalamic-somatosensory anatomy in trigeminal neuralgia. J Neurosurg. 2019:1–9.
71. Lee YJ, Moon HC, Tak S, Cheong C, Park YS. Atrophic changes and diffusion abnormalities of affected trigeminal nerves in trigeminal neuralgia using 7-T MRI. Stereotact Funct Neurosurg. 2019;97(3):169–75.

Medical Treatment in Trigeminal Neuralgia

Soonwook Kwon and Ju-Hong Min

1 Introduction

Trigeminal neuralgia (TN) mainly occurs unilaterally and is a very severe pain distributed in the second and third division of the trigeminal nerve. The nature of pain is electric shock-like, shooting, stabbing, or sharp, and is induced by spontaneous or innocuous stimuli [1]. In International Classification of Headache Disorders, 3rd edition, TN was classified into idiopathic, classic, and secondary TN; idiopathic and classic TNs were subdivided into purely paroxysmal and concomitant continuous pain subtypes.

Medical treatment is the first choice in treating TN, and drug response was up to 75%. When a physician decides on a medication, it is necessary to consider drug–drug interactions and the underlying disease. Microvascular decompression, rhizotomy, or radiosurgery may be applied if medication is insufficient or not tolerable. In 2008, American Academy of Neurology and the European Federation of Neurological Societies developed the first guideline on trigeminal neuralgia management [2]. After that the knowledge of the diagnosis, clinical features, imaging, and treatment of TN has been further updated, and the European Academy of Neurology (EAN) published the recommendation in 2019 [3]. Table 1 summarizes the medical treatment for TN suggested by the EAN guideline. In this chapter, medical treatment for TN was described with a focus on idiopathic or classic TN.

S. Kwon
Department of Neurology, Inha University School of Medicine, Incheon, Republic of Korea

J.-H. Min (✉)
Department of Neurology, Samsung Medical Center, Sungkyunkwan University School of Medicine, Seoul, Republic of Korea

Department of Neurology, Neuroscience Center, Samsung Medical Center, Seoul, Republic of Korea

Department of Health Sciences and Technology, SAIHST, Sungkyunkwan University, Seoul, Republic of Korea

Table 1 Summary of European Academy of Neurology guideline on pharmacological treatment of trigeminal neuralgia

Idiopathic or classic TN (primary TN)
Management of acute exacerbation
• In-hospital treatment may be necessary for titration of anti-epileptic drugs and rehydration. • Intravenous lidocaine (5 mg/kg over 60 min) or phenytoin/fosphenytoin • Opioids are not usually effective.
Management of long-term therapy
• First-line drugs: Carbamazepine (200–1200 mg/day) or oxcarbazepine (300–1800 mg/day) • Alternatively, lamotrigine, gabapentin, botulinum toxin type A, pregabalin, baclofen, and phenytoin may be used either as monotherapy or combined • Dosages should be adjusted according to pain level and side effects
Secondary TN
• Medical treatment of patients with secondary TN should be similar to those with primary TN

TN trigeminal neuralgia

K. Park, K. R. Cho (eds.), *Trigeminal Neuralgia*, https://doi.org/10.1007/978-981-19-9171-4_8

2 Management for Long-Term Therapy (Table 2)

2.1 First-Line Treatment

2.1.1 Carbamazepine

Carbamazepine (CBZ) is the drug of choice and has been approved by the FDA for the treatment of TN [3]. It binds to the alpha subunit of the voltage-gated sodium channels (VGSC), and thereby inhibition of action potentials, reduction of synaptic transmission, and stabilization of the membrane potential in hyperexcitable neurons [4, 5]. CBZ is metabolized by the cytochrome P-450 system and the half-life is 0.5 h.

Burke et al. reported a clinical trial of (RCT) including 70 patients with TN in 1966. After 2 weeks, compared to patients treated with placebo, those treated with CBZ showed a 58% improvement in pain (58% vs. 26%, $p < 0.01$) [6]. In Cochrane Library, CBZ was significantly better than placebo, with a relative benefit of 6.1 (3.9–9.7) and the numbers needed to treat to benefit (NNT) of 1.7 (1.5–2.0) [7]. In a recent real-world report regarding the efficacy and tolerability, a total of 354 patients ($n = 254$, classic TN; $n = 60$, secondary TN; and $n = 40$, idiopathic TN) were enrolled and the responder rates were 88.3% with CBZ and 90.9% with oxcarbazepine. In classic TN, the refractory rate (6%) was lower compared to idiopathic (15%) or secondary TN (27%). Somnolence and ataxia were common reasons for treatment interruption or dosage reduction [8].

The initial dose starts at 100 mg and is increased by 100 mg every 3 days until the pain is relieved and administered in 2–3 divided doses. The maintenance dose is 600–1200 mg per day in two or three divided doses. It is effective in about 70% of patients, and if there is no pain for more than 1 month, the dose can be reduced by 100 mg per week [9].

Adverse events are reported in about 40–60% of patients. Common side effects include somnolence, dizziness, nausea, vomiting, diplopia, ataxia, elevation of liver enzymes, and hyponatremia, which were more severe in elderly patients [7, 10]. Since severe adverse effects such as leukopenia, aplastic anemia, Stevens-Johnson syndrome occur rarely, routine complete blood count (CBC), serum electrolyte, and liver function tests should be checked.

Table 2 Long-term medical treatment in TN

Drugs	Initial dose	Maintenance dose	Adverse effects
Carbamazepine	100 mg/day	600–1200 mg/day	Somnolence, dizziness, nausea, vomiting, diplopia, ataxia, elevation of liver enzymes, hyponatremia, leukopenia, aplastic anemia, Stevens-Johnson syndrome
Oxcarbazepine	150 mg/day	400–1200 mg/day	Similar to carbamazepine
Lamotrigine	25 mg/day	150–400 mg/day	Sleepiness, dizziness, headache, vertigo, skin rash and ataxia, Steve-Johnson syndrome
Gabapentin	300 mg/day	2400 mg/day	Mild somnolence, dizziness, headache, confusion, nausea, ankle edema, hyperlipidemia, and weight gain
Baclofen	10 mg/day	60–80 mg/day	Drowsiness, dizziness, weakness, fatigue, nausea, hypotension, and constipation
Clonazepam	0.5–1.0 mg/day	20 mg/day	Drowsiness, weight gain, motor impairment, confusion, and psychomotor agitation
Valproate	250 mg/day	1000–3000 mg/day	Nausea, vomiting, anorexia, increased liver enzyme, hepatitis, hepatic encephalopathy, weight gain, tremor, teratogenicity, and hair loss
Phenytoin	100 mg/day	300–600 mg/day	Nystagmus, sedation, dizziness, nausea, vomiting, ataxia, skin rash, gingival hyperplasia, hirsutism, folate deficiency, agranulocytosis, anemia, and thrombocytopenia

2.1.2 Oxcarbazepine

Although few studies are available, compared to CBZ, the effect of oxcarbazepine (OXC) is similar and the side effects are lesser, so it is used as an alternative drug in TN. OXC also blocks the VGSC and is metabolized by cytosolic enzymes with lower potential for drug interaction and its half-life is 9 h [11, 12].

Liebel et al. reported the efficacies of CBZ and OXC in 48 typical TN patients; both groups experienced a 50% or greater reduction in the frequency of pain attacks per week, after 4–6 weeks of treatment [13]. In the long-term follow-up of a small cohort, OXC was also effective in TN [14].

The initial daily dose is 150 mg and is increased by 150 mg every 3 days until the pain is relieved. The maintenance dose is 400–1200 mg per day in two or three divided doses. The side effects of OXC are similar to those of CBZ but show less memory disturbance and fatigue. Older patients over 65 years of age do not differ significantly from younger patients, but vomiting, dizziness, nausea, and somnolence may occur more frequently [15, 16]. As CBZ, it is necessary to routinely check for CBC, electrolyte, especially sodium, and liver function test.

2.2 Other Medications

For TN that is not controlled with carbamazepine or oxcarbazepine, it could be changed to other medication such as lamotrigine or gabapentin, or add-on therapy, but the clinical effect is still uncertain.

2.2.1 Lamotrigine

Lamotrigine acts by blocking sodium channel thereby preventing anomalous discharge of trigeminal axons [17]. Canavero et al. reported the effectiveness of lamotrigine in patients with TN, which was not a RCT [18]. In this study, lamotrigine (150–600 mg) was administered to 21 patients with TN, who discontinued CBZ due to ineffectiveness, partial effectiveness, or adverse side effects. They showed 100% pain relief in 7 patients, almost complete remission in 7 patients, and partial control in 3 patients, whereas side effects were shown in 30% of the patients, of which skin rash (21%) was the most common. In a double-blind, placebo-controlled crossover trial, patients with TN who did not respond to taking CBZ or phenytoin for more than a month were treated with lamotrigine 400 mg and showed higher efficacy than the placebo group by 85% [19].

The initial daily dose is 25 mg and is increased by 25 mg every 3 days until pain is relieved. The maintenance dose is 150–400 mg per day in two or three divided doses. The common side effects of lamotrigine are sleepiness, dizziness, headache, vertigo, skin rash, and ataxia. Steve-Johnson syndrome (SJS) has been reported in 1 in 10,000 patients and slow titration of lamotrigine can help prevent SJS [20].

2.2.2 Gabapentin

Gabapentin is a drug that has been widely used for a long time in various pain syndromes, including fibromyalgia, diabetic neuropathy, and postherpetic neuralgia [21]. Gabapentin binds with the alpha2-delta subunit of voltage-dependent calcium channels and increases rates of γ-aminobutyric acid (GABA) synthesis and inhibits GABA degradation. The neurotransmitter GABA is thought to inhibit central pain [22–25].

In 1998, Zakrzewska et al. reported that gabapentin (900–2400 mg) was used in seven patients who developed TN due to multiple sclerosis, and full recovery in six patients was observed [26]. A retrospective study showed that gabapentin, treated with 100–2400 mg divided three times a day, was effective in relieving or reducing paroxysmal pain in nearly half of the 92 patients within 1–3 weeks without serious adverse effects [27].

The initial daily dose is 300 mg and is gradually increased by 300 mg every 2–3 days as tolerated. If necessary, it can be administered up to 2400 mg [28]. The advantage of gabapentin is that it can be increased relatively quickly to an appropriate dose, and has less drug interaction with other drugs, no hepatotoxicity, and no known idiosyncratic skin reactions. Mild somnolence, dizziness, headache, confusion, nausea, ankle edema, hyperlipidemia, and weight gain was reported as side effects of gabapentin [29]. However, in patients with impaired renal function, caution is needed, since gabapentin is exclusively eliminated renally.

2.2.3 Pregabalin

Pregabalin has similar mechanisms with gabapentin, but with some improvement in pharmacokinetics [30]. Pregabalin is completely absorbed and eliminated by the kidneys unbound or metabolized by plasma proteins. The effect of pregabalin on diabetic neuropathy, and postherpetic neuralgia, was well-known [31, 32]. A prospective, open-label study showed the efficacy of pregabalin in TN [33]. A total of 53 patients, including 14 patients with concomitant facial pain were treated with pregabalin at 75 mg and increased by 75–150 mg weekly. After 8 weeks, the intensity and frequency of attack were reduced by more than 50%; 13 patients (25%) showed complete remission, 26 patients (50%) were improved, and others were similar to before drug administration. In addition, pregabalin was less effective in patients with concomitant facial pain.

Common side effects of pregabalin are dizziness and drowsiness, which usually improve after 2 weeks. Others include headache, dry mouth, and peripheral edema.

2.2.4 Pimozide

Pimozide is an orally active antipsychotic drug that blocks dopamine receptors in neurons and is mainly used as the treatment for Tourette's syndrome [34]. In a randomized, double-blind crossover trial over 24 weeks, 48 patients with TN were administered 2–12 mg of pimozide [35]. The degree of pain reduction was higher in patients receiving pimozide than in patients receiving CBZ. (78.4% vs. 49.7%) Because of adverse effects such as cardiac arrhythmia and parkinsonism, pimozide is rarely used.

2.2.5 Baclofen

Baclofen is a skeletal muscle relaxant and inhibits excitatory neurotransmission by activating GABAB receptors [36]. In a double-blind crossover study, baclofen was effective in 7 out of 10 patients and in the open-label study, it was effective in 37 out of 50 patients (74%), and 25 patients received concurrent administration of CBZ or phenytoin [37].

Treatment can be started at a dose of 10 mg a day and maybe gradually increased by 10–20 mg every 3 days as tolerated. For maximum efficacy, the dose can be increased to 60–80 mg a day in 3 or 4 divided doses [38]. When baclofen is used with CBZ, the dose of carbamazepine may be reduced to 500 mg a day to maintain the potential synergistic effect [37]. Adverse effects of baclofen are drowsiness, dizziness, weakness, fatigue, nausea, hypotension, and constipation. Abrupt cession of baclofen could cause withdrawal symptoms such as agitation, insomnia, confusion, delusions, hallucinations, seizures, visual changes, psychosis, dyskinesia, high fever, and increased convulsions [39].

2.2.6 Clonazepam

Clonazepam modulates the action of GABA by binding to GABA-A receptors in the central nervous system thereby enhancing neuroinhibitory activity [40]. Clonazepam is used to treat panic disorder, epilepsy, and anxiety with or without agoraphobia. A study of a case series showed the effect of clonazepam in patients with TN [41]. Clonazpem 8 mg was initially administered to seven patients in which five out of them were treated with phenytoin or CBZ, but the effect was not sufficient, and the dose was reduced to 4 mg within 10 days, and the effect was evaluated after 1 month. Five of seven patients had complete remission, one patient had a partial response, but one patient showed no improvement. Marked drowsiness was the main side effect in the first week but improved after 2–3 weeks. Chandra reported the efficacy of clonazepam was 68.4% in CBZ-resistant patients and Smirne et al. reported that clonazepam is effective in preventing pain attacks in about 64% of patients with TN without severe complications [42, 43].

The initial dose is 0.5–1.0 mg per day in divided doses. The dose may be increased by 0.5–1 mg every 3–7 days, up to about 20 mg per day, if patients are tolerable [44]. The most common side effect is drowsiness, which usually improves over time. Other side effects are weight gain, motor impairment, confusion, and psychomotor agitation.

2.2.7 Valproate

Valproic acid is used to treat epilepsy, migraine, and bipolar disorders. There are several mechanisms for the action of valproic acid. Mainly, it increases GABA activity in the central nervous system by blocking the breakdown of GABA [45]. Other mechanisms include enhancing the synthesis of GABA, and changes in pre and postsynaptic receptor reaction to GABA. Valproic acid was effective in patients with TN, who were ineffective or intolerable to CBZ, clonazepam, and phenytoin and its long-term effect was also suggested [46]. When used with baclofen, it controls pain attack by reducing excitatory transmitter release, specifically substance P, modulating nociceptive stimulation of trigeminal neurons [47].

The initial daily dose is 250 mg per day and is increased up to 1000–3000 mg per day. Drug interactions should be considered when valproic acid is used with drugs such as clonazepam, carbamazepine, and primidone. The common side effects of valproate are nausea, vomiting, anorexia, increased liver enzyme, hepatitis, hepatic encephalopathy, weight gain, tremor, teratogenicity, and hair loss [48].

2.2.8 Phenytoin

Phenytoin blocks sodium channels in nerve cell membranes, reducing electrical signal propagation and stabilizing cell membranes. In 1960, Braham et al. suggested phenytoin as the treatment for TN, showing varying degrees of effectiveness in 70% of TN patients at 300–600 mg per day [49]. Blom commented that a dose of 400–600 mg caused more side effects, but a dose of 300 mg/day was less effective. Among patients whose pain cannot be controlled with carbamazepine monotherapy, 8–20% can benefit from phenytoin combination therapy.

The initial dose starts at 100 mg per day and can be increased to 100–200 mg three times a day [44]. The side effects are nystagmus, sedation, dizziness, nausea, vomiting, ataxia, skin rash, gingival hyperplasia, hirsutism, folate deficiency, agranulocytosis, anemia, and thrombocytopenia.

2.2.9 Botulinum Toxin Type A

Botulinum toxin type A (BTX) contributes to pain relief by reducing the secretion of inflammatory and excitatory neurotransmitters such as substance P, CGRP, and glutamate by inhibiting SNARE-medicated exocytosis [50]. BTX is widely used for headache control in patients with chronic migraine and shorter disease duration is associated with good early results [51]. Chuan-Jie et al. reported that among 42 patients, the BTX group (75 U/1.5 mL intradermal and/or submucosal injection) reported a decrease in pain within 2 weeks and a decrease in attack frequency within 1 week compared to the placebo group with statistical significance. In both groups with 75 U or 25 U BTX, visual analog scale showed a significant difference from 1 week and was maintained until 8 weeks compared to the placebo group [52, 53]. Common side effects of BTX are facial asymmetry, edema, pain, and bruising of injection site which are usually reversible within few days to weeks.

3 Management for Acute Exacerbation

Acute exacerbations are uncontrolled to result in very high-frequency attacks that may require hospitalization, fluid therapy, and pain control before adjustment of oral preventive medications [54]. There is no RCT on the management of acute exacerbation but administration of intravenous fosphenytoin and lidocaine showed effectiveness. Fosphenytoin is a prodrug of phenytoin and has less cardiovascular toxicity than phenytoin. Cheshire reported improvement in most of the three patients with TN exacerbation when fosphenytoin was administered at a dose of 11–18 mg/kg phenytoin for 20 min and maintained for up to 2 days [55]. Shusaku et al. reported that pain intensity decreased after administration of fosphenytoin in most patients within 24 h, and that it could be used as a rescue therapy for acute exacerbation before surgery

[56]. Lidocaine is an amino amide-type local anesthetic and antiarrhythmic drug. In a RCT, 5 mg/kg of lidocaine was infused into patients with TN for 60 min. Compared to placebo, intravenous lidocaine was more effective to reduce the intensity of pain, the allodynia, and the hyperalgesia [57]. Intravenous magnesium sulfate (30 mg/kg over 30 min) which blocks the N-methyl-D-aspartate receptor and inhibits the calcium ion influx to the neuron cell, rapidly reduced pain in patients with refractory TN [58].

4 Investigating Medications

Eslicarbazepine is an active metabolite and an extended-release formulation of OXC. It selectively interacts with the inactive state of VGSCs and inhibits Cav3.2 calcium channels with greater affinity than CBZ [59]. Although the safety and efficacy of eslicarbazepine are not well established, there have been some reports showing its effectiveness in patients with TN and other neuropathy with similar side effects compared to CBZ [60, 61]. Vixotrigine was discovered in 2006 as a new selective Nav1.7 channel blocker and is used to treat depression, bipolar disorder, and substance disorders. In a double-blind, placebo-controlled, randomized withdrawal phase 2a trial, it failed to prove the effect statistically but the time to treatment failure, number of attacks, and mean daily pain score were improved compared to the placebo group. Most common side effects were headache and dizziness [62]. Calcitonin gene-related peptide (CGRP) antagonist is an emerging medication for migraine and 4 CGRP antagonists for ligand (galcanezumab, fremanezumab, and eptinezumab) and receptor (erenumab) were approved by FDA [63–66]. Previously, some papers reported that CGRP levels are elevated in blood, cerebrospinal fluid, and plasma in patients with TN, and blocking CGRP receptors improves mechanical allodynia [67, 68]. Eliot et al. reported retrospective case series which showed the probability of pain and mood improvement by erenumab in patients with medication-resistant TN [69].

5 Conclusion

TN is well controlled with first-line treatments, such as CBZ and OXC, but some patients need second-line drugs or combination therapy because of side effects or ineffectiveness. When administering medications, patient's underlying medical conditions or the medications they are taking, should be considered. Recently, drugs that improve the pharmacological properties of existing drugs or reduce side effects are being developed, and new drugs such as CGRP antagonists are also being developed. There is a need for studies that suggest the efficacy and adverse effects in patients with TN.

References

1. Headache classification Committee of the International Headache Society (IHS). The international classification of headache disorders, 3rd edition. Cephalalgia. 2018;38:1–211.
2. Cruccu G, Gronseth G, Alksne J, et al. AAN-EFNS guidelines on trigeminal neuralgia management. Eur J Neurol. 2008;15:1013–28.
3. Bendtsen L, Zakrzewska JM, Abbott J, et al. European academy of neurology guideline on trigeminal neuralgia. Eur J Neurol. 2019;26:831–49.
4. Gambeta E, Chichorro JG, Zamponi GW. Trigeminal neuralgia: an overview from pathophysiology to pharmacological treatments. Mol Pain. 2020;16:1744806920901890.
5. Yang YC, Huang CS, Kuo CC. Lidocaine, carbamazepine, and imipramine have partially overlapping binding sites and additive inhibitory effect on neuronal Na+ channels. Anesthesiology. 2010;113:160–74.
6. Burke WJ, Grant JM, Selby G. The treatment of trigeminal neuralgia: a clinical trial of carbamazepine ("Tegretol"). Med J Aust. 1965;1:494–8.
7. Wiffen PJ, Derry S, Moore RA, et al. Carbamazepine for acute and chronic pain in adults. Cochrane Database Syst Rev. 2011:CD005451.
8. Di Stefano G, De Stefano G, Leone C, et al. Real-world effectiveness and tolerability of carbamazepine and oxcarbazepine in 354 patients with trigeminal neuralgia. Eur J Pain. 2021;25:1064–71.
9. van Kleef M, Lataster A, Narouze S, et al. Evidence-based interventional pain medicine according to clinical diagnoses. 2. Cluster headache. Pain Pract. 2009;9:435–42.
10. Bennetto L, Patel NK, Fuller G. Trigeminal neuralgia and its management. BMJ. 2007;334:201–5.
11. Beydoun S, Alarcon F, Mangat S, et al. Long-term safety and tolerability of oxcarbazepine in

painful diabetic neuropathy. Acta Neurol Scand. 2007;115:284–8.
12. Farrokh S, Tahsili-Fahadan P, Ritzl EK, et al. Antiepileptic drugs in critically ill patients. Crit Care. 2018;22:153.
13. Langohr JTLM-D. Oxcarbazepine in the treatment of idiopathic trigeminal neuralgia. Nervenheilkunde. 2001;20:461–5.
14. Zakrzewska JM, Patsalos PN. Long-term cohort study comparing medical (oxcarbazepine) and surgical management of intractable trigeminal neuralgia. Pain. 2002;95:259–66.
15. Tentolouris-Piperas V, Lee G, Reading J, et al. Adverse effects of anti-epileptics in trigeminal neuralgiform pain. Acta Neurol Scand. 2018;137:566–74.
16. Kutluay E, McCague K, D'Souza J, et al. Safety and tolerability of oxcarbazepine in elderly patients with epilepsy. Epilepsy Behav. 2003;4:175–80.
17. Lunardi G, Leandri M, Albano C, et al. Clinical effectiveness of lamotrigine and plasma levels in essential and symptomatic trigeminal neuralgia. Neurology. 1997;48:1714–7.
18. Canavero S, Bonicalzi V. Lamotrigine control of trigeminal neuralgia: an expanded study. J Neurol. 1997;244:527.
19. Zakrzewska JM, Chaudhry Z, Nurmikko TJ, et al. Lamotrigine (lamictal) in refractory trigeminal neuralgia: results from a double-blind placebo controlled crossover trial. Pain. 1997;73:223–30.
20. Wiffen PJ, Derry S, Moore RA. Lamotrigine for acute and chronic pain. Cochrane Database Syst Rev. 2011:CD006044.
21. Bialer M. Why are antiepileptic drugs used for nonepileptic conditions? Epilepsia. 2012;53(Suppl 7):26–33.
22. Laird MA, Gidal BE. Use of gabapentin in the treatment of neuropathic pain. Ann Pharmacother. 2000;34:802–7.
23. Magnus L. Nonepileptic uses of gabapentin. Epilepsia. 1999;40(Suppl 6):S66–72. discussion S73–64
24. Taylor CP, Gee NS, Su TZ, et al. A summary of mechanistic hypotheses of gabapentin pharmacology. Epilepsy Res. 1998;29:233–49.
25. Taylor CP. Emerging perspectives on the mechanism of action of gabapentin. Neurology. 1994;44:S10–6. discussion S31-12
26. Khan OA. Gabapentin relieves trigeminal neuralgia in multiple sclerosis patients. Neurology. 1998;51:611–4.
27. Cheshire WP Jr. Defining the role for gabapentin in the treatment of trigeminal neuralgia: a retrospective study. J Pain. 2002;3:137–42.
28. Al-Quliti KW. Update on neuropathic pain treatment for trigeminal neuralgia. The pharmacological and surgical options. Neurosciences (Riyadh). 2015;20:107–14.
29. Canavero S, Bonicalzi V. Drug therapy of trigeminal neuralgia. Expert Rev Neurother. 2006;6:429–40.
30. Guay DR. Pregabalin in neuropathic pain: a more "pharmaceutically elegant" gabapentin? Am J Geriatr Pharmacother. 2005;3:274–87.
31. Rosenstock J, Tuchman M, LaMoreaux L, et al. Pregabalin for the treatment of painful diabetic peripheral neuropathy: a double-blind, placebo-controlled trial. Pain. 2004;110:628–38.
32. Dworkin RH, Corbin AE, Young JP Jr, et al. Pregabalin for the treatment of postherpetic neuralgia: a randomized, placebo-controlled trial. Neurology. 2003;60:1274–83.
33. Obermann M, Yoon MS, Sensen K, et al. Efficacy of pregabalin in the treatment of trigeminal neuralgia. Cephalalgia. 2008;28:174–81.
34. Colvin CL, Tankanow RM. Pimozide: use in Tourette's syndrome. Drug Intell Clin Pharm. 1985;19:421–4.
35. Lechin F, van der Dijs B, Lechin ME, et al. Pimozide therapy for trigeminal neuralgia. Arch Neurol. 1989;46:960–3.
36. Evenseth LSM, Gabrielsen M, Sylte I. The GABAB Receptor-Structure, Ligand Binding and Drug Development. Molecules. 2020;25:3093.
37. Parekh SSK, Kotdawalla H. Baclofen in carbamazepine resistent trigeminal neuralgia—a double blind clinical trial. Cephalalgia. 1989;9(10_suppl):392–3.
38. Fromm GH, Terrence CF, Chattha AS, et al. Baclofen in trigeminal neuralgia: its effect on the spinal trigeminal nucleus: a pilot study. Arch Neurol. 1980;37:768–71.
39. Coffey RJ, Ridgely PM. Abrupt intrathecal baclofen withdrawal: management of potentially life-threatening sequelae. Neuromodulation. 2001;4:142–6.
40. Riss J, Cloyd J, Gates J, et al. Benzodiazepines in epilepsy: pharmacology and pharmacokinetics. Acta Neurol Scand. 2008;118:69–86.
41. Caccia MR. Clonazepam in facial neuralgia and cluster headache. Clinical and electrophysiological study. Eur Neurol. 1975;13:560–3.
42. Chandra B. The use of clonazepam in the treatment of tic douloureux (a preliminary report). Proc Aust Assoc Neurol. 1976;13:119–22.
43. Smirne S, Scarlato G. Clonazepam in cranial neuralgias. Med J Aust. 1977;1:93–4.
44. Green MW, Selman JE. Review article: the medical management of trigeminal neuralgia. Headache. 1991;31:588–92.
45. Johnston D. Valproic acid: update on its mechanisms of action. Epilepsia. 1984;25(Suppl 1):S1–4.
46. Peiris JB, Perera GL, Devendra SV, et al. Sodium valproate in trigeminal neuralgia. Med J Aust. 1980;2:278.
47. Nimisha Desai KS, Gandhi I. Baclofen sodium valproate combination in carbamazepine resistant trigeminal neuralgia: a double blind clinical trial. Cephalalgia. 1991;11:321–2.
48. Nanau RM, Neuman MG. Adverse drug reactions induced by valproic acid. Clin Biochem. 2013;46:1323–38.

49. Braham J, Saia A. Phenytoin in the treatment of trigeminal and other neuralgias. Lancet. 1960;276:892–3.
50. Burstein R, Blumenfeld AM, Silberstein SD, et al. Mechanism of action of OnabotulinumtoxinA in chronic migraine: a narrative review. Headache. 2020;60:1259–72.
51. Lee MJ, Lee C, Choi H, et al. Factors associated with favorable outcome in botulinum toxin a treatment for chronic migraine: a clinic-based prospective study. J Neurol Sci. 2016;363:51–4.
52. Wu CJ, Lian YJ, Zheng YK, et al. Botulinum toxin type A for the treatment of trigeminal neuralgia: results from a randomized, double-blind, placebo-controlled trial. Cephalalgia. 2012;32:443–50.
53. Zhang H, Lian Y, Ma Y, et al. Two doses of botulinum toxin type a for the treatment of trigeminal neuralgia: observation of therapeutic effect from a randomized, double-blind, placebo-controlled trial. J Headache Pain. 2014;15:65.
54. Bendtsen L, Zakrzewska JM, Heinskou TB, et al. Advances in diagnosis, classification, pathophysiology, and management of trigeminal neuralgia. Lancet Neurol. 2020;19:784–96.
55. Cheshire WP. Fosphenytoin: an intravenous option for the management of acute trigeminal neuralgia crisis. J Pain Symptom Manag. 2001;21:506–10.
56. Noro S, Seo Y, Honjo K, Okuma M, Asayama B, Amano Y, Kyono M, Sako K, Nakamura H. Intravenous fosphenytoin therapy for rescue of acute trigeminal neuralgia crisis in patients awaiting neurosurgical procedures: a cross-sectional study. J Clin Neurosci. 2021;94:59–64.
57. Stavropoulou E, Argyra E, Zis P, et al. The effect of intravenous lidocaine on trigeminal neuralgia: a randomized double blind placebo controlled trial. ISRN Pain. 2014;2014:853826.
58. Soleimanpour H, Aghamohammadi D, Ghaffarzad A, et al. Novel treatment in refractory tic douloureux. J Clin Anesth. 2014;26:495–6.
59. Soares-da-Silva P, Pires N, Bonifacio MJ, et al. Eslicarbazepine acetate for the treatment of focal epilepsy: an update on its proposed mechanisms of action. Pharmacol Res Perspect. 2015;3:e00124.
60. Sanchez-Larsen A, Sopelana D, Diaz-Maroto I, et al. Assessment of efficacy and safety of eslicarbazepine acetate for the treatment of trigeminal neuralgia. Eur J Pain. 2018;22:1080–7.
61. Alcantara Montero A, Sanchez Carnerero CI. Eslicarbazepine acetate for neuropathic pain, headache, and cranial neuralgia: evidence and experience. Neurologia. 2019;34:386–95.
62. Zakrzewska JM, Palmer J, Morisset V, et al. Safety and efficacy of a Nav1.7 selective sodium channel blocker in patients with trigeminal neuralgia: a double-blind, placebo-controlled, randomised withdrawal phase 2a trial. Lancet Neurol. 2017;16:291–300.
63. Silberstein SD, Dodick DW, Bigal ME, et al. Fremanezumab for the preventive treatment of chronic migraine. N Engl J Med. 2017;377:2113–22.
64. Stauffer VL, Dodick DW, Zhang Q, et al. Evaluation of Galcanezumab for the prevention of episodic migraine: the EVOLVE-1 randomized clinical trial. JAMA Neurol. 2018;75:1080–8.
65. Dodick DW, Goadsby PJ, Silberstein SD, et al. Safety and efficacy of ALD403, an antibody to calcitonin gene-related peptide, for the prevention of frequent episodic migraine: a randomised, double-blind, placebo-controlled, exploratory phase 2 trial. Lancet Neurol. 2014;13:1100–7.
66. Goadsby PJ, Reuter U, Hallstrom Y, et al. A controlled trial of Erenumab for episodic migraine. N Engl J Med. 2017;377:2123–32.
67. Qin ZL, Yang LQ, Li N, et al. Clinical study of cerebrospinal fluid neuropeptides in patients with primary trigeminal neuralgia. Clin Neurol Neurosurg. 2016;143:111–5.
68. Michot B, Bourgoin S, Viguier F, et al. Differential effects of calcitonin gene-related peptide receptor blockade by olcegepant on mechanical allodynia induced by ligation of the infraorbital nerve vs the sciatic nerve in the rat. Pain. 2012;153:1939–48.
69. Parascandolo E, Levinson K, Rizzoli P, et al. Efficacy of Erenumab in the treatment of trigeminal neuralgia: a retrospective case series. Neurol Clin Pract. 2021;11:227–31.

Part II

Microvascular Decompression

Anesthetic Management of Microvascular Decompression for Trigeminal Neuralgia

Ji-Hye Kwon and Jeong Jin Lee

1 Preoperative Management

Preoperative evaluation followed the general anesthesia procedure, such as medical history review, laboratory tests, and airway evaluation. Careful evaluation of the cervical spine is helpful in considering the patient's position during surgery. Obtaining information about the history of opioid and nonopioid analgesic use, which is known as a risk factor for post-craniotomy pain, can help manage acute or chronic postoperative pain. Traditionally, fasting for at least 8 h beforehand has been recommended, but recently, preoperative carbohydrate loading has been shown to be beneficial for enhanced recovery after surgery in patients undergoing craniotomy, similar to the evidence in other specialties [1, 2].

2 Intraoperative Management

In addition to general monitoring, such as electrocardiography, oxygen saturation monitoring, and noninvasive blood pressure (BP) monitoring, neuromuscular monitoring, which evaluates the degree of muscle relaxation, is mounted on the ulnar nerve and adductor pollicis muscle, and bispectral index (BIS) monitoring is performed to evaluate the depth of anesthesia.

Total intravenous anesthesia (TIVA) using propofol and remifentanil or balanced anesthesia using volatile anesthetics and opioids can be performed, but most are selected considering the effect on IONM. Anesthesia induction was initiated with a bolus intravenous injection of thiopental or propofol and an opioid analgesic such as remifentanil, fentanyl, or sufentanil. After confirming that the eyelid reflex had disappeared, neuromuscular blocking agents (NMBAs) such as rocuronium or vecuronium should be injected to establish optimal intubation conditions. The concentration of the anesthetic agent should be titrated to maintain a target BIS value of 40–60. Due to the fact that a sudden change in BP is possible, arterial catheterization is required. Arterial BP should be controlled to be within 20% of the preoperative value measured on the day before surgery.

During microsurgery, unexpected bucking or straining can have fatal consequences; therefore, the patient should never move. Prevention can be achieved by continuous intravenous infusion of NMBA or by careful titration of appropriate concentrations of analgesics and anesthetics. However, for MVD surgery, complete muscle relaxation should be avoided because facial nerve electromyography (FNEMG) monitoring is essential to prevent facial nerve damage. If no NMBA is used during surgery, deeper anesthesia is required, but extreme hypotension and brady-

J.-H. Kwon · J. J. Lee (✉)
Department of Anesthesiology and Pain Medicine, Samsung Medical Center, Sungkyunkwan University School of Medicine, Seoul, Republic of Korea
e-mail: jjeong.lee@samsung.com

K. Park, K. R. Cho (eds.), *Trigeminal Neuralgia*, https://doi.org/10.1007/978-981-19-9171-4_9

cardia may occur. This problem can be alleviated by the injection of inotropic agents.

2.1 Positioning

Most MVD surgeries can be performed using the park-bench position (3/4 side prone position). The risks related to this position include the potential for brachial plexus injuries, stretch injuries, pressure palsies, and ventilation-perfusion (V/Q) mismatch. Careful positioning and padding can help prevent injuries. Special attention is required for positioning the patient's dependent arm because of the potential danger of axillary artery compression and brachial plexus injury. The use of a chest roll placed under the dependent upper thorax may decrease this risk. Padding at the elbow may decrease the risk of upper extremity neuropathy, and padding under the hard surface at the fibular head may decrease the risk of peroneal neuropathy. Avoiding the inappropriate use of padding (e.g., padding too tightly) also decreases the risk of perioperative neuropathy [3].

Excessive neck flexion can cause venous obstruction or cervical spine damage, which can lead to increased intracranial pressure (ICP), swelling of the upper airways, or quadriplegia. Preexisting cervical stenosis can cause damage to the cervical spine. Problems of excessive neck flexion can be avoided by ensuring that there is a two-finger gap between the mentum of the mandible and the sternal notch, and that airway pressure does not rise during head fixation under controlled ventilation with a fixed tidal volume. The patient's face can be difficult to access during MVD surgery because the operating table rotates and the patient's head is 90° or 180° away from the anesthesia machine. Therefore, patients should be checked carefully for signs of obstruction such as discoloration of the face, lips, or tongue before rotating the table, and the corrugated tube and monitoring lines should be carefully secured before the start of the operation.

The lateral position under general anesthesia and mechanical ventilation may worsen the V/Q mismatch, ventilation going mainly to the upper lung, and perfusion to the lower lung. Applying PEEP and a low inspiratory fraction of oxygen during anesthesia can prevent VQ mismatch and postoperative atelectasis [3, 4].

2.2 Anesthesia for Intraoperative Neuromonitoring

The essential IONM during MVD surgery for TN is FNEMG and brain stem auditory evoked potential (BAEP). Each of them helps to detect and prevent the seventh or eighth CN damage early. Anesthesiologists should be aware of the anesthetic and non-anesthetic factors that affect IONM [5].

Due to the fact that EMG waves are influenced by NMBA, this requires that the patient is not paralyzed or is in a constant state of incomplete paralysis. However, if muscle relaxants are omitted, there is a risk of body movement (BM) or patient-ventilator desynchronization (PVA). Huang et al. recommended that T1% should be maintained in the range of 30–60% of the control (T0), while TOF% should be maintained at a range of 20–30% to monitor facial nerve EMG without BM or PVA [6]. In general, IV anesthetics are preferred in this case because volatile anesthetics affect FN EMG more than IV anesthetics at the same depth of anesthesia [7].

Facial nerve-triggered EMG and the lateral spreading response (LSR) are considered to be effective diagnostic tools for complete decompression and also an important prognostic factor in MVD surgery for HFS [8]. However, in the case of TN, LSR was not a prognostic factor. Recently, the blink reflex has been described as a useful intraoperative technique to monitor the sensory part of the trigeminal nerve. They described that seven patients whose R1 disappeared during the surgery all experienced facial numbness postoperatively, while of the 86 patients whose R1 remained, only two patients had facial numbness. General anesthesia may have affected this reflex. In this study, BR was successfully elicited in 93 of 103 cases (90.29%) during MVD surgery under general anesthesia using intravenous propofol and remifentanil without additional muscle relaxants after intubation, although the preoperative blink reflex was normal. They suspected that anesthesia was the main cause of the discrepancy and that, in some cases, craniotomy was performed quickly and the muscle relaxants and inhalation anesthetics had not yet been fully metabolized. There are still a few reports about this monitoring, and further evaluation is needed [9].

Evoked potentials (Eps) of brainstem origin (i.e., BAEPs and subcortical portions of SSEPs) are considered less prone to modification by anesthetics than cortical potentials (i.e., the cortical portion of SSEPs and VEPs). BAEPs are almost always entirely unaffected by anesthetics [5].

2.3 Trigeminal Arrhythmia

The TCR refers to changes in the autonomic nervous system, such as bradycardia or asystole, when the sensory branches of the trigeminal nerve are manipulated. This phenomenon is known to occur because sensory trigeminal neurons and motor vagus neurons are adjacent to each other in the brainstem. When stimulation activates the sensory nucleus of the trigeminal nerve in the fourth ventricle floor, small internal nerve fibers of the reticular formation connect premotor neurons in the nucleus ambiguus and the dorsal motor nucleus of the vagus nerve. A reflex pathway activates cardioinhibitory parasympathetic vagal neurons to complete the reflex arc (Fig. 1). TCR is present in all craniomaxillofacial surgeries. TCR may be subtyped depending on the trigger points: central TCR triggered by stimulation of the intracranial course of the trigeminal nerve, that is, from the Gasserian ganglion to the brainstem, and peripheral TCR caused by the stimulation of the trigeminal nerve along the extracranial pathway to the Gasserian ganglion. Peripheral TCR is further subdivided into the ophthalmocardiac reflex (OCR) and maxillomandibulocardiac reflex (MCR) depending on the branches of the affected trigeminal nerve. Peripheral stimulation co-activates vagal and sympathetic nerves, resulting in both sympathetically mediated peripheral vasoconstriction (hypertension) and parasympathetically mediated bradycardia. This is in contrast to central stimulation of the TCR, where profound activation of the cardiac vagal branch and distinct inhibition of the inferior cardiac sympathetic nerve is observed and usually manifests as bradycardia and hypotension. Since central TCR may occur during MVD surgery for TN, hypotension and bradycardia are the main manifestations [10].

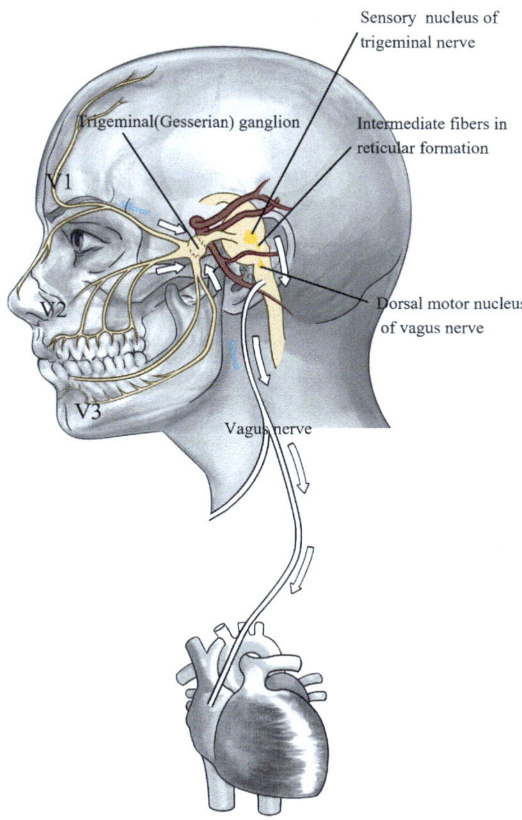

Fig. 1 Trigemino-cardiac reflex (TCR) pathway. When afferent stimulation activates the sensory nucleus of the trigeminal nerve in the fourth ventricle floor, small internuncial nerve fibers of the reticular formation connect premotor neurons in the nucleus ambiguus and the dorsal motor nucleus of the vagus nerve. A reflex pathway activates cardioinhibitory parasympathetic vagal neurons and efferent vagal nerve to complete the reflex arc. V1: ophthalmic branch of the trigeminal nerve, V2: maxillary branch of the trigeminal nerve, V3: mandibular branch of the trigeminal nerve

In a review of 28 patients who underwent MVD for TN, intraoperative TCR occurred in

18%, where the patients' HR (46% from baseline) and MABP (57% from baseline) decreased significantly during preparation around the trigeminal nerve. One patient developed a 33 s lasting asystole, which returned to a normal cardiac rhythm within 83 s after the surgical manipulation was discontinued. TCR occurred upon separating microvascular structures from the sensorial radix of the trigeminal nerve in all cases. This means that the trigeminal pathway forms the afferent pathway of the autonomic response [11]. Therefore, the surgeon should notify the anesthesiologist if he directly approaches the nerve or any of its branches. Direct trauma to the nervous tissue should be minimized as smooth and gentle manipulations are less likely to evoke TCR. The preemptive administration of atropine or glycopyrrolate for the prevention of TCR is controversial. Intraoperative factors such as light anesthesia, hypercapnia, hypoxia, and acidosis should be corrected before the beginning of surgical manipulation, as they potentiate TCR. A thorough and constant monitoring of the HR and MABP during the surgical procedure allows the surgeon to immediately interrupt his surgical maneuvers once hemodynamic deterioration from TCR occurs. This has mostly been shown to be sufficient in causing a cessation of the reflex and in restoring normal HR and BP levels, without the need to administer anticholinergics. However, administration of anticholinergics may be required in some cases where bradycardia is severe or persists despite termination of the stimulus. After the heart rate is restored, the surgeon can continue the surgery with gentle manipulation [12].

2.4 Cranial Nerve Dysfunction and Respiratory Center Injury

Surgery in the posterior fossa can injure vital circulatory and respiratory brainstem centers and cranial nerves or their nuclei. Such injuries may occur as a result of direct surgical trauma, ischemia from retraction, or other interruptions in the blood supply. Cranial nerve dysfunction, particularly of nerves IX, X, and XII, can result in a loss of control and patency of the upper airway. EMG of the lower cranial nerves during surgery can help detect the risk of cranial nerve injury. Abnormal cardiovascular responses can result from irritation of the lower portion of the pons and the upper medulla. These areas are most often stimulated during procedures on the fourth ventricle floor. Isolated damage to respiratory centers may rarely occur without preceding circulatory signs during surgery. Therefore, abrupt onset of bradycardia and hypotension, tachycardia and hypertension, or bradycardia and hypertension as well as ventricular dysrhythmias should alert the anesthesiologist to the possibility of such an injury. Meticulous attention to the electrocardiogram and direct transduction of arterial pressure during manipulation in this region are necessary to provide the surgeon with an immediate warning of the risk of damage to the adjacent cranial nerve nuclei and respiratory centers [13].

2.5 Pneumocephalus and Cerebrospinal Fluid Leakage

Although the sitting position notably increases the likelihood of pneumocephalus, this can also occur in the park-bench or prone positions [14]. Air enters the subarachnoid space because cerebrospinal fluid (CSF) is lost during surgery. In patients with cerebral atrophy, CSF drainage is marked; air can replace CSF on the surface of the brain and in the lateral ventricles. Expansion of pneumocephalus following dural closure can compress the brain. Postoperative pneumocephalus can cause delayed awakening and continued impairment of neurological function [15]. Due to these concerns, nitrous oxide is rarely used for sitting craniotomies [13]. The surgeon sometimes asks for the induction of a Valsalva maneuver (VM) to confirm a watertight dural closure. If the dural closure is not tight, CSF is expelled following an increase in ICP, and the air is sucked inside the cranium to equalize the ICP, opening up the possibility of pneumocephalus. In addition, forceful or prolonged VM can be associated with profound and complicated physiological responses, and significant complications can occur. Therefore, clinicians should be well-acquainted with its applied physiology and judiciously use it to avoid the complications associated with it [16]. When we used high-dose volatile anesthetics, which are potent cerebral vasodilators, the brain could bulge out after dural opening, and an infusion of mannitol or application of hyperventilation was mandatory. However, during TIVA anesthesia, infusing mannitol or applying hyperventilation to reduce ICP during surgery should be performed in consultation with the surgeon [17].

2.6 Venous Air Embolism

Venous air embolism (VAE) is a very rare complication that can occur when the pressure within an open vein is sub-atmospheric. It may occur in any surgical position (or during any procedure) when the wound is above the level of the heart. If the patient undergoes MVD surgery in a sitting or semi-sitting position, the risk of VAE should be considered. A recent study examining the angle of head elevation that caused clinically significant VAE involved 13 patients who underwent MVD surgery in a semi-sitting position [18]. The most sensitive monitoring modalities are precordial Doppler and transesophageal echocardiography. An abrupt decrease in end-tidal CO_2 is another indicator of air embolism. When air embolism is detected, anesthesiologists should warn surgeons to stop surgery and apply saline or water-soaked gauze. Aspiration of air from the right atrium through a central venous catheter and changing the patient's position to head-down and right-side-up to prevent air from traveling to the coronary or cerebral artery is another step [13, 17].

3 Postoperative Management

3.1 Extubation and Airway Management

Most patients awake immediately after surgery, and extubation is possible. However, in rare cases, lower cranial nerve dysfunction, respiratory center injury, or macroglossia may occur. If there is suspicion of a circulatory center injury (i.e., severe hypertension, bradycardia, or arrhythmia during the operation), this should be taken into account during planning for extubation and postoperative care.

The posterior fossa is a relatively small space, and its compensatory latitudes are even more limited than those of the supratentorial space. Relatively little swelling can result in disorders of consciousness, respiratory drive, and cardiomotor function. Abnormal respiration after MVD is more likely to occur when the brainstem injury is the result of vessel occlusion or hematoma, which can develop in a delayed manner, rather than direct mechanical damage caused by retraction or dissection in the brainstem. In a retrospective analysis of 46 patients (0.66% of 6974 cases of MVD) who presented with a decline in consciousness after waking up from the anesthesia, 15 patients (0.2%) died. The authors reported that mortality is significantly higher in trigeminal cases with cerebellar hematoma, and immediate hematoma evacuation plus ventricular drainage could give the patient a greater chance of survival [19].

Continuous monitoring of BP, pulse, respiration, and blood oxygen saturation during the immediate postoperative period is mandatory. The patient's consciousness and pupillary changes should also be closely observed. If a patient shows a sudden increase in BP accompanied by bradycardia and unconsciousness, slow and deep breathing or even arrest, decreased oxygen saturation, dilated pupils, and diminished or absent light reflex, the possibility of infarction, swelling, or bleeding in the cerebellum or brainstem should be considered. Immediate communication with the neurosurgeon is required, an emergent head computed tomography scan should be considered, and other immediate actions should be taken as necessary [20].

3.2 Macroglossia

Abnormal swelling of the tongue is a rare postoperative complication that is often associated with serious airway obstruction and prolonged intubation. Risk factors for macroglossia include a surgery duration of more than 8 h, type of surgery (i.e., suboccipital and/or posterior fossa craniotomies and spine surgeries), and patient position (i.e., prone, park-bench, or sitting). The etiology of macroglossia is multifactorial, and possible mechanisms include local mechanical tongue compression interfering with venous and/or lymphatic drainage, regional venous thrombosis, and/or local trauma. Prevention, awareness of the possibility, and early recognition are the best forms of treatment. Therefore, excessive fluid infusion should be avoided. Complications include airway obstruction, reintubation, difficult reintubation, prolonged intubation, intensive care unit stay, and tongue necrosis. Early airway management should be considered if macroglossia develops after extubation. Airway management may be difficult and a surgical airway may be required. Other supportive treatments may be required, such as placing the patient in a head-up position, preventing further tongue compression, steroids, keeping the tongue moist to prevent desiccation, and administering analgesics as needed [21].

3.3 Nausea and Vomiting

Patients frequently experience postoperative nausea and vomiting (PONV) after MVD of the cranial nerves. MVD and acoustic neuroma resection were associated with an increased likelihood of PONV compared with craniotomy performed for other tumor resections since the surgery is near the vomiting center [22]. The risk was also higher among patients who underwent MVD for TN than among those treated for hemifacial spasm. Female sex was more susceptible to PONV, and the use of a volatile agent increased the risk of PONV. Intravenous anesthesia and prophylactic antiemetic agents such as ondansetron, ramosetron, and metoclopramide can prevent PONV. However, despite the use of intraoperative prophylactic ondansetron, the overall incidence of PONV (nausea, emesis, or both) was reported to be 60% during the first 24 h after surgery. The application of a prophylactic transdermal scopolamine patch may also help to prevent PONV. It may be necessary to administer a combination of antiemetics to decrease the incidence of PONV after retromastoid craniotomy [23]. When vomiting occurs, the patient's head should be rotated to one side to avoid aspiration, and symptomatic treatment should be provided.

3.4 Postoperative Pain

Postoperative pain after craniotomy has been undermanaged for numerous reasons; however, adequate treatment of postoperative pain in these patients is essential to avoid pain-related complications [24, 25]. Post-craniotomy pain is known to be more frequent in patients who underwent infratentorial procedures than those submitted to a supratentorial approach, and the subtemporal and suboccipital surgical approach yielded the highest incidence of postoperative pain [24, 26]. Hence, it is common that patients who undergo MVD surgery complain of severe pain after surgery despite the relatively small incision size. Preoperative pain, preoperative use of opiates, and depression related to pain are also possible risk factors for post-craniotomy pain, [27, 28] which is the reason why the importance of postoperative pain in patients with TN is emphasized. It is challenging to provide pain relief while preserving neurological function. In an effort to improve the traditional therapeutic approach using low-dose opioids, multimodal analgesia has been proposed. The combined use of nonopioid analgesics, such as acetaminophen or gabapentinoids, has been shown to improve pain control and reduce opioid consumption without losing clinical neurologic examination [29].

Scalp nerve blocks or scalp infiltration with local anesthetics are beneficial for acute postoperative pain. Scalp nerve block for MVD surgery targeting the greater auricular, posterior auricular, and lesser occipital nerves can be performed (Fig. 2a) [29]. The greater auricular nerve is issued from the superficial cervical plexus and wraps around the posterior border of the sternocleidomastoid muscle at the level of the cricoid cartilage.

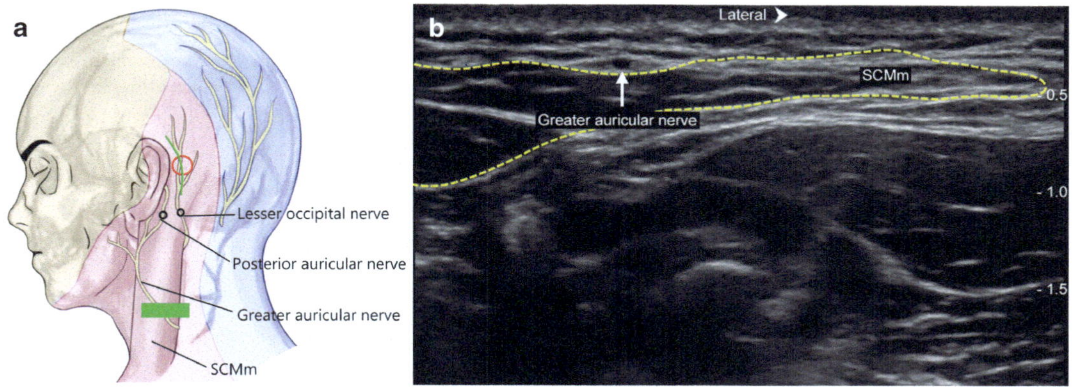

Fig. 2 (**a**) Schematic illustration of the innervation of scalp nerves on the incision line and craniotomy site of MVD surgery. Green line represents the incision line and red circle represents craniotomy. Black circles represent posterior auricular and lesser occipital nerve block and green rectangle represents ultrasound probe during greater auricular nerve block. (**b**) Ultrasound image of the greater auricular nerve. Greater auricular nerve (white arrow) can be identified by confirming that it runs medially over the sternocleidomastoid muscle as the ultrasound probe moves cephalad. SMCm; sternocleidomastoid muscle

It runs superficially over the muscle, and its dorsal branch ascends and supplies the scalp posteriorly to the ear. Ultrasonography-guided block can be performed subcutaneously (identified with in-plane or out-of-plane approach) with 2–3 mL of the chosen solution (Fig. 2b) [30]. The posterior auricular branches of the greater auricular nerves are blocked 1–2 cm posterior to the ear at the level of the tragus. The lesser occipital nerve arises from the second cervical nerve, although the third cervical nerve also gives some fibers and innervates the lateral portion of the posterior scalp and upper auricle. Unlike other scalp nerves, this nerve is difficult to identify with ultrasonography; thus, anatomical landmarks are used to block it: the nerve is 2.5 cm lateral to the occipital artery over the occiput and branches into the medial and lateral parts at approximately the midpoint between the inion and the inter-mastoid line.

3.5 Postoperative Delirium (PODE)

PODE is a common complication of MVD surgery among patients with primary cranial nerve disorders and has been reported to occur in approximately one-quarter of patients (24.2%). Old age, male sex, a history of hypertension, preoperative carbamazepine (CBZ) therapy (especially long-term high-dose therapy), postoperative sleep disturbance, and tension pneumocephalus were associated with developing PODE after MVD procedures. Patients with these risk factors should be closely monitored. In addition, the dosage of CBZ should be gradually lowered prior to surgery [15].

4 Anesthetic Management of Radiofrequency Ablation (RFA) for TN

Percutaneous radiofrequency ganglion/rootlet ablation is a highly effective procedure for the treatment of TN. For a successful procedure, both a skilled surgeon and a skilled anesthesia team are essential. With precise awareness of detailed steps, the anesthesiologist must be able to sedate the patient deeply but safely during canalization of the foramen ovale, as needed for lesion generation, and be able to rapidly wake the patient for intraoperative sensory testing. Various anesthetic strategies for RFA have been described, including ganglion block under monitored anesthetic care using propofol, remifentanil, and dexmedetomidine [31]. However, monitored anesthetic care is frequently associated with respiratory insufficiency. Various techniques have been recently introduced to reduce the risk of respiratory depression. The use of a high-flow nasal cannula (HFNC) can improve patient oxygenation [32] and monitor the oxygen reserve index (ORi) to detect hypoxia earlier [33, 34]. Combined HFNC and ORi monitoring may provide adequate oxygen reserves in patients undergoing RFA for TN.

Perçutaneous procedures for TN have long been regarded as the riskiest procedure for TCR. The incidence of TCR depends on the type of percutaneous procedure and the stimulus used. Studies on percutaneous procedures for trigeminal pain suggest that mechanical stimulation (balloon compression) carries the highest risk for TCR, and preoperative atropine administration can significantly reduce (but not completely eliminate) the occurrence of this reflex [10].

References

1. Liu B, Wang Y, Liu S, Zhao T, Zhao B, Jiang X, et al. A randomized controlled study of preoperative oral carbohydrate loading versus fasting in patients undergoing elective craniotomy. Clin Nutr. 2019;38(5):2106–12. https://doi.org/10.1016/j.clnu.2018.11.008.
2. Stumpo V, Staartjes VE, Quddusi A, Corniola MV, Tessitore E, Schröder ML, et al. Enhanced recovery after surgery strategies for elective craniotomy: a systematic review. J Neurosurg. 2021:1–25. https://doi.org/10.3171/2020.10.Jns203160.
3. Rozet I, Vavilala MS. Risks and benefits of patient positioning during neurosurgical care. Anesthesiol Clin. 2007;25(3):631–53., x. https://doi.org/10.1016/j.anclin.2007.05.009.
4. Park J, Min JJ, Kim SJ, Ahn JH, Kim K, Lee JH, et al. Effects of lowering inspiratory oxygen fraction during microvascular decompression on postoperative gas exchange: a pre-post study. PLoS One. 2018;13(11):e0206371. https://doi.org/10.1371/journal.pone.0206371.
5. Nunes RR, Bersot CDA, Garritano JG. Intraoperative neurophysiological monitoring in neuroanesthesia. Curr Opin Anaesthesiol. 2018;31(5):532–8. https://doi.org/10.1097/aco.0000000000000645.
6. Huang H, Jiang H, Liu J, Chen J, Qiu L, Wang J, et al. Facial nerve monitoring under different levels of neuromuscular blockade with Cisatracurium Besilate in parotid tumour surgery. Biomed Res Int. 2021;2021:5655061. https://doi.org/10.1155/2021/5655061.
7. Jellish WS, Leonetti JP, Buoy CM, Sincacore JM, Sawicki KJ, Macken MP. Facial nerve electromyographic monitoring to predict movement in patients titrated to a standard anesthetic depth. Anesth Analg. 2009;109(2):551–8. https://doi.org/10.1213/ane.0b013e3181ac0e18.
8. Kong DS, Park K, Shin BG, Lee JA, Eum DO. Prognostic value of the lateral spread response for intraoperative electromyography monitoring of the facial musculature during microvascular decompression for hemifacial spasm. J Neurosurg. 2007;106(3):384–7. https://doi.org/10.3171/jns.2007.106.3.384.
9. Ying T, Bao B, Yuan Y, Zhong W, Zhu J, Tang Y, et al. Blink reflex monitoring in microvascular decompression for trigeminal neuralgia. Neurol Res. 2021;43(7):591–4. https://doi.org/10.1080/01616412.2021.1900705.
10. Chowdhury T, Mendelowith D, Golanov E, Spiriev T, Arasho B, Sandu N, et al. Trigeminocardiac reflex: the current clinical and physiological knowledge. J Neurosurg Anesthesiol. 2015;27(2):136–47. https://doi.org/10.1097/ANA.0000000000000065.
11. Schaller B. Trigemino-cardiac reflex during microvascular trigeminal decompression in cases of trigeminal neuralgia. J Neurosurg Anesthesiol. 2005;17(1):45–8.
12. Sandu N, Chowdhury T, Meuwly C, Schaller B. Trigeminocardiac reflex in cerebrovascular surgery: a review and an attempt of a predictive analysis. Expert Rev Cardiovasc Ther. 2017;15(3):203–9. https://doi.org/10.1080/14779072.2017.1286983.
13. Butterworth Iv JF, Mackey DC, Wasnick JD. Anesthesia for neurosurgery. In: Morgan & Mikhail's clinical anesthesiology, 6th ed. McGraw-Hill Education: New York, NY; 2018.
14. Toung TJ, McPherson RW, Ahn H, Donham RT, Alano J, Long D. Pneumocephalus: effects of patient position on the incidence and location of aerocele after posterior fossa and upper cervical cord surgery. Anesth Analg. 1986;65(1):65–70.
15. He Z, Cheng H, Wu H, Sun G, Yuan J. Risk factors for postoperative delirium in patients undergoing microvascular decompression. PLoS One. 2019;14(4):e0215374. https://doi.org/10.1371/journal.pone.0215374.
16. Haldar R, Khandelwal A, Gupta D, Srivastava S, Rastogi A, Singh PK. Valsalva maneuver: its implications in clinical neurosurgery. Neurol India. 2016;64(6):1276–80. https://doi.org/10.4103/0028-3886.193832.
17. Gracia I, Fabregas N. Craniotomy in sitting position: anesthesiology management. Curr Opin Anaesthesiol. 2014;27(5):474–83. https://doi.org/10.1097/aco.0000000000000104.
18. Kurihara M, Nishimura S. Estimation of the head elevation angle that causes clinically important venous air embolism in a semi-sitting position for neurosurgery: a retrospective observational study. Fukushima J Med Sci. 2020;66:67–72.

19. Xia L, Liu MX, Zhong J, Dou NN, Li B, Sun H, et al. Fatal complications following microvascular decompression: could it be avoided and salvaged? Neurosurg Rev. 2017;40(3):389–96. https://doi.org/10.1007/s10143-016-0791-y.
20. Lee JJ. Anesthetic management of MVD. In: Park K, Park JS, editors. Hemifacial spasm: a comprehensive guide. Singapore: Springer; 2020. p. 111–8.
21. Brockerville M, Venkatraghavan L, Manninen P. Macroglossia in neurosurgery. J Neuroanesthesiol Crit Care. 2017;04(02):78–84. https://doi.org/10.4103/jnacc-jnacc-64.16.
22. Tan C, Ries CR, Mayson K, Gharapetian A, Griesdale DE. Indication for surgery and the risk of postoperative nausea and vomiting after craniotomy: a case-control study. J Neurosurg Anesthesiol. 2012;24(4):325–30. https://doi.org/10.1097/ANA.0b013e3182611a30.
23. Meng L, Quinlan JJ. Assessing risk factors for postoperative nausea and vomiting: a retrospective study in patients undergoing retromastoid craniectomy with microvascular decompression of cranial nerves. J Neurosurg Anesthesiol. 2006;18(4):235–9.
24. Gottschalk A, Berkow LC, Stevens RD, Mirski M, Thompson RE, White ED, et al. Prospective evaluation of pain and analgesic use following major elective intracranial surgery. J Neurosurg. 2007;106(2):210–6. https://doi.org/10.3171/jns.2007.106.2.210.
25. Durieux ME, Himmelseher S. Pain control after craniotomy: off balance on the tightrope? J Neurosurg. 2007;106(2):207–9. https://doi.org/10.3171/jns.2007.106.2.207.
26. De Benedittis G, Lorenzetti A, Migliore M, Spagnoli D, Tiberio F, Villani RM. Postoperative pain in neurosurgery: a pilot study in brain surgery. Neurosurgery. 1996;38(3):466–9. discussion 9–70. https://doi.org/10.1097/00006123-199603000-00008.
27. Klimek M, Ubben JF, Ammann J, Borner U, Klein J, Verbrugge SJ. Pain in neurosurgically treated patients: a prospective observational study. J Neurosurg. 2006;104(3):350–9. https://doi.org/10.3171/jns.2006.104.3.350.
28. Rimaaja T, Haanpää M, Blomstedt G, Färkkilä M. Headaches after acoustic neuroma surgery. Cephalalgia. 2007;27(10):1128–35. https://doi.org/10.1111/j.1468-2982.2007.01410.x.
29. Galvin IM, Levy R, Day AG, Gilron I. Pharmacological interventions for the prevention of acute postoperative pain in adults following brain surgery. Cochrane Database Syst Rev. 2019;2019(11):CD011931. https://doi.org/10.1002/14651858.CD011931.pub2.
30. Zetlaoui PJ, Gauthier E, Benhamou D. Ultrasound-guided scalp nerve blocks for neurosurgery: a narrative review. Anaesth Crit Care Pain Med. 2020;39(6):876–82. https://doi.org/10.1016/j.accpm.2020.06.019.
31. Ghali MGZ, Viswanathan A, Burchiel KJ. Trigeminal ganglion/rootlets ablation for pain. In: Functional neurosurgery and neuromodulation. Elsevier; 2019.
32. Renda T, Corrado A, Iskandar G, Pelaia G, Abdalla K, Navalesi P. High-flow nasal oxygen therapy in intensive care and anaesthesia. Br J Anaesth. 2018;120(1):18–27. https://doi.org/10.1016/j.bja.2017.11.010.
33. Fleming NW, Singh A, Lee L, Applegate RL 2nd. Oxygen reserve index: utility as an early warning for desaturation in high-risk surgical patients. Anesth Analg. 2021;132(3):770–6. https://doi.org/10.1213/ane.0000000000005109.
34. Scheeren TWL, Belda FJ, Perel A. The oxygen reserve index (ORI): a new tool to monitor oxygen therapy. J Clin Monit Comput. 2018;32(3):379–89. https://doi.org/10.1007/s10877-017-0049-4.

Intraoperative Neurophysiological Monitoring for Trigeminal Neuralgia in Microvascular Decompression

Sang-Ku Park

1 Introduction

We would like to explain intraoperative neurophysiological monitoring in trigeminal neuralgia during microvascular decompression surgery.

First, brainstem auditory evoked potentials (BAEPs) are tested to determine whether there is damage to the auditory nerve in trigeminal neuralgia surgery, BAEPs monitoring during intraoperative neurophysiological monitoring (INM) and hearing, warning criteria, and other methods of preservation hearing are explained in detail to help the cochlear nerve test during surgery.

Second, in trigeminal neuralgia surgery, what kind of tests were used to determine whether the patient's pain control was successful during surgery was examined.

In the trigeminal nerve somatosensory evoked potential (SEP) test, the V2 and V3 regions, above and below the lip, are electrically stimulated and detected as a waveform formed in the sensory cortex of the opposite brain changes and characteristics of the waveform have been described.

The masseter reflex test is the H masseter reflex that returns through the trigeminal motor nucleus in the midbrain along the motor fibers of the trigeminal nerve when electrical stimulation is applied to the masseter nerve changes and characteristics of the waveform have been described.

The blink reflex test is a reflex that returns through the sensory nucleus (Vm) and nucleus of the spinal tract (Vs) of the midbrain and pons along the V1 travel path of the trigeminal nerve by applying electrical stimulation to the supraorbital nerve. Changes and characteristics of the waveform have been described.

Third, the characteristic free-running electromyography (EMG) waveforms in patients with trigeminal neuralgia were examined.

S.-K. Park (✉)
Department of Neurosurgery, Konkuk University Medical Center, Konkuk University School of Medicine, Seoul, Republic of Korea
e-mail: 20200476@kuh.ac.kr

2 Brainstem Auditory Evoked Potentials (BAEPs)

1. Brainstem Auditory Evoked Potentials (BAEPs)
   - 1.1 BAEPs monitoring during INM and hearing
   - 1.2 Warning Criteria
   - 1.3 Other methods of preservation hearing
2. Trigeminal nerve SEP
   - 2.1 Optimal test of T-SEP method
3. Masseter Reflex
   - 3.1 Optimal test of Masseter Reflex method
4. Blink Reflex
   - 4.1 Optimal test of Blink Reflex method
5. Free-running EMG
   - 5.1 Optimal electrode insertion method for Trigeminal nerve EMG measurement

K. Park, K. R. Cho (eds.), *Trigeminal Neuralgia*, https://doi.org/10.1007/978-981-19-9171-4_10

2.1 BAEPs Monitoring during INM and Hearing

Hearing loss is one of the most common complications of MVD surgery. In general, hearing loss after surgery is about 1.9% (0.2–3.9%) [1]. These reasons are caused by excessive stretching of CN VIII, direct trauma, manipulation of the labyrinth artery, or AICA [2–4].

Anatomically, the more cerebellar traction is, the more hearing loss can occur. According to our study, 106 (6.98%) of 1518 patients with hemifacial spasm had functional hearing changes. Among them, hearing loss was permanent in 12 patients (0.79%), and the BAEP waveform changed immediately after cerebellar traction in 7 of these 12 patients [5]. In the past, the incidence rate was as high as 1%–23.8% [6].

Of course, in trigeminal neuralgia, the trigeminal nerve and the auditory nerve are far apart, so the probability of hearing loss is lower than that of hemifacial spasm, but there are cases in which a change in hearing occurs after surgery. The reason for this may be that the surgical operation is inexperienced, but it may also be that the method of testing BAEPs is not smooth.

In general, BAEPs are tested in an outpatient laboratory at a 10 Hz stimulation rate and 1000–4000 time average. This standard was also proposed by the American Clinical Neurophysiology Society (ACNS) in 2006. When examining a non-anesthetized patient, the EMG response caused by unconscious movement or tension is included in the waveform, so this standard is used for testing. It is very reasonable to do. However, according to the ACNS recommendation, if a stimulation frequency of 10 Hz and an averaging frequency of 1000 are applied, it takes 100 s to obtain a waveform of one BAEPs.

If it is an outpatient examination performed to check the presence or absence of a disease, even if it takes a long time, it is not a problem if an accurate waveform can be obtained. However, it is necessary to quickly check whether there is nerve damage that occurs suddenly during surgery, and it is IONM to prevent this situation. Therefore, if it takes a relatively long time to obtain BAEPs, there is a risk of missing an opportunity to detect damage to major nerves late and to recover them.

If the BAEPs test is performed during surgery as the standard of ACNS, it is observed that the BAEPs waveform is measured well without any abnormality while completing 1000 or more averaging times, and then the waveform is suddenly lost and observed when the next test is performed.

Wave loss is observed when the averaging time is completed and the next inspection is started after completing the averaging time without any change in the waveform that can serve as a warning standard. We hypothesized that this phenomenon was caused by the averaging process being too long or the stimulation rate being too slow. For example, if there were normal waveforms up to 800 times during 1000 BAEPs tests, and auditory nerve damage waveforms occurred during the remaining 200 times and were included in the averaging process, then the waveforms that have been tested for 1000 times are the normal and damaged auditory nerve waveforms. I wondered how it would be reflected.

So, I tried to shorten the test time. Similarly, many other researchers have tried to shorten the test time to less than 30 s by changing the stimulation frequency and averaging times [7–9].

We reported that it was possible to obtain reliable BAEPs when a stimulation frequency of 43.9 Hz and an average frequency of 400 were applied, and the time required to obtain one interpretable BAEPs was reduced to less than 10 s. We called this method Real-time BAEPs [10]. This new rapid test method made it possible to quickly discriminate the degree of auditory nerve damage caused by surgery within 10 s, and it was found that waveform changes occur very frequently within 10 s.

Two methods of stimulation are possible, condensation and dilution depending on the initial movement of the transducer diaphragm. In IONM, the alternating polarity stimulation method that alternately uses condensation and dilution is used to generate noise waves. Stimulation artifacts should be minimized so that wave I can be observed well.

2.2 Warning Criteria

In the past, there was a case where even an extension of 0.5 ms in wave V latency was dangerous [11]. Of course, the case of a complete loss of wave V is recognized as dangerous in the past or present [11–13].

The standard applied worldwide is 1.0-ms prolongation and greater than 50% decrease in amplitude of the wave V [14–17]. The reason for this is that the American Clinical Neurophysiology Society suggested guidelines [18].

If BAEPs wave loss occurs during surgery, the brain retractor is first removed to eliminate anything that affects the cochlear nerve. Then, warm saline irrigation or papaverine is administered to improve the unsuspicious blood flow of the surrounding blood vessels or direct nerve damage. In order to recover more quickly, move the bed so that the patient's head is lowered to raise the blood pressure in the head.

When the real-time BAEPs method was applied to surgery, it was frequently observed that the latency and amplitude of the waveform change within 10 s. Even if there is no problem in the latency period, wave V latency may be extended to less than 1 ms with just dura open, and it is very slow and continuously extended to 3 ms.

However, it was found that the amplitude rapidly decreased or disappeared by more than 50% within 10 s of a single test. Therefore, the cochlear nerve damage can be more accurately discriminated only when the test is performed within 10 s [19] (Fig. 1).

2.2.1 BAEPs Changes of Mechanism

The cause of waveform change during surgery can be divided into traumatic mechanical damage caused by direct external damage to the auditory nerve and vascular circulation damage caused by the influence of perforator blood vessels related to the cochlear nerve [21].

Traumatic mechanical damage is a direct injury to the cochlear nerve by a brain retractor or suction tip. In this case, a change occurs in the BAEPs waveform. When it is very weakly affected, the interpeak latency of waveforms I-III-V is prolonged, and when it is affected slightly more strongly, the amplitude of waveform V decreases by more than 50%. If it is very seriously affected, all the waveforms except the wave I will be lost.

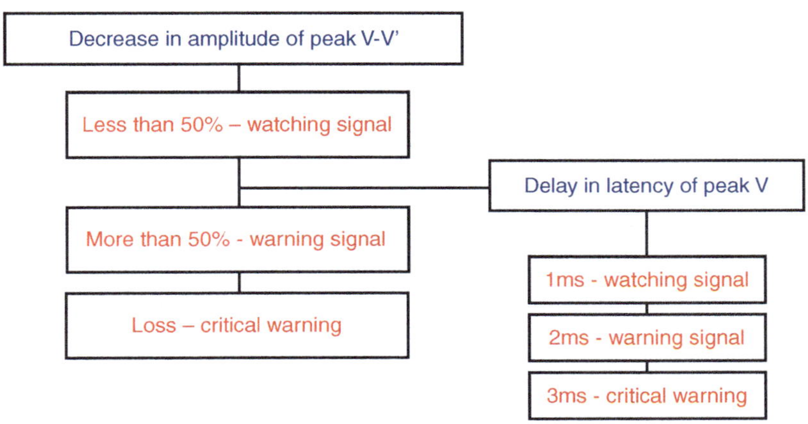

Fig. 1 Correlation of amplitude and latency in warning criteria. Warning criteria applied when using real-time BAEP. The relationship between latency and amplitude is presented separately based on wave V. In real-time BAEP tests, latency changes were always observed first, followed by amplitude changes. In addition, latency change was observed slowly and continuously, and amplitude changes suddenly decreased by more than 50% within 10 s. © Springer Nature Singapore Pte Ltd. 2021. Sang-Ku Park, Byung-Euk Joo, Kwan Park. Intraoperative Neurophysiological Monitoring in Hemifacial Spasm A Practical Guide. https://doi.org/10.1007/978-981-16-1327-2 [20]

Since the well-known warning criteria of 1.0-ms prolongation and greater than 50% decrease in amplitude of wave V are well observed, it can be appropriately treated during surgery.

However, in rare cases, there is no change in any waveform, and then all the waveforms except the I waveform are suddenly lost. In this case, the cochlear nerve is severely affected in a short period of time.

However, even if the operation was completed with the loss of the waveform, the hearing after surgery is usually normal in many cases. The reason for this is that the time of damage to the auditory nerve was quickly detected within 10 s to prevent further damage, and it is thought that a considerable amount of time is required for the damaged auditory nerve to recover. Therefore, even if the BAEPs waveform is not recovered until the end of the operation, there are cases where the hearing is normal after the operation. If the timing of the damage to the auditory nerve could not be detected within 10 s and the test method was performed after 1–2 min, most of the patients who lost the BAEPs waveform during surgery will have hearing loss after surgery.

Among patients who experienced BAEPs wave loss due to traumatic mechanical damage, low-frequency hearing loss occurs very occasionally after surgery, which is presumed to be due to the anatomical structure of the cochlear nerve and cochlear (Fig. 2).

Vascular circulation damage is the occurrence of vasospasm in peripheral arterial vessels affecting the auditory nerve. In this case, the BAEPs waveform loses all waveforms including the I waveform.

Waveform I of BAEPs originates from cochlear. In other words, as a problem occurs in the blood circulation of the arterial blood vessels related to the auditory nerve, there is a problem in the blood supply not only to the cochlear nerve itself but also to the cochlear and vestibular organs.

When such vascular circulation damage occurs, the previously known warning criteria of 1.0-ms prolongation and greater than 50% decrease in amplitude of wave V are not observed.

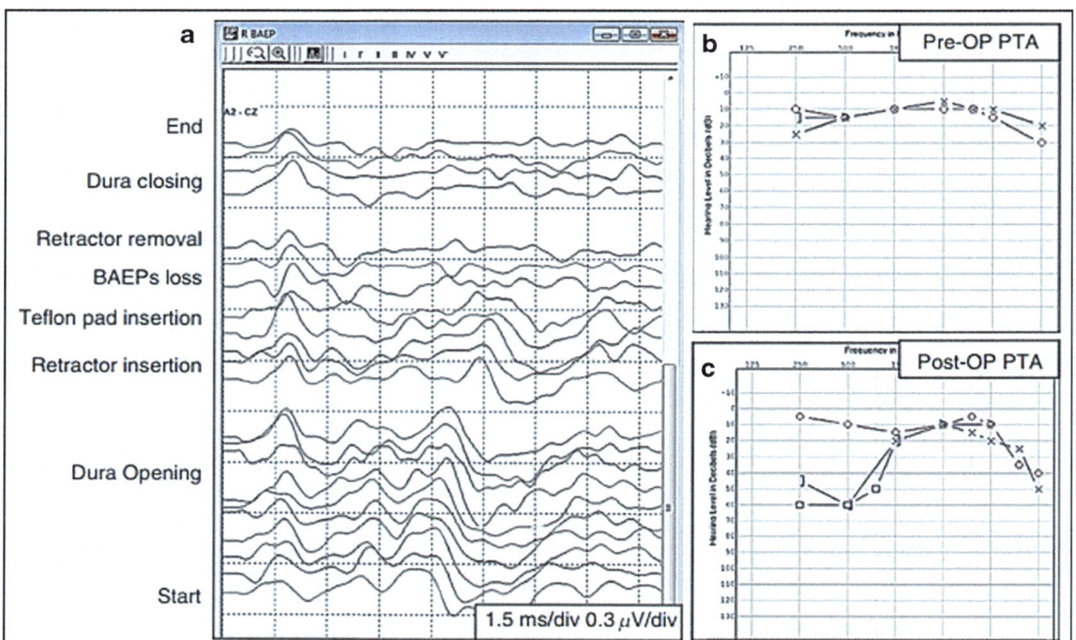

Fig. 2 When the BAEPs waveform is lost due to the brain retractor, Stack wave of BAEPs (**a**), pre-operation pure tone audiometry (**b**), post-operation pure tone audiometry (**c**). © Springer Nature Singapore Pte Ltd. 2021. Sang-Ku Park, Byung-Euk Joo, Kwan Park. Intraoperative Neurophysiological Monitoring in Hemifacial Spasm A Practical Guide. https://doi.org/10.1007/978-981-16-1327-2 [20]

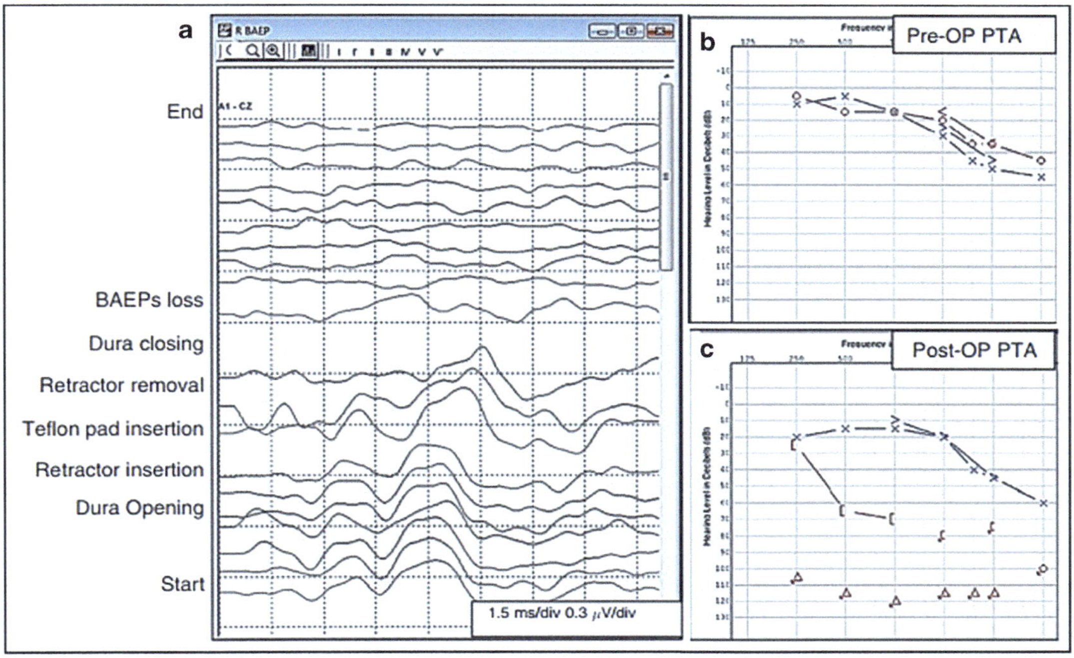

Fig. 3 When all BAEPs are lost without Wave I, Stack wave of BAEPs (**a**), pre-operation pure tone audiometry (**b**), post-operation pure tone audiometry (**c**). © Springer Nature Singapore Pte Ltd. 2021. Sang-Ku Park, Byung-Euk Joo, Kwan Park. Intraoperative Neurophysiological Monitoring in Hemifacial Spasm A Practical Guide. https://doi.org/10.1007/978-981-16-1327-2 [20]

Characteristically, it is observed that there is no reproducibility with a large amplitude as if the waveform is dancing. Then, the waveform is observed reproducibly as a flat wave. The reason for this is thought to be that the reproducibility of the waveform is lost due to the inconsistent blood supply to the auditory nerve, as it is observed that vasospasm is generated in the blood vessel itself and vibrates when a failure occurs in the blood vessel supplying blood to the auditory nerve.

When vascular circulation damage occurred and the operation was completed without recovery until the end of the operation, in our experience, total hearing loss accompanied by vestibulopathy occurred in all patients (Fig. 3).

2.3 Other Methods of Preservation Hearing

Level-specific (LS) CE-Chirp® brainstem auditory evoked potentials is a fast stimulation method that can rapidly detect intraoperative hearing loss within 10–15 s with an alternate polarity stimulation rate of 41.1 Hz and an average time of 400–800 method. This test method can also prevent a lot of hearing loss after surgery [22].

In recent years, the number of surgeries with endoscopy is increasing brain retraction can be omitted and the offending site can be observed in high quality. Therefore, it is advantageous to decompress the offending vessel and nerve more clearly [23, 24]. In addition, since there is little change during BAEP monitoring, it is possible to more stably preserve the cochlear nerve during surgery [25].

3 Trigeminal Nerve Somatosensory Evoked Potentials

3.1 Optimal Test of T-SEP Method

Long-latency trigeminal nerve somatosensory evoked potentials (SEP) were recorded from the scalp after simultaneously stimulating second and third branches of the trigeminal nerve.

The trigeminal nerve SEP waveform is well observed in the state of general anesthesia than in the awake state because there is no interference caused by the facial muscle contraction of the patient.

Trigeminal nerve SEP was recorded with an average latency of 12.4 ms and an average amplitude of 5.7 μV different patients have different amplitudes and different latency periods. However, it is maintained well during surgery [26].

The stimulus intensity ranged from 7 to 16 mA using a stimulation duration of 2 ms and a pulse rate of 4.7 Hz for stimulation, in order to activate the V2,3 region more, the waveform can be measured better when stimulated with biphasic polarity amplifier input 160, Notch filter off, band pass 50–4 K Hz.

Recordings were performed with subdermal needle electrodes placed at C5 or C6 unilateral on the side of the surgery, with Fpz as reference (according to the international 10–20 System).

Electrical stimulation should be stimulated with an intensity of around 10 mA to ensure smooth waveform formation.

In general, N14, P19, and N27 waveforms are mainly formed (Fig. 4), but sometimes several highly reproducible waveforms are formed even after the N27 waveform (Fig. 5).

The amplitude of trigeminal nerve SEP is observed to vary from person to person. Therefore, it is difficult to evaluate the amplitude. However, since it has an absolute latency period,

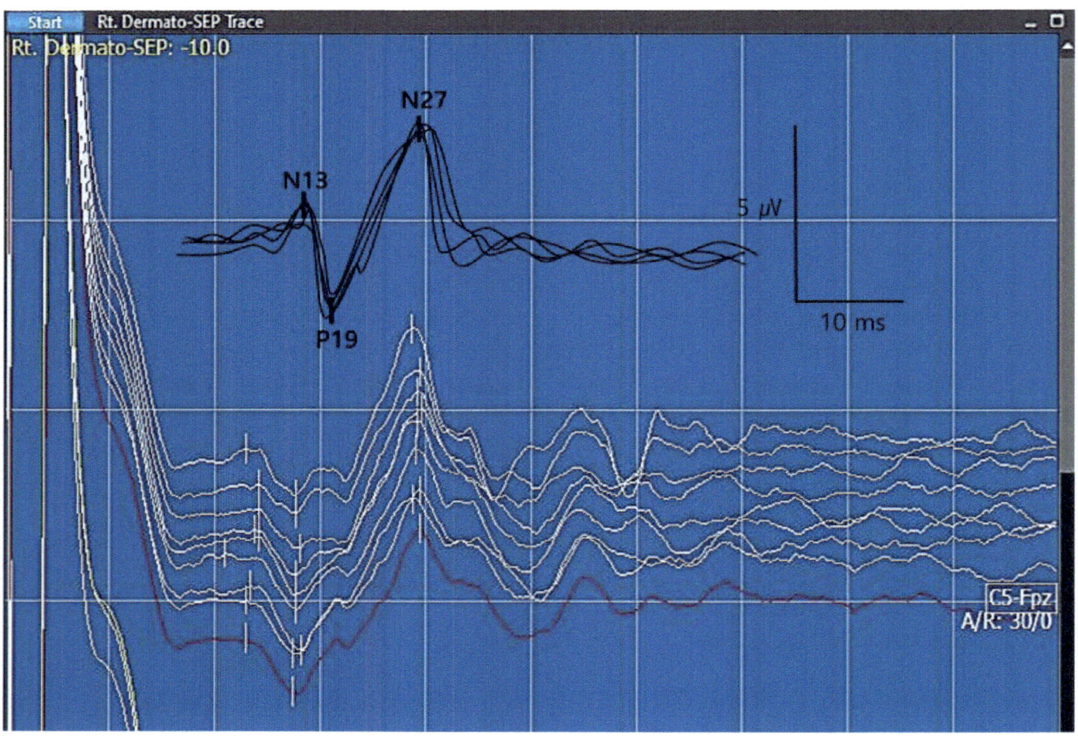

Fig. 4 Trigeminal nerve SEP waveform measured during surgery

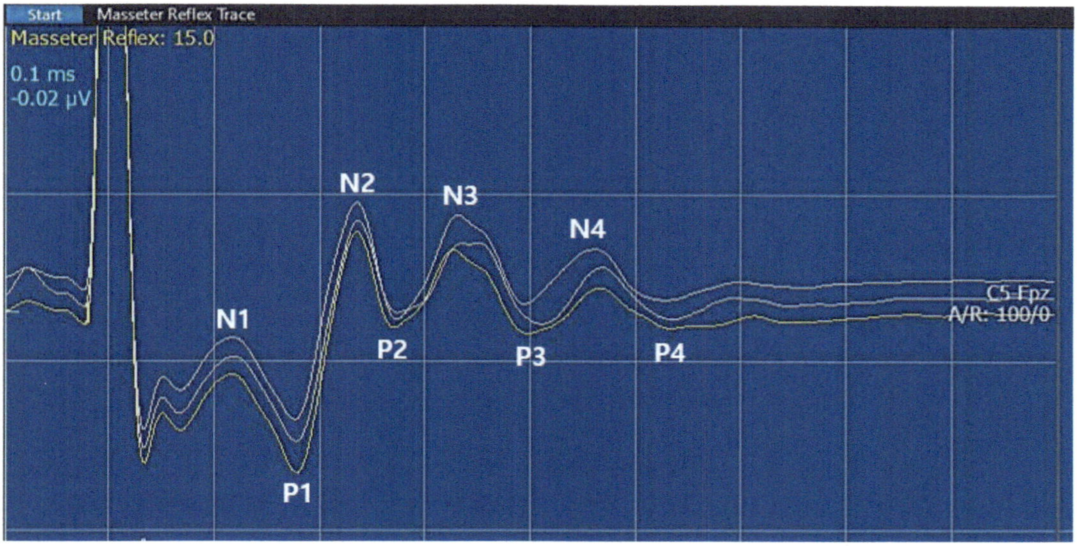

Fig. 5 Highly reproducible multiple waveform shapes after N14, P19, and N27 waveforms

the function of the trigeminal nerve can be evaluated by changing the latency period.

When it comes to the injury of the V1 or V2 branch, the existing method of SEP study for the trigeminal nerve, which stimulates the mental branch, is considered to be inappropriate to evaluate the true site of injury.

That is, in the case of trigeminal nerve SEP, evaluation should be limited to V3 types.

The induced waveform varies according to the stimulation site and the position of the recording electrode. Even with the same stimulation location, stimulation artifacts can be directly generated by complex muscle action potentials following facial muscle stimulation, even if the position of the recording electrode is constant, it is difficult to obtain a constant waveform because the homunculus area for facial proprioception is different and wide for each individual.

And there is anatomical variation between individuals. Therefore, sensitivity and specificity are lowered depending on the patient, in particular, it cannot be a good test for trigeminal neuralgia surgery because there is no significant difference in the waveform before and after Teflon insertion during surgery [27–33].

4 Masseter Reflex

4.1 Optimal Test of Masseter Reflex Method

When electrical stimulation is applied to the masseter nerve, the H masseter reflex with a latency of 5.4 ± 1.3 ms is measured, returning via the trigeminal motor nucleus in the midbrain along the motor fibers of the trigeminal nerve.

From the trigeminal mesencephalic nucleus, fibers descend to the mid-pons to monosynaptically activate the jaw-closing motoneurons of the ipsilateral masseter muscle [34].

In brainstem surgery, masseter reflex can be a useful test to detect trigeminal nerve and upper brainstem damage, and in the presence of trigeminal neuralgia, H masseter reflex with increased excitability of masseter reflex is measured (Fig. 6) [35, 36].

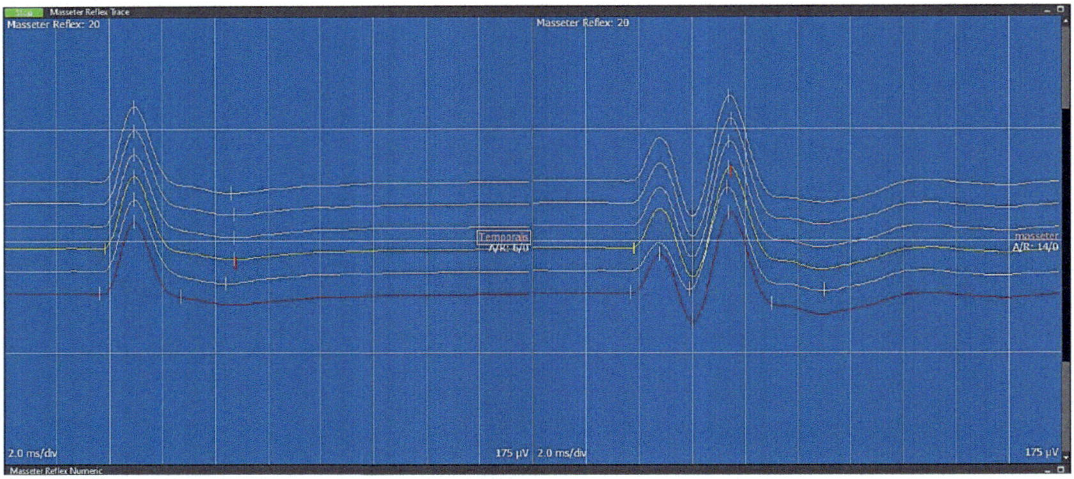

Fig. 6 H masseter reflex waveform measured in the masseter muscle

It is not always measured in all patients with trigeminal neuralgia. Even when it is measured during surgery, it cannot be a good test for trigeminal neuralgia surgery because there is no significant difference in the waveform before and after Teflon insertion.

5 Blink Reflex

5.1 Optimal Test of Blink Reflex Method

The blink reflex (BR) is elicited by the electrical stimulation of the supraorbital nerve and consists of two responses, the early ipsilateral response (R1) and the late bilateral response (R2).

R1 is the result of activation of an oligosynaptic arc that includes trigeminal afferents, pontine connections in the trigeminal sensory nucleus, the motor nucleus of the facial nerve, the facial nerve, and the orbicularis oculi muscle.

R2 is a bilateral response with the same afferent and efferent pathways as R1, but it results from complex polysynaptic connections within the pons and medulla oblongata.

Even if the patient is sleepy, the measurement of the Blink reflex waveform is not smooth. However, it has been thought that waveform measurement is impossible under general anesthesia because it is a more serious condition. Meanwhile, a method that can measure waveforms even under general anesthesia was developed, making it possible to measure waveforms even during surgery (Fig. 7) [37].

A train of 1–8 constant current stimuli or double train, with an interstimulus interval of 2 ms, a duration of 0.3–0.5 ms, an intensity of 2–20 mA, and a train repetition rate at 0.4 Hz frequency, inter-train the test is performed with an interval range of 20–40 ms.

Stimulates the supraorbital nerve and records from the orbicularis oculi muscle on the same side. The test waveform is measured with an R1 latency range of 8.9–16.5 ms, and the amplitude is observed very differently depending on the patient. The R2 waveform is not observed due to the effect of anesthesia.

If R1 is well observed and maintained during surgery, it means that there is no abnormality in trigeminal nerve (V1) function. When R1 is lost during surgery, most of the facial numbness occurs after surgery [38].

It is not always measured in all patients with trigeminal neuralgia. Even when it is measured during surgery, it cannot be a good test for trigeminal neuralgia surgery because there is no significant difference in the waveform before and after Teflon insertion (Figs. 8 and 9).

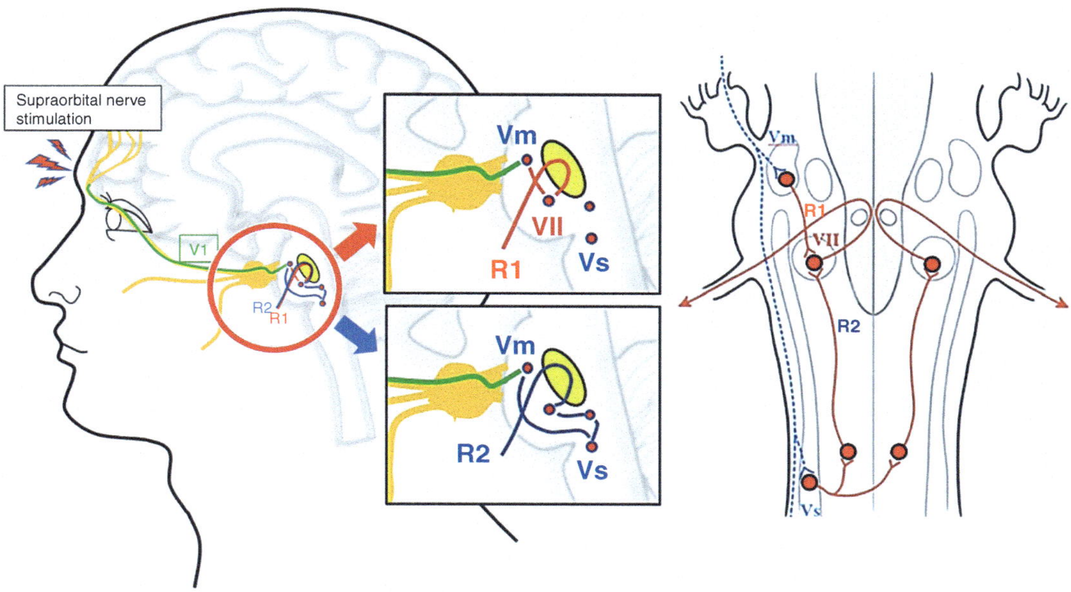

Fig. 7 Anatomy and waveforms of the blink reflex. The afferent limb of the blink reflex is mediated by sensory fibers of the supraorbital branch of the ophthalmic division of the trigeminal nerve, which synapses with both the main sensory nucleus (Vm) in the mid-pons and the nucleus of the spinal tract (Vs) in the medulla. The earlier R1 response is mediated by a disynaptic connection between the Vm nucleus and the ipsilateral facial motor nucleus (VII). The later R2 response are mediated by multisynaptic pathway between the Vs nucleus and both ipsilateral and contralateral facial nucleus (VII)

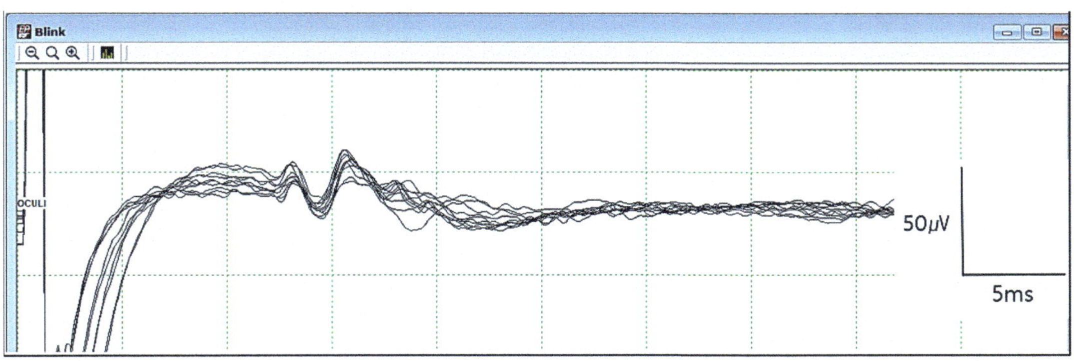

Fig. 8 R1 waveform of blink reflex test measured during surgery

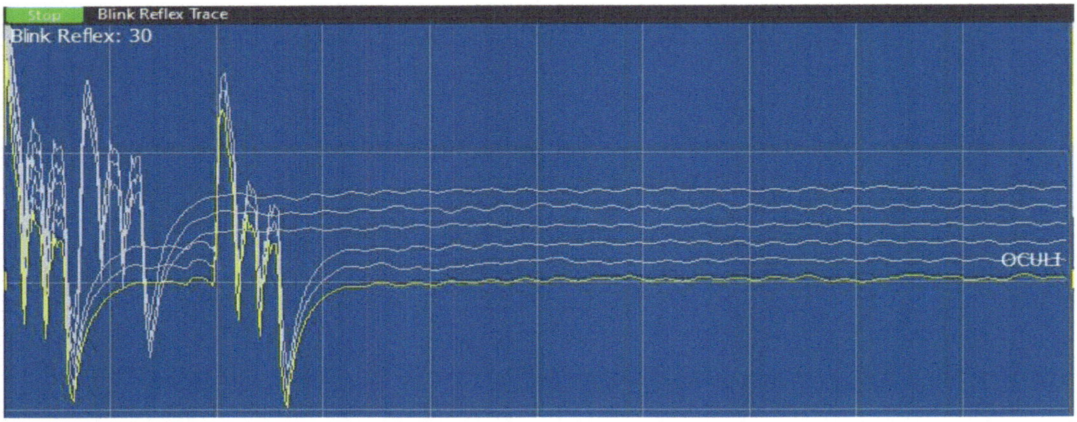

Fig. 9 There are cases where the waveform cannot be observed even when measured by train or double train

6 Free-Running Electromyography

6.1 Optimal Electrode Insertion Method for Trigeminal Nerve EMG Measurement

The trigeminal nerve is a sensory nerve and consists of three nerves (Fig. 10), the Ophthalmic nerve (V1), the maxillary nerve (V2), the mandibular nerve (V3), and the Motor branch (Fig. 11a) branching from V3.

According to innervation, the sensory areas of the face are also divided into three groups. Motor nerves are responsible for the temporalis and masseter muscles.

Therefore, free-running EMG in the trigeminal nerve is specifically well observed in the temporalis muscle and the masseter muscle (Fig. 11b).

Trigeminal nerve EMG and facial nerve EMG show different latencies of compound muscle action potential (CMAP) generated by electrical stimulation and different free-running EMG waveforms [39–42]. When a motor branch is touched during trigeminal neuralgia surgery, a free-running EMG waveform can be observed, and it has the unique characteristic of showing a spike wave or a burst wave. Waveforms with continuous spike waves like the b-train wave are not observed. Waveforms observed for a short moment can be easily missed, so it must be observed very carefully (Fig. 12).

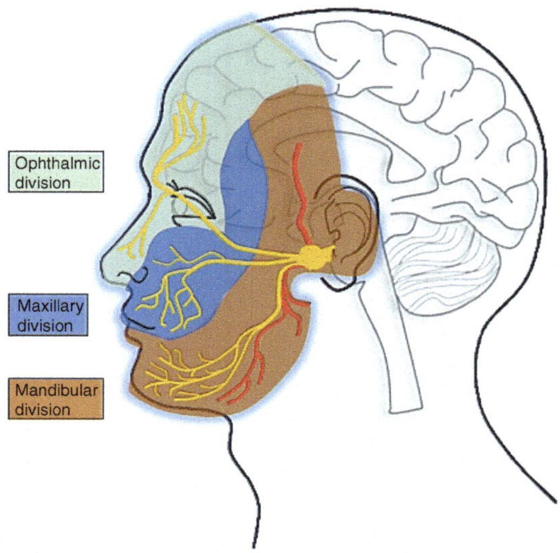

Fig. 10 Facial area division of trigeminal nerve

I will explain in detail how the trigeminal nerve EMG and the facial nerve EMG are observed as different shaped waveforms. The classification of EMG waveforms is as follows (Fig. 13).

The facial nerve consists of temporal branch, zygomatic branch, buccal branch, mandibular branch, and cervical branch, and is responsible for the frontalis, orbicularis oculi, orbicularis oris, and mentalis muscles (Fig. 14).

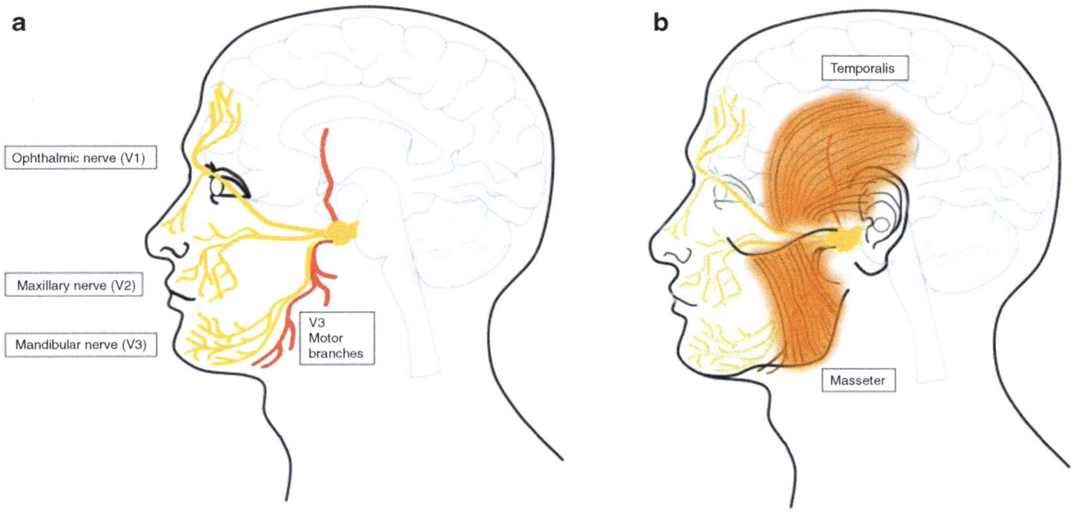

Fig. 11 Branches of the trigeminal nerve (**a**) and facial muscles (**b**)

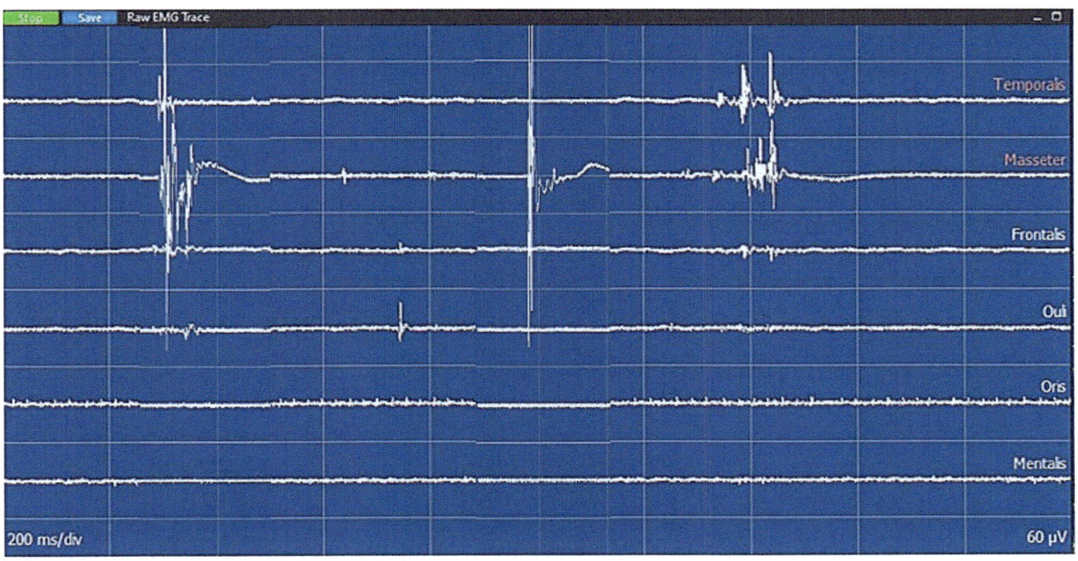

Fig. 12 Typical trigeminal nerve EMG waveform

Unlike the trigeminal nerve EMG, which is observed only in the form of a spike wave or a simple burst wave, in the facial nerve EMG, various waveforms such as spike, burst, and train are observed (Fig. 15).

In order to more clearly compare the EMG waveforms generated from the facial nerve and the trigeminal nerve, electrodes are inserted into the frontalis, orbicularis oculi, orbicularis oris, and mentalis muscles corresponding to the facial nerve, and electrodes are placed on the temporalis and masseter muscles corresponding to the trigeminal nerve. After insertion, we examined what kind of waveforms were observed when only the facial nerve was touched (Fig. 16).

Contrary to the above we examined what kind of waveforms were observed when only the trigeminal nerve was touched (Fig. 17).

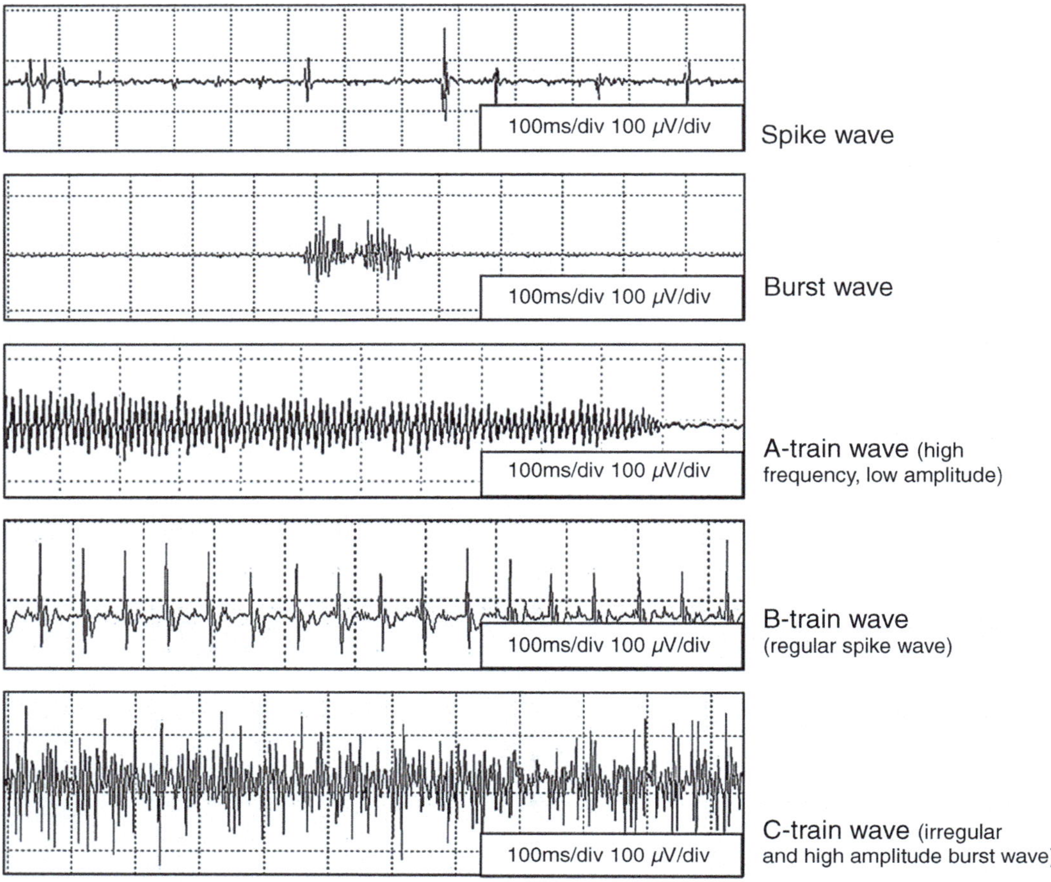

Fig. 13 The classification of EMG: Waveforms. © Springer Nature Singapore Pte Ltd. 2021. Sang-Ku Park, Byung-Euk Joo, Kwan Park. Intraoperative Neurophysiological Monitoring in Hemifacial Spasm A Practical Guide. https://doi.org/10.1007/978-981-16-1327-2 [20]

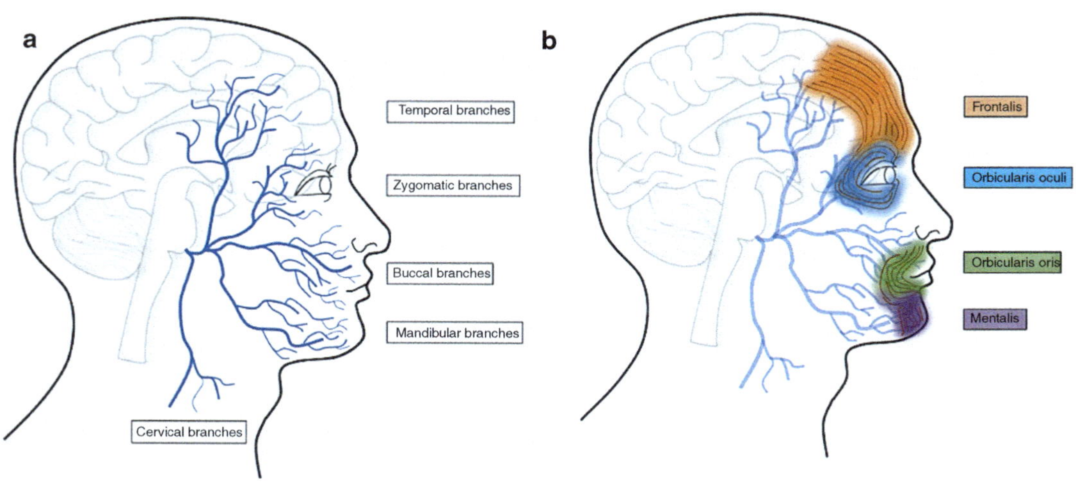

Fig. 14 Branches of the facial nerve (**a**) and facial muscles (**b**)

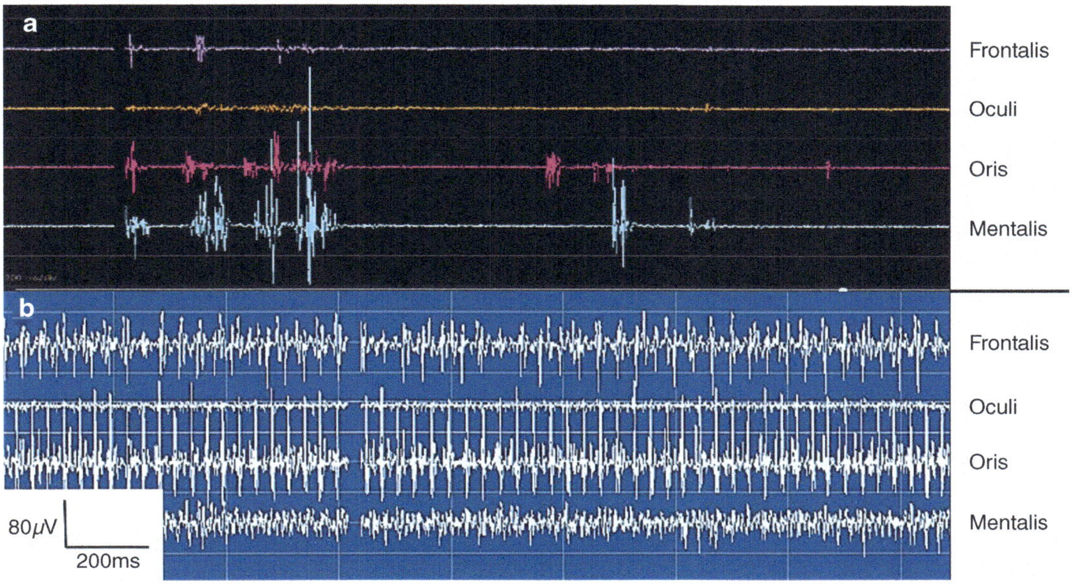

Fig. 15 A burst wave observed when the facial nerve is directly touched (**a**), and a b-train wave observed when the facial nerve is indirectly starched (**b**)

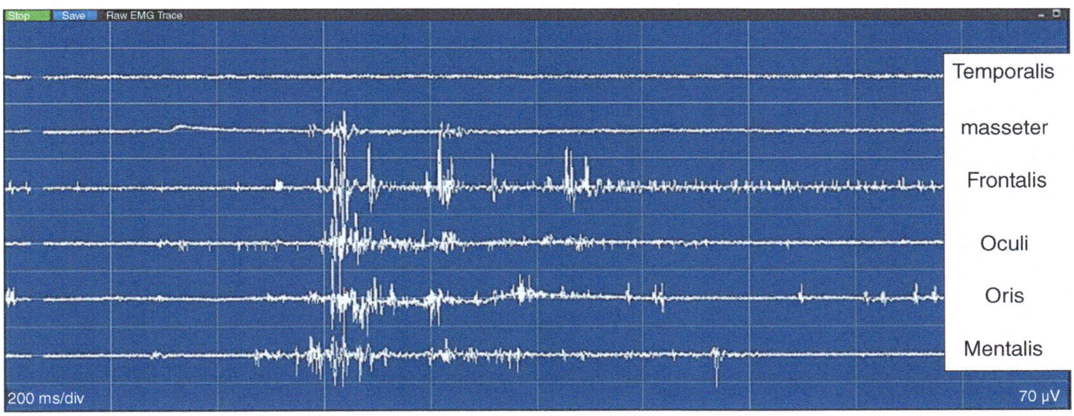

Fig. 16 Typical facial nerve EMG shapes

The facial nerve EMG is very seriously observed during saline irrigation, but the trigeminal nerve EMG is rarely observed (Fig. 18).

When performing surgery related to the trigeminal nerve, we sometimes observe EMG that occurs in mentalis. When the electrode is installed on the masseter muscle, it is not possible to choose the muscle correctly, so the mentalis waveform may be mixed into the free-running EMG.

The reason for this is that the mandibular nerve (V3) is in charge of the inner mylohyoid muscle under the chin and the anterior belly of digastric muscle, so free-running EMG waveforms are sometimes observed in mentalis.

Also, the medial pterygoid and lateral pterygoid muscles are included inside the masseter muscle, so very weak EMG waveforms are sometimes observed in the orbicularis oculi and orbicularis oris.

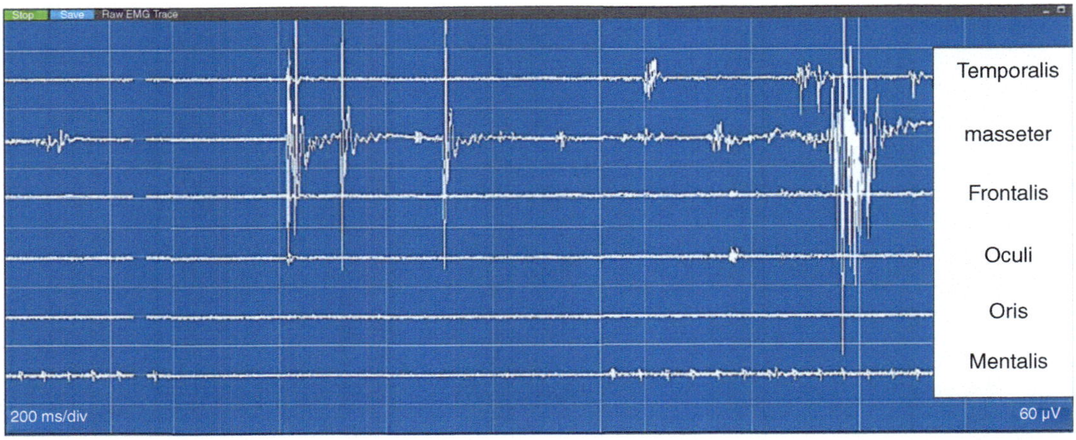

Fig. 17 Typical trigeminal nerve EMG shape

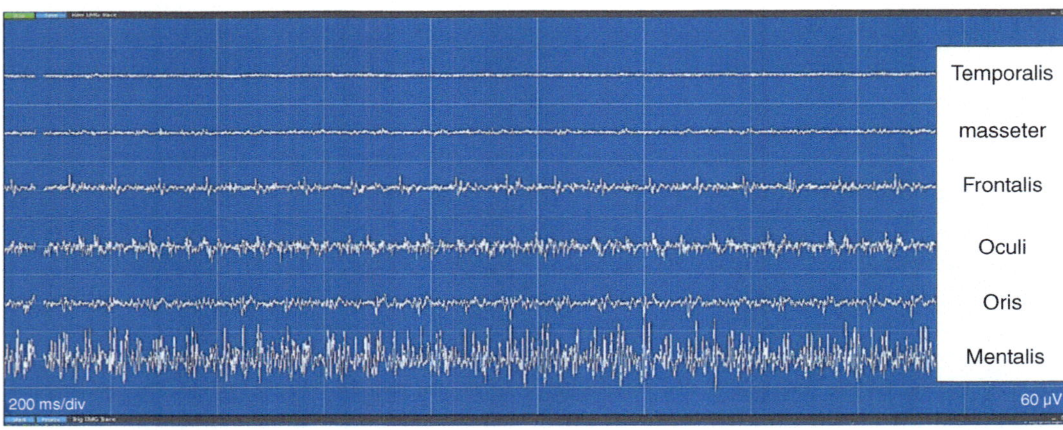

Fig. 18 EMG waveforms observed during saline irrigation

For this reason, sometimes the facial nerve EMG waveform may be observed when the trigeminal nerve is being operated surgically (Fig. 19).

The trigeminal nerve is involved in the temporalis and masseter muscles, and the facial nerve is involved in the frontalis, orbicularis oculi, orbicularis oris, and mentalis muscles.

In trigeminal nerve EMG, no wave like b-train wave is observed, and only burst wave is observed. However, in the facial nerve EMG, all types of EMG waveforms are observed, and in particular, b-train waves are observed very frequently.

However, sometimes b-train waves are observed in the temporalis and masseter muscles related to the trigeminal nerve. This reason is thought to be due to facial nerve involvement (Fig. 20).

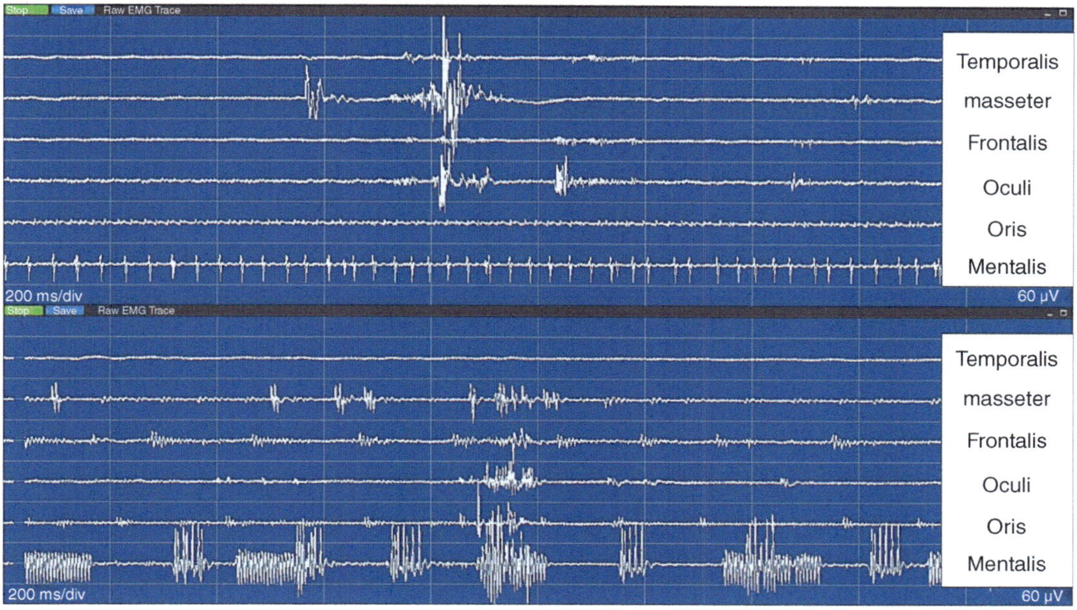

Fig. 19 Facial nerve EMG observed during trigeminal nerve surgery

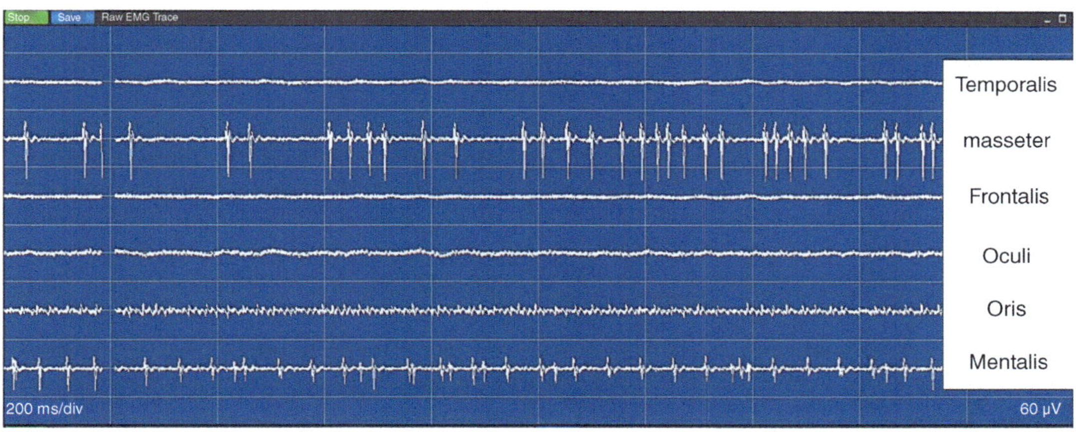

Fig. 20 B-train wave observed in the temporalis or masseter muscles related to the trigeminal nerve

References

1. Xia L, Zhong J, Zhu J, Wang YN, Dou NN, Liu MX, et al. Effectiveness and safety of microvascular decompression surgery for treatment of trigeminal neuralgia: a systematic review. J Craniofac Surg. 2014;25:1413–7.
2. Bartindale M, Kircher M, Adams W, Balasubramanian N, Liles J, et al. Hearing loss following posterior fossa microvascular decompression: a systematic review. Otolaryngol Head Neck Surg. 2018;158:62–75.
3. Park K, Hong SH, Hong SD, Cho YS, Chung WH, Ryu NG. Patterns of hearing loss after microvascular decompression for hemifacial spasm. J Neurol Neurosurg Psychiatry. 2009;80:1165–7.
4. Tomasello F, Esposito F, Abbritti RV, Angileri FF, Conti A, Cardali SM, et al. Microvascular decompression for trigeminal neuralgia: Technical refinement for complication avoidance. World Neurosurg. 2016;94:26–31.
5. Lee MH, Lee HS, Jee TK, Jo KI, Kong DS, Lee JA, et al. Cerebellar retraction and hearing loss after microvascular decompression for hemifacial spasm. Acta Neurochir. 2015;157:337–43.
6. Rizvi SS, Goyal RN, Calder HB. Hearing preservation in microvascular decompression for trigeminal neuralgia. Laryngoscope. 1999;109(4):591–4. https://doi.org/10.1097/00005537-199904000-00013.
7. James ML, Husain AM. Brainstem auditory evoked potential monitoring: when is change in wave V significant? Neurology. 2005;65:1551–5.
8. Thirumala PD, Carnovale G, Habeych ME, Crammond DJ, Balzer JR. Diagnostic accuracy of brainstem auditory evoked potentials during microvascular decompression. Neurology. 2014;83(19):1747–52.
9. Ying T, Thirumala P, Gardner P, Habeych M, Crammond D, Balzer J. The incidence of early postoperative conductive hearing loss after microvascular decompression of hemifacial spasm. J Neurol Surg B Skull Base. 2015;76(6):411–5.
10. Joo BE, Park SK, Cho KR, Kong DS, Seo DW, Park K. Real-time intraoperative monitoring of brainstem auditory evoked potentials during microvascular decompression for hemifacial spasm. J Neurosurg. 2016;125(5):1061–7.
11. Colletti V, Fiorino FG, Mocella S, Policante Z. ECochG, CNAP and ABR monitoring during vestibular schwannoma surgery. Audiology. 1998;37:27–37.
12. Grundy BL, Janetta PJ, Procopio PT, Lina A, Boston JR, Doyle E. Intraoperative monitoring of brain-stem auditory evoked potentials. J Neurosurg. 1982;57:674–81.
13. Schlake HP, Milewski C, Goldbrunner RH, Kindgen A, Riemann R, Helms J, Roosen K. Combined intraoperative monitoring of hearing by means of auditory brainstem responses (ABR) and transtympanic electrocochleography (ECochG) during surgery of intra- and extrameatal acoustic neurinomas. Acta Neurochir. 2001;143:985–95.
14. Radtke RA, Erwin CW, Wilkins RH. Intraoperative brainstem auditory evoked potentials: significant decrease in postoperative morbidity. Neurology. 1989;39:187–91.
15. Manninen PH, Patterson S, Lam AM, Gelb AW, Nantau WE. Evoked potential monitoring during posterior fossa aneurysm surgery: a comparison of two modalities. Can J Anaesth. 1994;41:92–7.
16. Raudzens PA, Shetter AG. Intraoperative monitoring of brain-stem auditory evoked potentials. J Neurosurg. 1982;57:341–8.
17. Watanabe E, Schramm J, Strauss C, Fahlbusch R. Neurophysiologic monitoring in posterior fossa surgery. II. BAEP-waves I and V and preservation of hearing. Acta Neurochir. 1989;98:118–28.
18. American Clinical Neurophysiology Society. Guideline eleven: guidelines for intraoperative monitoring of sensory evoked potentials. J Clin Neurophysiol. 1994;11:77–87.
19. Park SK, Joo BE, Lee S, Lee JA, Hwang JH, Kong DS, et al. The critical warning sign of real-time brainstem auditory evoked potentials during microvascular decompression for hemifacial spasm. Clin Neurophysiol. 2018;129(5):1097–102.
20. Park S-K, Joo B-E, Park K. Intraoperative neurophysiological monitoring in hemifacial spasm: a practical guide. Singapore: Springer nature; 2021. https://doi.org/10.1007/978-981-16-1327-2.
21. Joo B-E, Park S-K, Lee MH, Lee S, Lee J-a, Park K. Significance of wave I loss of brainstem auditory evoked potentials during microvascular decompression surgery for hemifacial spasm. Clin Neurophysiol. 2020;131(4):809–15. https://doi.org/10.1016/j.clinph.2019.12.409.
22. Mastronardi L, Caputi F, Cacciotti G, Scavo CG, Roperto R, Sufianov A. Microvascular decompression for typical trigeminal neuralgia: Personal experience with intraoperative neuromonitoring with level-specific-CE-Chirp® brainstem auditory evoked potentials in preventing possible hearing loss. Surg Neurol Int. 2020;11:388. https://doi.org/10.25259/SNI_702_2020. eCollection 2020.
23. Yadav YR, Parihar V, Ratre S. Endoscopic microvascular decompression for trigeminal neuralgia: is it what we should aim for? World Neurosurg. 2018;114:436–7.
24. Komatsu F, Imai M, Hirayama A, Hotta K, Hayashi N, Oda S, Shimoda M, Matsumae M. Endoscopic microvascular decompression with transposition for trigeminal neuralgia and Hemifacial spasm: technical note. J Neurol Surg A Cent Eur Neurosurg. 2017;78(3):291–5. https://doi.org/10.1055/s-0036-1592077.
25. Feng B-H, Zhong W-X, Li S-T, Wang X-H. Fully endoscopic microvascular decompression of the hemifacial spasm: our experience. Acta Neurochir. 2020;162:1081–7. https://doi.org/10.1007/s00701-020-04245-5.

26. Malcharek MJ, Landgraf J, Hennig G, Sorge O, Aschermann J, Sablotzki A. Recordings of long-latency trigeminal somatosensory-evoked potentials in patients under general anaesthesia. Clin Neurophysiol. 2011;122:1048–54.
27. Lee EC, Kim EJ, Park CH, Hong SE, Kim MO. Somatosensory evoked potentials from the three branches of the trigeminal nerve and clinical correlation. J Korean Assoc Electrodiagn Med. 2016;18(1):11–7.
28. Buettner UW, Petuch F, Scheglmann K, Stohr M. Diagnostic significance of cortical somatosensory evoked potentials following trigeminal nerve stimulation. Adv Neurol. 1982;32(339):1982.
29. Findler G, Feinsod M, Sahar AA. Trigeminal neurinoma with unusual presentation; report of a case with trigeminal somatosensory evoked responses. Surg Neurol. 1983;19:351.
30. Kountouris D, Fritz D, Fritz J, Blumm R, Greulich W, Gehlen W. Blink reflex & trigeminal nerve somatosensory evoked potentials: essentials in vascular brainstem diseases. Monogr Neural Sci. 1984;11:222.
31. Stohr M, Petrdch F, Scheglmann K. Somatosensory evoked potentials following trigeminal nerve stimulation in Trigeminal neuralgia. Ann Neural. 1981;9:63.
32. Wastell DG, Bennett AJ, Barker GR. Early experiences using trigeminal somatosensory evoked potentials to assess sensory deficit. Electroencephalogr Clin Neurophysiol. 1985;63:79.
33. Bennet AJ, Wastell DJ, Barker GR, Blackburn CW, Rood JP. Trigeminal somatosensory evoked potentials: a review of the literature as applicable to oral dysaesthesias. Int J Oral Maxillofac Surg. 1987;16:408.
34. Ulkatan S, Jaramillo AM, Téllez MJ, Goodman RR, Deletis V. Feasibility of eliciting the H reflex in the masseter muscle in patients under general anesthesia. Clin Neurophysiol. 2017;128:123–7. https://doi.org/10.1016/j.clinph.2016.10.092.
35. Svensson P, Macaluso GM, de Laat A, Wang K. Effects of local and remote muscle pain on human jaw reflexes evoked by fast stretches at different clenching levels. Exp Brain Res. 2001;139(4):495–502.
36. Te'llez MJ, Ulkatan S. Chapter 16. Bringing the masseter reflex into the operating room. In: Deletis V, Shils JL, Sala F, Seidel K, editors. Neurophysiology in neurosurgery a modern approach. 2nd ed. Cambridge: Academic; 2021. p. 255–60.
37. Deletis V, Urriza J, Ulkatan S, Fernandez-Conejero I, Lesser J, Misita D. The feasibility of recording blink reflexes under general anesthesia. Muscle Nerve. 2009;39:642–6. https://doi.org/10.1002/mus.21257.
38. Ying T, Bao B, Yuan Y, Zhong W, Zhu J, Tang Y, Li S. Blink reflex monitoring in microvascular decompression for trigeminal neuralgia. Neurol Res. 2021;43(7):591–4. https://doi.org/10.1080/01616412.2021.1900705. Epub 2021 Apr 15.
39. Ashram YA, Zohdy YM, Rayan TA, Badr-El-Dine MMK. Value of intraoperative monitoring of the trigeminal nerve in detection of a superiorly displaced facial nerve during surgery for large vestibular Schwannomas. Neurosurg Rev. 2022;45(2):1343–51. https://doi.org/10.1007/s10143-021-01646-7.
40. Acioly MA, Liebsch M, de Aguiar PH, Tatagiba M. Facial nerve monitoring during cerebellopontine angle and skull base tumor surgery: a systematic review from description to current success on function prediction. World Neurosurg. 2013;80(6):e271–300.
41. Vivas EX, Carlson ML, Neff BA, Shepard NT, McCracken DJ, Sweeney AD, et al. Congress of Neurological Surgeons systematic review and evidence-based guidelines on intraoperative cranial nerve monitoring in vestibular Schwannoma surgery. Neurosurgery. 2018;82(2):E44–6. https://doi.org/10.1093/neuros/nyx513.
42. Acioly MA, Liebsch M, de PHP A, Tatagiba M. Facial nerve monitoring during cerebellopontine angle and skull base tumor surgery: a systematic review from description to current success on function prediction. World Neurosurg. 2013;80(6):e271–300. https://doi.org/10.1016/j.wneu.2011.09.026. Epub 2011 Nov 1.

The Principal Surgical Techniques for Microvascular Decompression: Surgical Treatment for Trigeminal Neuralgia

Bong Jin Park and Chang Kyu Park

1 Introduction

Trigeminal neuralgia is caused by compression of blood vessels on the trigeminal nerve in 80–85% of cases. In this case, good results can be obtained by properly decompressing [1]. It is usually accessed to trigeminal nerve through the retrosigmoid approach. When the culprit vessel is identified, decompression is performed using decompressive materials such as Teflon. Sometimes a vein is the offending vessel, and sometimes the culprit vessel is not observed. In this case, rhizotomy or internal neurolysis is performed [2]. Nevertheless, the reasons for not performing invasive surgery are: (1) Various treatments other than surgery and good treatment results [3, 4]. (2) Surgical anatomy is unfamiliar and the operation field is narrow and deep. (3) There are factors that affect the difficulty of surgery, such as protrusion of petrosal bone and the route of superior petrosal vein. (4) The offending vessel was confirmed on the preoperative MR images and surgery was performed, but it is difficult to manage when there is no clear offender, or a small perforator or vein is the culprit vessel.

B. J. Park (✉) · C. K. Park
Department of Neurosurgery, Kyung Hee University Hospital, Kyung Hee University College of Medicine, Seoul, Republic of Korea
e-mail: hyunsong@khmc.or.kr

2 Surgical Anatomy

Most microvascular decompression (MVD) surgeries are performed using a retrosigmoid approach (RSA). In particular, RSA is sufficiently exposed to the trigeminal nerve and other lower cranial nerves and brainstem [5]. The position of the RSA is mostly lateral decubitus, and the head position may vary depending on the preference of the surgeon, but in most cases, it is better to rotate the temple parallel to the floor to the opposite side of the lesion and slightly bend the vertex toward the floor [6]. In addition, it is recommended to flexion around the cheeks and chin in an anterior-posterior plane to secure the surgical field of view. At this time, excessive flexion should not be done because the jugular vein may be compressed.

The skin incision is usually straight, but in some cases, it is curved. In this case, it is important to draw an incision by figuring out the positions of the mastoid tip and notch. Most of the sigmoid sinus travels along the posterior margin of the mastoid process and the transverse sinus travels along the line connecting the external auditory canal and inion, so it is important to check the skin incision using these anatomical marks (Fig. 1).

After a skin incision, it is recommended to properly stop bleeding using an electric cauterizer, which prevents visual field obstruction due to unexpected bleeding during microsurgery.

K. Park, K. R. Cho (eds.), *Trigeminal Neuralgia*, https://doi.org/10.1007/978-981-19-9171-4_11

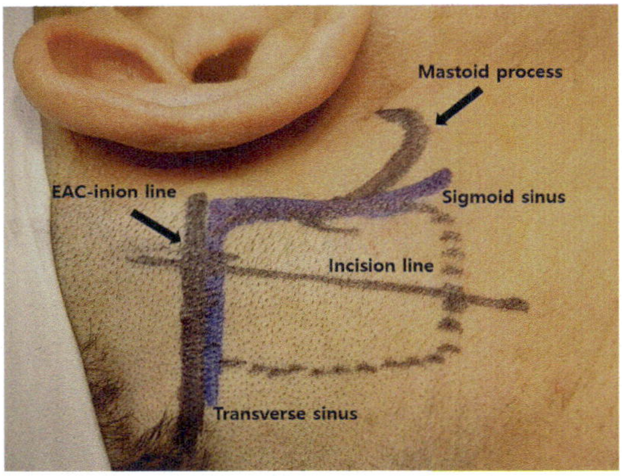

Fig. 1 A figure showing anatomical landmarks before surgery. The dotted line is the craniotomy line

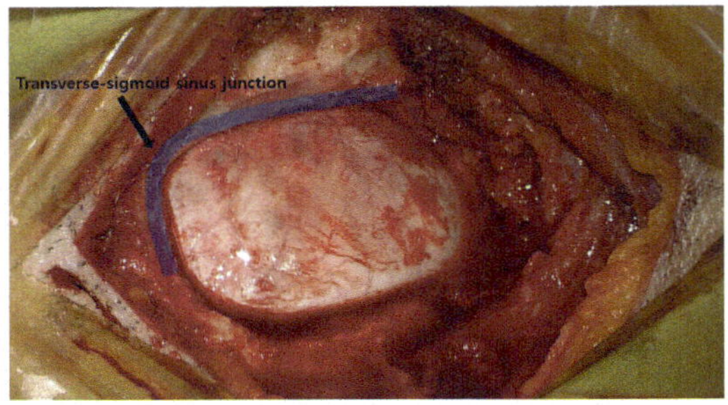

Fig. 2 Exposed dura after craniotomy. The blue sinus is artificially painted. Arrows indicate the transverse-sigmoid sinus junction

After this, the relevant muscle layers are dissected in turn. Most of the occipital artery ruptures during muscle dissection, which should be treated appropriately. Excessive bleeding may occur if the emissary vein is greatly developed when the skull base is exposed. In this case, it is important to find the exact bleeding point and block the pore. If the mastoid notch is confirmed and the asterion is observed, a sufficient surgical field can be obtained.

When performing the initial burr hole in the medio-caudal direction of the asterion, it is safe to prevent damage to the sinus. During craniotomy, it is better to proceed with the anterior margin of craniotomy until the lateral margin of the sigmoid sinus is visible, and the superior margin of craniotomy to proceed until the margin of the transverse sinus is observed. Eventually, if the transverse-sigmoid sinus junction is observed, the pontine cistern can be approached with the shortest distance (Fig. 2).

3 Making Surgical Field

3.1 Dural Incision and CSF Drainage

If the puncture is performed at the site of the cerebellum, the cerebrospinal fluid (CSF) drains naturally with good results [7]. When sufficient drainage is achieved, dural pulsation is observed as the subdural space is freed up. If CSF drainage is not sufficient after puncture, linear incision is performed at a point 1–2 mm away from the sinus margin as much as possible. After that, if the cerebellomedullary cistern is opened while retraction of the cerebellum on the caudal side, CSF drainage can be easily performed. In order to create an easy-to-operate field, most of the sideways Y-shaped incisions are made (Fig. 3).

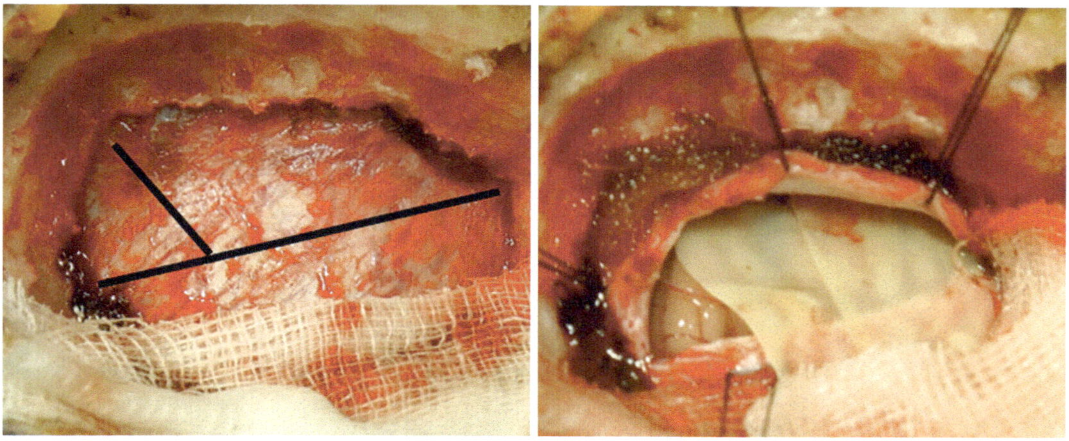

Fig. 3 The figure on the left is a schematic drawing for the dura incision line. One axis of the incision advances toward the transverse-sigmoid sinus junction, allowing brief access to the tentorium. The cerebellum was showed after Y shape dural opening

4 Basic Surgical Techniques

4.1 Microsurgical Dissection and Trigeminal Nerve Indentification

Slowly retract the cerebellum while advancing toward the medial. If you have a lot of experience, you can easily go up and check the tentorium, and if you follow it, you can check the superior petrosal vein (SPV) (Fig. 4). If the tentorium is not well-identified, it is better to check other cranial nerves first and then go to the trigeminal nerve. If cranial nerve (CN) VIII is detected from the beginning, it can sometimes be confused with the V nerve. In this case, it is necessary to check the caudal part and observe whether other lower cranial nerves are identified. If CN VIII is confirmed, CN V is mostly confirmed from the inside when entering the supero-medial direction.

Anatomically, an arachnoid membrane is formed between SPV and cranial nerve VIII, and it must be separated through micro-dissection (Fig. 5). If you forcefully try to remove this membrane, small blood vessels may be damaged, causing bleeding and sometimes infarction of the cranial nerve. It is important to remove the membrane around the SPV well because a retraction may be necessary if the space of the trigeminal nerve is insufficient (Fig. 6).

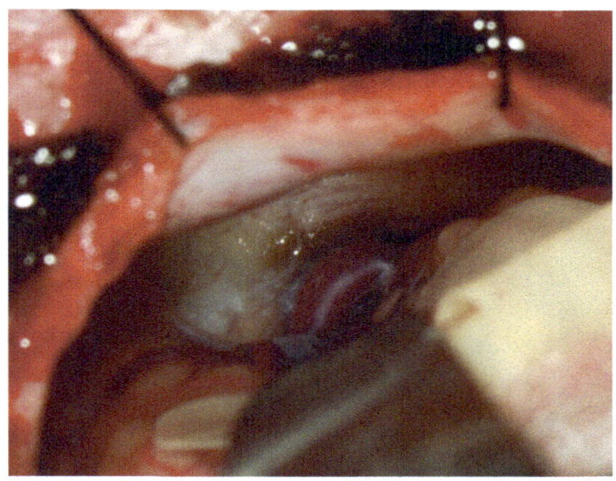

Fig. 4 A view of the petro-tentorial junction confirmed by pulling the cerebellum in the cephalic direction. Superior petrosal vein is observed downward

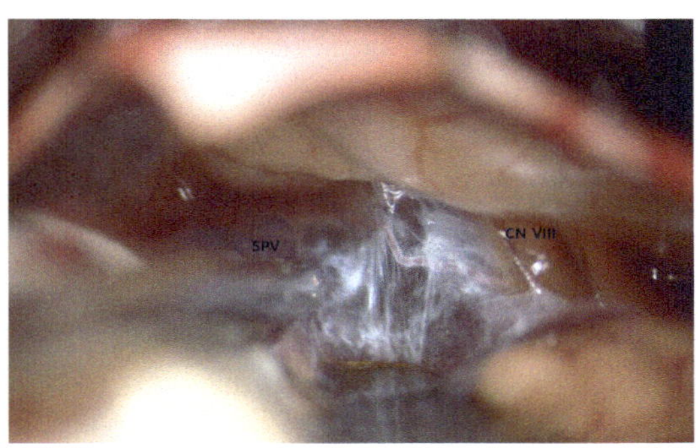

Fig. 5 An arachnoid membrane is formed between superior petrosal vein and cranial nerve VIII. It is observed that there are small blood vessels around the membrane

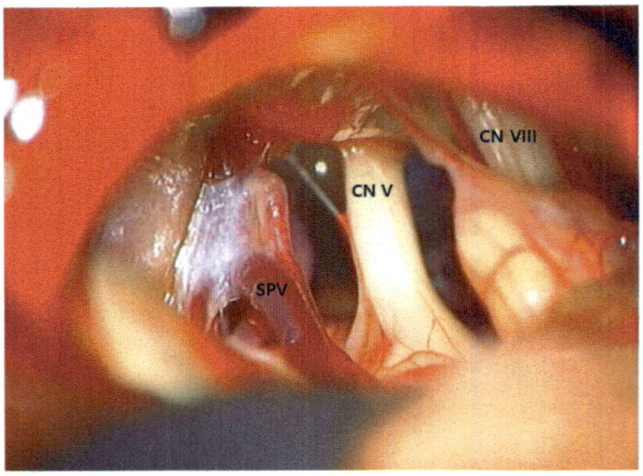

Fig. 6 After removal of the Arachnoid membrane, superior petrosal vein, cranial nerve V, and VIII were observed in one field of view

5 Neurovascular Decompression

5.1 Nerve Exploration

In trigeminal neuralgia, not only the root entry zone area of the nerve but also the contact of blood vessels anywhere in the nerve can cause symptoms, so the entire nerve should be looked at carefully. The reason is that, unlike other cranial nerves, the central myelin of the trigeminal nerve is not limited to the REZ, but is widely distributed in the nerve (Fig. 7). It is necessary to sufficiently retract the cerebellum to examine the root entry zone, and also carefully look around the Meckel's cave [8]. It is difficult to explore the inner side of the nerve in the view of the microscope, but it is necessary to examine the inner side even if the nerve is slightly set aside. For the efficiency of this search, it is necessary to search the preoperative image well. An endoscope is sometimes used to fully examine the nerve [9].

5.2 Neurovascular Decompression

The most important and basic principle is that all culprit vessels in contact with nerves should be isolated [10–12]. The etiology of trigeminal neuralgia is still unknown. Therefore, all blood vessels that may be the cause should take appropriate management. The nerve and surrounding blood vessels must be carefully separated. That makes it easier to decompress. This is a method of removing the contact between the nerve and the culprit vessel by inserting a substance between the nerve and the blood vessel. Teflon is most commonly used as a decompression substance (Fig. 8). However, if bleeding occurs at the decompression site or if there are many sites in contact with the dura due to excessive insertion, granulomas may form over time. These granulomas may also cause symptoms to recur [13, 14]. It is important to insert the right amount.

Due to the complications of these surgical techniques, surgical glue, or other surgical products such as Tachosil have recently been used without Teflon [15–17]. Those studies have been published recently, and although the initial effect is acceptable, the durability is controversial because there is not enough follow-up.

5.3 Complicated Cases

5.3.1 Venous Offender

Most of the offending vessels are known as arteries. However, studies on veins as culprit vessels are also being published steadily [18–20]. According to the study results, only veins were found as the offending vessels in 5–18% of cases [21]. And when symptoms recur or symptoms do not disappear after surgery, most of the studies suggest that veins are the cause. Although offending vein can also achieve good results with adequate decompression, there is a study reporting that good results can be obtained only when sacrificed [22]. But arguably, most surgeons say that the veins should be preserved as much as possible during surgery.

5.3.2 No Vascular Conflict

Partial sensory rhizotomy (PSR) may be performed when no clear offending vessels are observed in the surgical field or preoperative examination (Fig. 9). In the past, when anatomical knowledge about somatotrophy was lacking, it brought various results for postoperative pain relief and sensory impairment. However, these

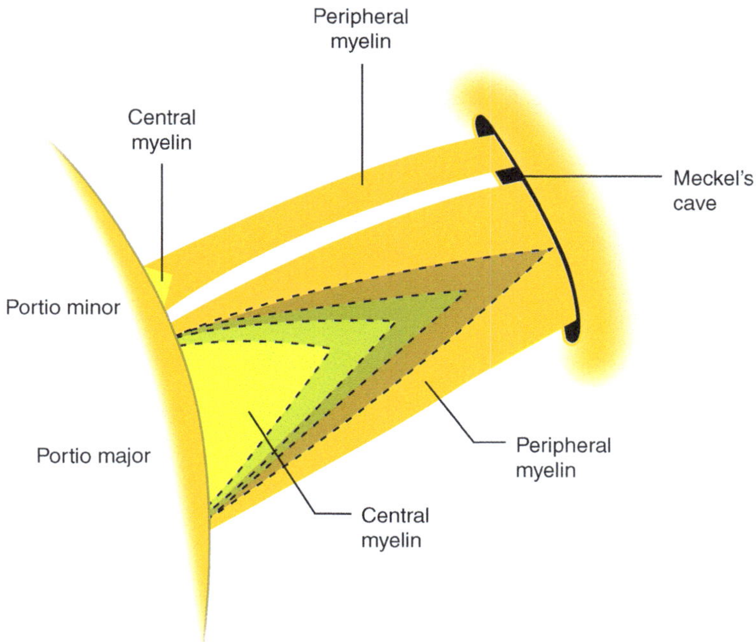

Fig. 7 Unlike other cranial nerves, the central myelin of the trigeminal nerve is widely distributed throughout the nerve

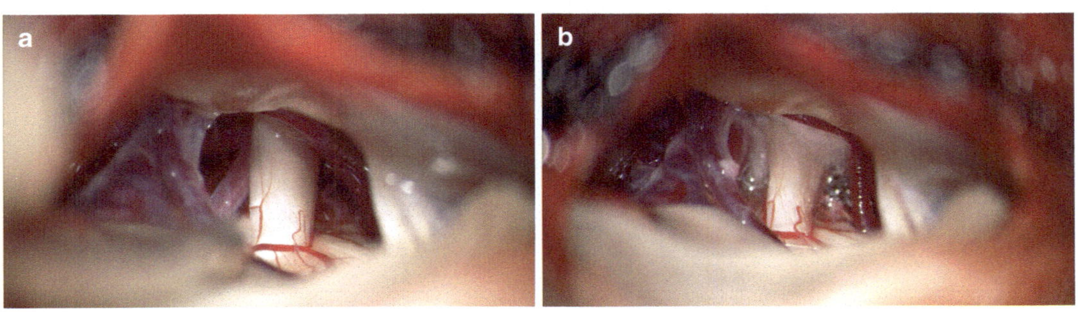

Fig. 8 The superior cerebellar artery (SCA) and vein are contacting both sides of the TN (**a**); Decompression of SCA and vein was done using Teflon (**b**)

shortcomings have been partially resolved through recent anatomical studies. According to a study recently published, as a result of performing PSR in the patient group including secondary trigeminal neuralgia, 86.4% of patients reported complete pain relief, and postoperative hypesthesia was reported in 22.7% [23]. However, another study reported 48% postoperative pain relief [24]. This difference is said to be due to the difference between the cross-sec-

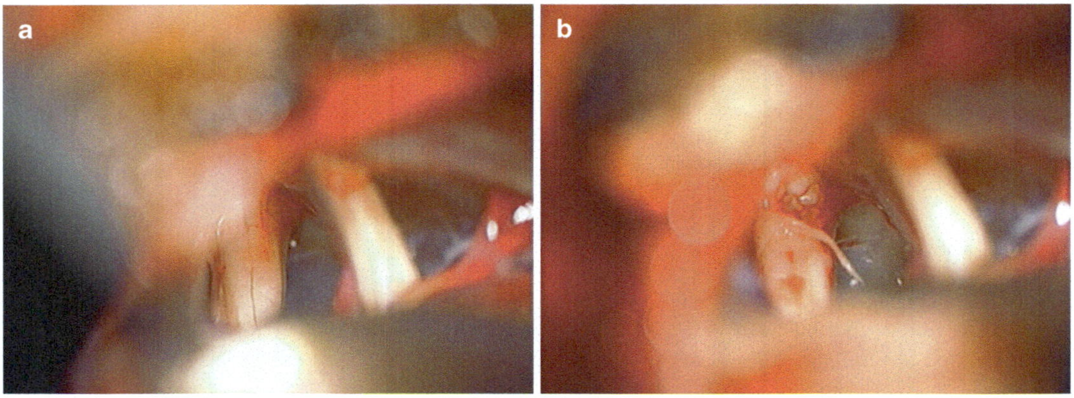

Fig. 9 In figure (**a**), there was no neurovascular contact. PSR is performed in the V2 region (**b**)

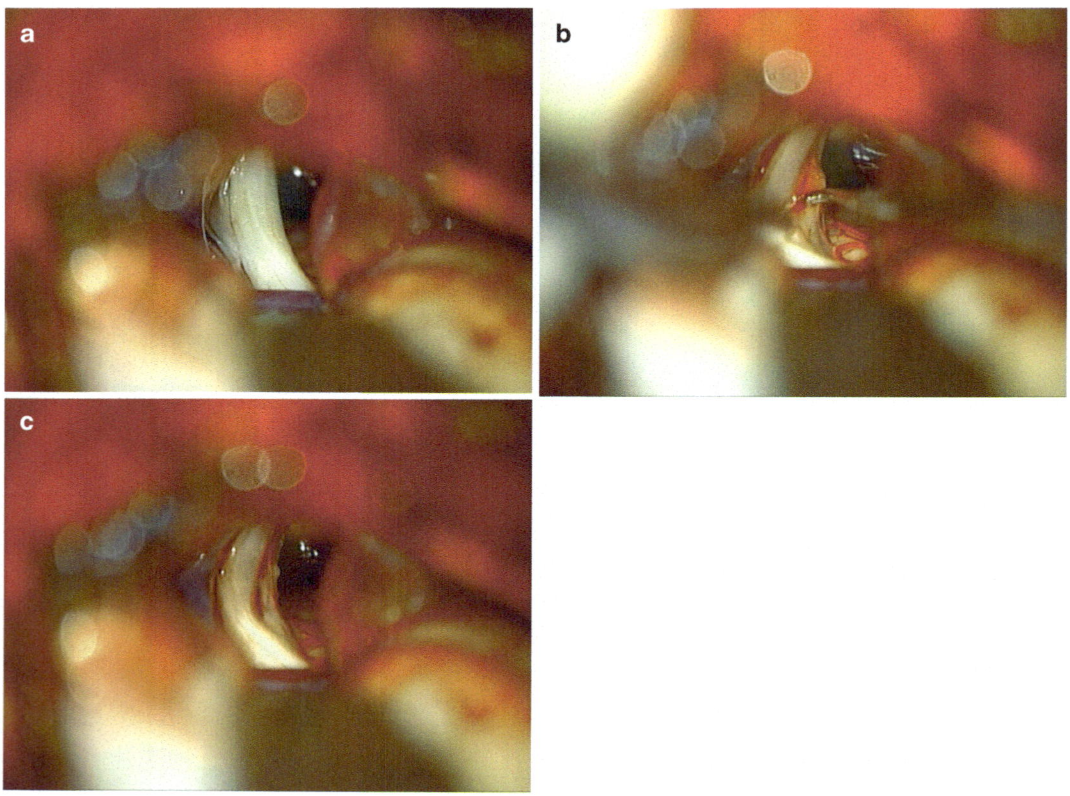

Fig. 10 Culprit vessels are not observed in surgical field (**a**); Nerve combing was performed using a blunt-tip probe for the V1, 2 region (**b**); Internal neurolysis performed (**c**)

tional area of the sensory root and the location of sectioning. As a result, the section of the ventrolateral two-thirds of the pars major of the trigeminal nerve at the pons provides favorable outcomes.

If there is no clear offender, internal neurolysis (nerve combing) can be performed. Usually, the trigeminal nerve itself is then longitudinally divided along its fibers, using a straight blunt-tip probe (Fig. 10). A study

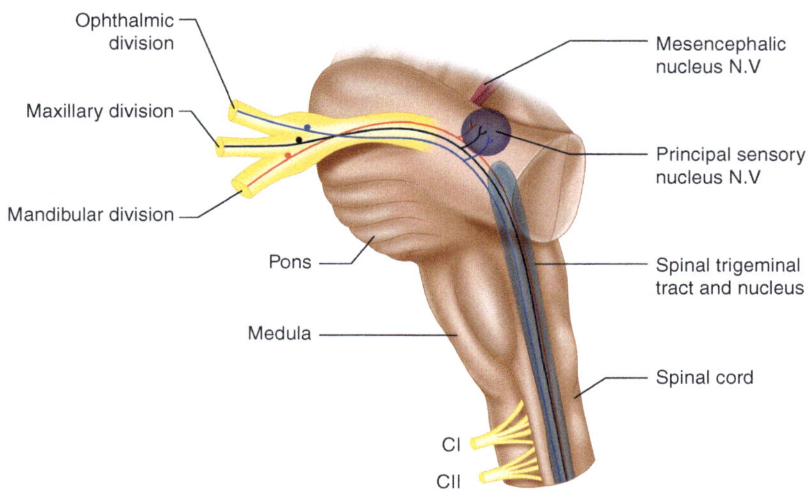

Fig. 11 Sensory nerve fibers coming from each region undergo medial rotation before entering the pons through the REZ

reported that as a result of internal neurolysis [25], 100% of asymptomatic patients were obtained immediately after surgery. And thereafter, they reported 91.3% of pain relief. Eleven percent of patients presented severe facial numbness immediately after surgery, which improved 6 months after surgery. Moreover, another study reported the long-term outcome of internal neurolysis [26]. A 47% pain-free rate was reported 5 years after surgery. Most patients (96%) experienced facial numbness or hypesthesia, but these symptoms did not affect the patient's quality of life.

In order to perform PSR or internal neurolysis, an accurate understanding of the travel and rotation of the trigeminal nerve is required. Root fiber entering the spinal trigeminal tract have a definite topographic organization. In the spinal trigeminal nucleus, the ophthalmic division is located most ventral, fibers of the mandibular division are most dorsal, but it internally rotates through the REZ. The positions of V1, V2, and V3 in the fifth nerve in the cisternal portion are determined by the rotation of nerves. Based on this rationale, PSR or IN is performed according to the pain area (Fig. 11).

6 The Unexpected Complications during Surgery

6.1 Cerebellar Swelling

The cerebellum may prolapse due to sudden pressure changes when the dura is opened after craniotomy in a state where the jugular vein was compressed in the surgical position, the abdominal pressure rises, or other conditions where the intracranial pressure may rise. It has already been found through previous studies that the movement of the neck induces compression of the jugular vein [27]. In the cerebral venous drainage system, when the patient is in the supine position, the main venous drainage route is the jugular vein, so it is more important to have a surgical position in which the jugular vein is not compressed. Especially if the patient's neck is short or thick, this situation should be more careful. In order to prevent such a case, it is good to drain the CSF by opening the dura mater slightly from the cistern. If CSF drainage does not occur and cerebellar edema progresses gradually, it is recommended to

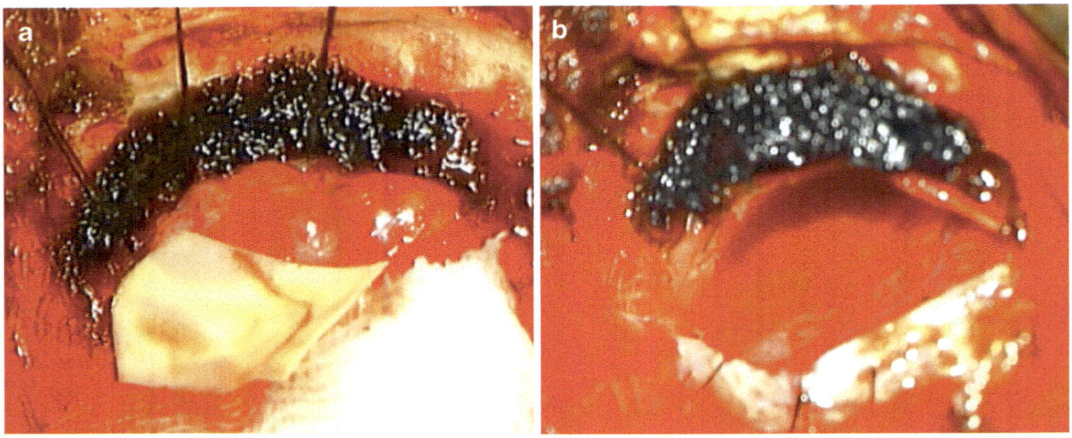

Fig. 12 The figure on the left shows the sudden herniation of the cerebellum (**a**). Space created after cerebrospinal fluid drainage by traction of the cerebellum (**b**)

puncture the cerebellomedullary cistern after boldly retracting the cerebellum. This is because the pontine cistern is far from approachable and there is SPV, so it may cause another problem while blindly performing traction. Once the CSF has been adequately drained, the original surgical purpose can be achieved (Fig. 12).

6.2 Sudden Hemorrhage

Bleeding may be observed suddenly in the visual field during surgery, usually while looking at the microscope. Especially in elderly patients, abrupt drainage of CSF can cause supratentorial subdural hemorrhage, in which case a large amount of CSF may be gushed out or bleeding may occur. In this case, the first important thing is to secure the surgical field of view. When fibrin lumps are deposited in the nerve area due to bleeding, the division of blood vessels and nerves becomes unclear and it is difficult to dissect, making it difficult to perform an accurate operation. In this case, sufficient saline irrigation is required to prevent fibrin deposition. Even if it takes time, it is better to perform irrigation until a sufficient field of view is secured. Bleeding due to the rupture of small blood vessels (usually small veins) often stops spontaneously after sufficient irrigation. If blood flows inside the epidural area, it is recommended to correct the cause of the bleeding.

7 Conclusion

Surgical treatment, including MVD, for TN is different from other treatments in that it directly manages the cause of the disease. As with any other skull base surgery, there are several risks associated with surgery. However, if you acquire enough anatomical knowledge and deal with unexpected situations resolutely, you can control morbidity well. It is important to understand the preoperative image. If appropriate management for the culprit vessels (including rhizotomy) is applied, the surgical outcome can be significantly improved.

References

1. Kang IH, Park BJ, Park CK, Malla HP, Lee SH, Rhee BA. A clinical analysis of secondary surgery in trigeminal neuralgia patients who failed prior treatment. J Korean Neurosurg Soc. 2016;59(6):637–42.
2. Oh IH, Choi SK, Park BJ, Kim TS, Rhee BA, Lim YJ. The treatment outcome of elderly patients with idiopathic trigeminal neuralgia: micro-vascular decompression versus gamma knife radiosurgery. J Korean Neurosurg Soc. 2008;44(4):199–204.

3. Lee JK, Choi HJ, Ko HC, Choi SK, Lim YJ. Long term outcomes of gamma knife radiosurgery for typical trigeminal neuralgia-minimum 5-year follow-up. J Korean Neurosurg Soc. 2012;51(5):276–80.
4. Seo HJ, Park CK, Choi MK, Ryu J, Park BJ. Clinical outcome of percutaneous trigeminal nerve block in elderly patients in outpatient clinics. J Korean Neurosurg Soc. 2020;63(6):814–20.
5. Tan LA, Gerard CS, Ahuja SK, Moftakhar R. Retrosigmoid approach for resection of cerebellopontine angle meningioma and decompression of the trigeminal nerve. Neurosurg Focus. 2014;36(1 Suppl):1.
6. Wang XW, Fu XJ, Dong SY. The retrosigmoid approach surgery of trigeminal never. Lin Chuang Er Bi Yan Hou Ke Za Zhi. 2000;14(3):116–7.
7. Park CK, Lee SH, Rhee BA, Choi SK. Puncture of cerebellar horizontal fissure for Retrosigmoid approach: a prospective and quantitative analysis. Oper Neurosurg (Hagerstown). 2017;13(6):689–92.
8. Kumon Y, Sakaki S, Kohno K, Ohta S, Ohue S, Miki H. Three-dimensional imaging for presentation of the causative vessels in patients with hemifacial spasm and trigeminal neuralgia. Surg Neurol. 1997;47(2):178–84.
9. Balansard CF, Meller R, Bruzzo M, Chays A, Girard N, Magnan J. Trigeminal neuralgia: results of microsurgical and endoscopic-assisted vascular decompression. Ann Otolaryngol Chir Cervicofac. 2003;120(6):330–7.
10. Barker FG 2nd, Jannetta PJ, Bissonette DJ, Larkins MV, Jho HD. The long-term outcome of microvascular decompression for trigeminal neuralgia. N Engl J Med. 1996;334(17):1077–83.
11. Lee SH, Koh JS, Lee CY. Trigeminal neuralgia caused by an anomalous posterior inferior cerebellar artery from the primitive trigeminal artery: case report. Cerebellum. 2011;10(2):199–203.
12. Park CK, Choi HJ, Lee SH, Rhee BA. Trigeminal neuralgia caused by persistent primitive trigeminal artery. J Korean Neurosurg Soc. 2014;56(3):278–80.
13. Chen J, Lee S, Lui T, Yeh Y, Chen T, Tzaan W. Teflon granuloma after microvascular decompression for trigeminal neuralgia. Surg Neurol. 2000;53(3):281–7.
14. Rzaev DA, Kulikova EV, Moysak GI, Voronina EI, Ageeva TA. Teflon granuloma after microvascular decompression of the trigeminal nerve root in a patient with recurrent trigeminal neuralgia. Zh Vopr Neirokhir Im N N Burdenko. 2016;80(2):78–83.
15. Abi-Aad KR, Turcotte E, Patra DP, Welz ME, Maiti T, Hess R, et al. Vascular transposition of the superior cerebellar artery using a fenestrated clip and fibrin glue in trigeminal neuralgia: 2-dimensional operative video. Oper Neurosurg (Hagerstown). 2020;19(1):E50–e1.
16. Otani N, Toyooka T, Fujii K, Kumagai K, Takeuchi S, Tomiyama A, et al. "Birdlime" technique using TachoSil tissue sealing sheet soaked with fibrin glue for sutureless vessel transposition in microvascular decompression: operative technique and nuances. J Neurosurg. 2018;128(5):1522–9.
17. Otani N, Toyooka T, Takeuchi S, Tomiyama A, Wada K, Mori K. Novel technical variations and increased adhesive strength in the "Birdlime" transposition technique for microvascular decompression. World Neurosurg. 2018;116:e460–e8.
18. Kasuya H, Tani S, Kubota Y, Yokosako S, Ohbuchi H, Arai N, et al. Characteristics and management of the offending veins in microvascular decompression surgery for trigeminal neuralgia. Neurosurg Rev. 2021;44(4):2337–47.
19. Lee SH, Levy EI, Scarrow AM, Kassam A, Jannetta PJ. Recurrent trigeminal neuralgia attributable to veins after microvascular decompression. Neurosurgery. 2000;46(2):356–61. discussion 61–2.
20. Oishi M, Fukuda M, Noto Y, Kawaguchi T, Hiraishi T, Fujii Y. Trigeminal neuralgia associated with the specific bridging pattern of transverse pontine vein: diagnostic value of three-dimensional multifusion volumetric imaging. Stereotact Funct Neurosurg. 2011;89(4):226–33.
21. Soni P, Potter T, Soni PP, Estemalik E, Recinos PF, Kshettry VR. Outcomes of microvascular decompression for trigeminal neuralgia with purely venous compression: a systematic review and meta-analysis. Clin Neurol Neurosurg. 2020;198:106230.
22. McLaughlin MR, Jannetta PJ, Clyde BL, Subach BR, Comey CH, Resnick DK. Microvascular decompression of cranial nerves: lessons learned after 4400 operations. J Neurosurg. 1999;90(1):1–8.
23. Terrier LM, Amelot A, François P, Destrieux C, Zemmoura I, Velut S. Therapeutic failure in trigeminal neuralgia: from a clarification of trigeminal nerve Somatotopy to a targeted partial sensory Rhizotomy. World Neurosurg. 2018;117:e138–e45.
24. Young JN, Wilkins RH. Partial sensory trigeminal rhizotomy at the pons for trigeminal neuralgia. J Neurosurg. 1993;79(5):680–7.
25. Li MW, Jiang XF, Niu C. Efficacy of internal Neurolysis for trigeminal neuralgia without vascular compression. J Neurol Surg A Cent Eur Neurosurg. 2021;82(4):364–8.
26. Ko AL, Ozpinar A, Lee A, Raslan AM, McCartney S, Burchiel KJ. Long-term efficacy and safety of internal neurolysis for trigeminal neuralgia without neurovascular compression. J Neurosurg. 2015;122(5):1048–57.
27. Gooding CA, Stimac GK. Jugular vein obstruction caused by turning of the head. AJR Am J Roentgenol. 1984;142(2):403–6.

Pitfalls and Pearls in Microvascular Decompression for Trigeminal Neuralgia

Minsoo Kim and Kwan Park

1 Setting for Operative Room

It is important to individually set the operating room environment according to the type of surgery, required personnel, and equipment. In case of microvascular decompression (MVD) for trigeminal neuralgia (TN), there must be enough space on the back of the patient for the operator to access the surgical field of view from various angles. The intraoperative neurophysiologic monitoring (IONM) technologists may need to approach the patient's face to ensure stable monitoring during surgery.

Figure 1 is the schema of the authors' operating room setting. The patient's head faces the opposite side of the anesthesiologist and anesthetist, and the scrub nurse and scrub table are positioned on the right side of the patient's body regardless of the direction of the lesion. A mayo stand is used to give the operator immediate access to the necessary instruments, and the surgical microscope is always positioned on the left side of the patient's body. The IONM technologist is positioned to face the operator, allowing immediate and active communication. Although our protocol has the disadvantage of positioning the patient's head away from the anesthesiologist, we believe that MVD can be performed safely because the patient's head position is constant, and the possibility of intraoperative bleeding is low.

M. Kim
Department of Neurosurgery, Gangneung Asan Hospital, Gangneung, Gangwon-do, Korea

K. Park (✉)
Department of Neurosurgery, Konkuk University Medical Center, Konkuk University School of Medicine, Seoul, Republic of Korea
e-mail: kwanpark@skku.edu

K. Park, K. R. Cho (eds.), *Trigeminal Neuralgia*, https://doi.org/10.1007/978-981-19-9171-4_12

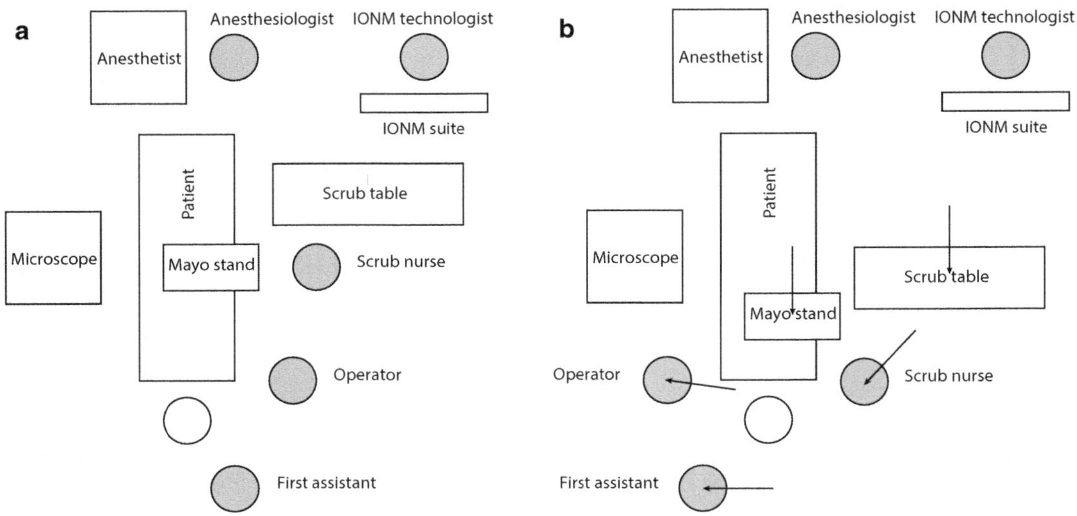

Fig. 1 Operative setting for microvascular decompression for trigeminal neuralgia. Layout for operative room for surgery of right (**a**) and left side (**b**). The difference in the positions of the staff depending upon the side of surgery are indicated in arrows

2 Patient Positioning and Preparation

Although positions such as the lateral, prone, or sitting position can be used [1–3], authors prefer lateral park-bench position [4–6]. The shoulder of the side of the lesion must be positioned away from the operator as it obstructs the operator's hand when taking a true-lateral position. The shoulder and upper limb on the opposite side should be unsupported by the operating table because the range of rotation and tilt of the patient's head is widened.

Authors prefer to raise the patient's upper body and elevate the vertex from the floor such that the angle between the superior-inferior axis of the head and the floor was approximately 10° [4]. Raising the patient's upper body and vertex facilitated venous return, reducing bleeding during the surgical approach. Additionally, less cerebellar bulging through the craniotomy window reduced the risk of cerebellar cortical injury, and as the cerebrospinal fluid could be released from the lateral cerebellomedullary cistern rather than cisterna magna, craniotomy in the inferior direction could be minimized (Fig. 2). As authors did not require access inferiorly to reach the foramen magnum or cisterna magna, the risk of bleeding from the venous plexus near the foramen magnum could be avoided.

The head was not rotated to the contralateral side from the affected side, and the anterior-posterior axis of the head was maintained parallel to the floor. A neutral position or rotation to the side of the lesion of the head facilitates cerebellar retraction by gravity in patients undergoing MVD for TN. This provides wider access to Meckel's cave without the risk of injury from the introduction of brain retractors. Additionally, raising the patient's upper body does not require preoperative lumbar drainage before surgery.

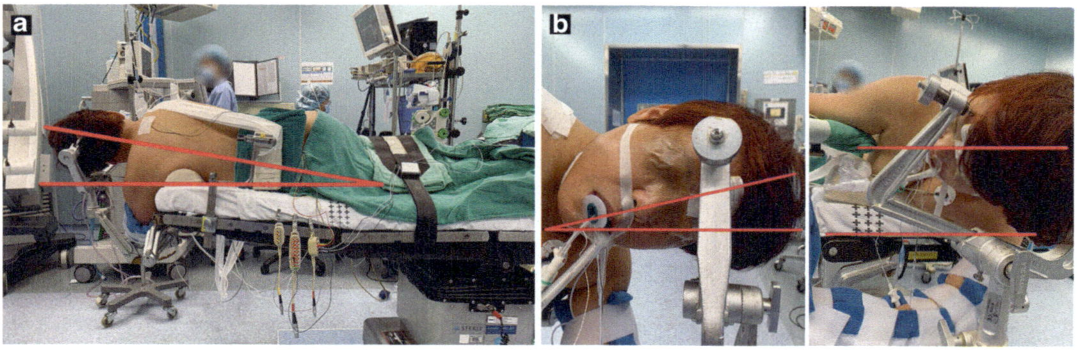

Fig. 2 Patient positioning during microvascular decompression for trigeminal neuralgia (from M Kim et al. with permission [4]). (**a**) The patient's upper body and vertex are elevated from the floor such that the angle between the vertex and the floor is approximately 10°. (**b**) the head is not rotated to the contralateral side from the affected side, and the anterior-posterior axis of the head is maintained parallel to the floor

3 Craniotomy

Two types of craniotomies are possible for the MVD for TN—the infratentorial lateral supracerebellar approach or the conventional lateral suboccipital approach [7]. The infratentorial lateral supracerebellar approach has several advantages: (a) The risk of perioperative complication related to facial and vestibulocochlear nerve is reduced because the trajectory of this approach is distant from the nerve complex; (b) The medial surface of the trigeminal nerve and its relationship to the superior cerebellar artery is clearly visible in this approach; (c) The Meckel's cave is also clearly visible without disturbance of the suprameatal tubercle.

The key point during the craniotomy is to sufficiently expose the junction of the sigmoid and transverse sinus. Because the upper limit of the surgical field is the reflected dural leaflet, insufficient craniotomy narrows the surgical field of view and induces excessive cerebellar retraction in the inferior direction.

Since the authors do not drain cerebrospinal fluid from the cisterna magna, the lower margin of the craniotomy need not extend close to the foramen magnum. However, the operator should remember that insufficient craniotomy windows may duce the operation more difficult and increase surgical morbidity. Figure 3 illustrates bony landmarks and expected craniotomy margin for MVD for TN.

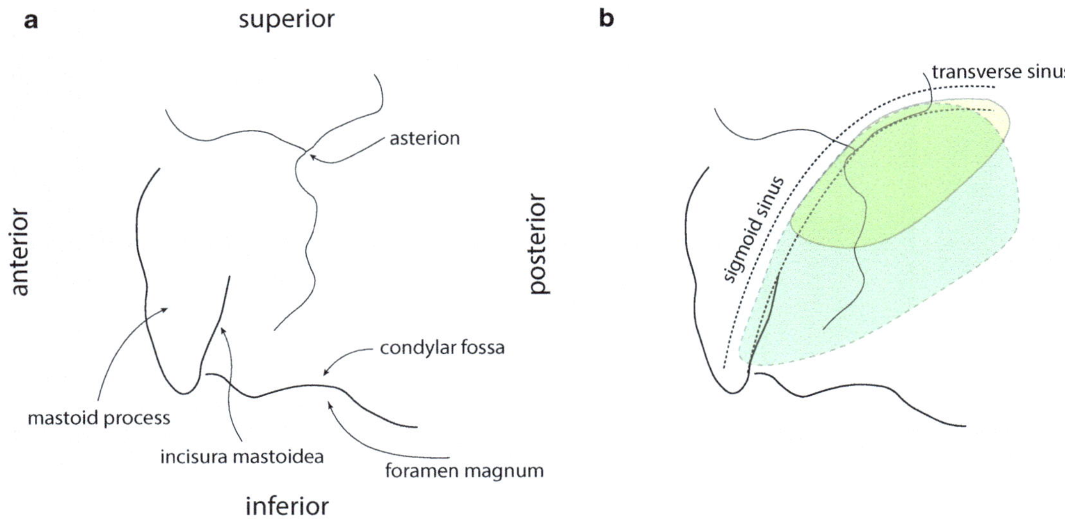

Fig. 3 Bony landmarks and expected area of craniotomy for microvascular decompression for trigeminal neuralgia. (**a**) anatomical landmarks for retromastoid suboccipital approach; (**b**) the areas of bony openings for infratentorial lateral supracerebellar approach (yellow) and conventional retrosigmoid lateral suboccipital approach (green). Transverse and sigmoid sinuses are marked in dotted lines

4 Epidural Bleeding Control and Dural Opening (Fig. 4)

To prevent influx of bleeding from the epidural space into the intracranial space, authors place a hemostatic agent along the craniotomy margin. After durotomy, a piece of Gelfoam (absorbable gelatin sponge, Pharmacia & Upjohn Company LLC, North Peapack, New Jersey, United States) is used to prevent blood from flowing into the intracranial space at the border of the dural leaflets to act like a dam. Another method of preventing blood from pooling at the caudal end of the craniotomy site can also be used using a silicone tube and a vacuum suction system.

The authors performed durotomy parallel to the sigmoid sinus and transverse sinus. However, in order to sufficiently secure the upper limit of the surgical field of view, an incision close to the junction of the transverse and sigmoid sinus is added. After pulling the dural leaflet to apply proper tension using 4-0 silk and a rubber band, they are secured to the surgical drape.

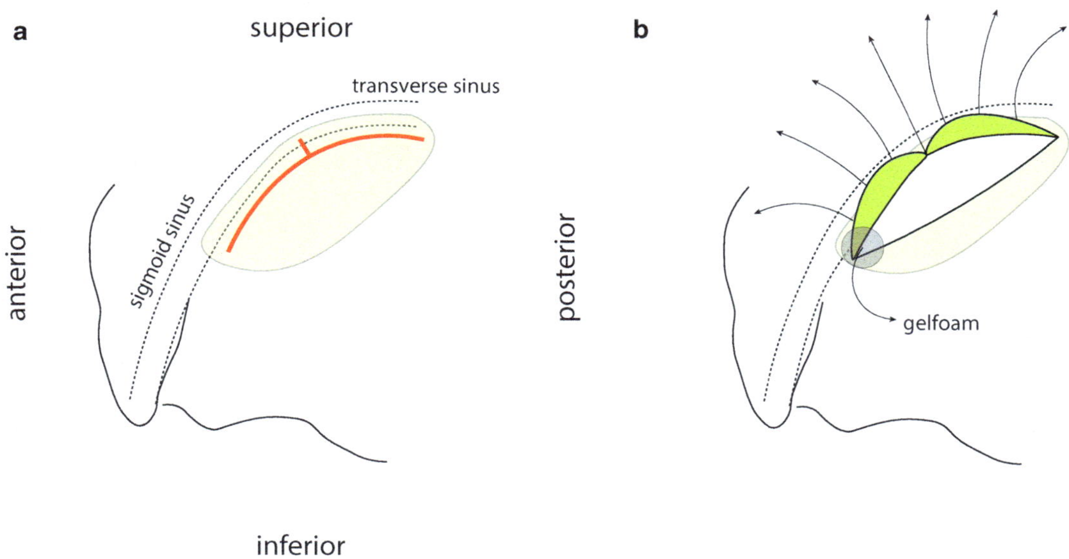

Fig. 4 Durotomy and prevention of blood influx to intracranial space. (**a**) Red lines indicate the incision lines of durotomy. A short incision to the junction of transverse-sigmoid sinus is essential for the wider view of surgical field. (**b**) Dural leaflets are tacked up using 4-0 silk. The junction of transverse-sigmoid sinus needs to be tightly tacked up. A piece of Gelfoam is placed to prevent influx of blood

5 Entering Intracranially

After opening the dura, gentle retraction of the posterior portion of the tentorial cerebellar surface allows access to the trigeminal nerve through the space between the cerebellum and tentorium.

In the case of the conventional lateral suboccipital approach, the cerebrospinal fluid is drained from the lateral cerebellomedullary cistern. In the infratentorial lateral supracerebellar approach, the cerebrospinal fluid is drained between the tentorium and the tentorial cerebellar surface. At this time, gentle retraction is important because rupture of the bridging vein draining from the cerebellar surface to the tentorial sinus may occur; therefore, authors use a retractor only in exceptional cases. The authors' positioning, which allows raising the patient's upper body and elevating vertex, is also useful because vascular structures such as superior petrosal vein become less tense, reducing its susceptibility to vascular injury by manipulation, as well no lumbar drainage is needed. Usually, the neurovascular structures are rarely coagulated or divided during the procedure and were instead dissected free from the arachnoid adhesions using micro-bayonet forceps and micro-scissors.

6 Approach to the Superior Petrosal Vein

Manipulating the superior petrosal vein is very important in accessing the trigeminal nerve. Several veins drain into the superior petrosal sinus, inferior petrosal sinus, jugular bulb, marginal sinus, or sigmoid sinus from veins of the anterolateral surface of the pons, posterior surface of the midbrain, and petrosal cerebellar surface near the flocculus [3, 8]. Among them, the superior petrosal vein often obscures the trigeminal nerve in the surgical field and often becomes the culprit vessel of trigeminal neuralgia. Moreover, the superior petrosal vein may rupture during cerebellar retraction. There are studies that perioperative complication occurs after sacrifice of the superior petrosal vein [9–13]. Conversely, there are studies that preemptive ligation of superior petrosal vein does not increase complications [14, 15].

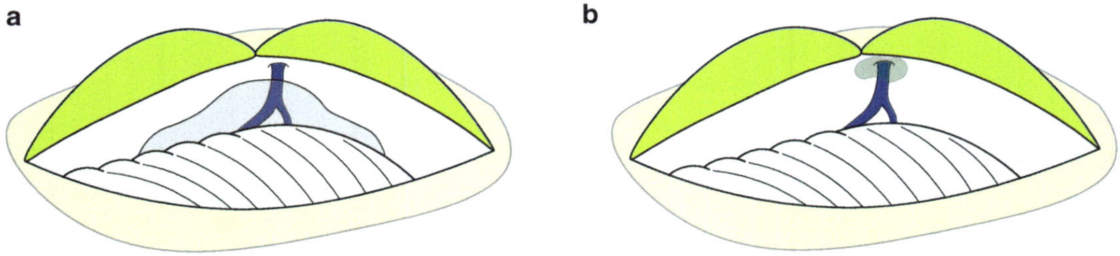

Fig. 5 Covering the opening of the superior petrosal sinus with fibrin glue to prevent bleeding from stretch injury. (**a**) superior petrosal veins (blue) entering superior petrosal sinus and covering arachnoid membrane (gray). Extensive dissection of arachnoid membrane is essential during the surgery. (**b**) After sufficient dissection of arachnoid membrane, fibrin glue (green) can be applied before decompression of the trigeminal nerve to the opening of superior petrosal sinus to prevent the vascular rupture resulting from stretch injury in selected cases

In the cases of the authors, preemptive control nor posthemorrhagic coagulation of superior petrosal vein was not performed during more than 300 MVD for TN [4]. As described above, elevation of upper body and vertex from the floor loosen the superior petrosal vein, reduce susceptibility to vascular injury by manipulation, and keep the working corridor wide.

In cases presenting with a high likelihood of superior petrosal vein rupture during decompression of culprit vessel, authors cover and seal the superior petrosal vein along its trajectory with fibrin glue (Tisseel, Baxter Healthcare Corp., Deerfield, Illinois, United States) before decompression. Covering the opening of the superior petrosal sinus at the tentorial side when applying the glue is important because the junction of the vessels is more invulnerable to stretching injury. However, care must be taken to avoid immersing small vessels other than the superior petrosal vein in the glue because of the risk of unexpected vascular injury resulting from adhesion to the surrounding tissues or stretching (Fig. 5).

7 Management of a Bleeding Superior Petrosal Vein

Bleeding of the superior petrosal vein is treated in several ways depending on the location of vascular rupture. In the authors' experience, the junction of the superior petrosal vein and sinus is the most frequent location of tearing. Authors control the bleeding without coagulation or sectioning of the injured vein, by raising the patient's vertex and padding a piece of Surgicel (knitted fabric of oxidized regenerated cellulose, Ethicon, Bridgewater, New Jersey, United States) on the avulsed site. Next, a small piece of Gelfoam was inserted into adjacent cisterns to act as barriers for blood accumulation and clot formation. These sponges were removed after the whole procedure.

A relatively small number of cases show bleeding from the main trunk of the superior petrosal vein. Elevating the patient's upper body and vertex is the key to hemostasis in these cases as well. In most cases, bleeding from superior petrosal vein is self-limiting as gentle compression of the bleeding focus with a neurosurgical pattie controlled the bleeding. Although ligation of a superior petrosal vein is a justifiable surgical technique, authors recommend preservation of the superior petrosal vein whenever possible.

8 Approach to Trigeminal Nerve and Neurovascular Decompression

Care should be taken not to injure trochlear nerve running along the tentorial incisura during approach to the trigeminal nerve, because even light touch to trochlear nerve may result in postoperative diplopia. Through appropriate dissection of arachnoid membrane, trigeminal nerve and surrounding vascular structures are revealed. Since neurovascular compression in any part of the trigeminal nerve, from the Meckel's cave to the root entry zone, may cause trigeminal neuralgia, it is important to thoroughly inspect the whole segment of trigeminal nerve, especially the medial surface.

In cases without any evidence of arterial compression, discoloration or indentation of the trigeminal nerve by vein or thick arachnoid trabeculae adhered to the nerve can be the pathology.

Interposition and transposition techniques are possible to detach the culprit structure from the trigeminal nerve. In almost all cases, the authors performed the interposition technique by inserting Teflon felt (polytetrafluoroethylene, The Chemours Company, Wilmington, Delaware, United States) between the culprit vessel and the trigeminal nerve. Authors could achieve Barrow Neurological Institute score I-II in 269 patients (78.2%) among 344 patients, and III-IV in 58 (16.9%) [4].

Authors apply fibrin glue on the Teflon felt after confirming that no vessel is in contact with the trigeminal nerve, then cover the large-diameter bled vessels with fibrin glue to prevent delayed bleeding [6].

References

1. Jannetta PJ. Microsurgical approach to the trigeminal nerve for tic Douloureux. Prog Neurol Surg. 1976;7:180–200. https://doi.org/10.1159/000428328:180-200.
2. Kondo A. Follow-up results of microvascular decompression in trigeminal neuralgia and hemifacial spasm. Neurosurgery. 1997;40(1):46–51. discussion 51–42.
3. Matsushima T, Rhoton AL Jr, de Oliveira E, Peace D. Microsurgical anatomy of the veins of the posterior fossa. J Neurosurg. 1983;59(1):63–105.
4. Kim M, Park SK, Lee S, Lee JA, Park K. Prevention of superior petrosal vein injury during microvascular decompression for trigeminal neuralgia: operative nuances. J Neurol Surg B Skull Base. 2021;83(Suppl 2):e284–90.
5. Lee S, Park SK, Lee JA, et al. A new method for monitoring abnormal muscle response in hemifacial spasm: a prospective study. Clin Neurophysiol. 2018;129(7):1490–5.
6. Lee S, Park SK, Joo BE, Lee JA, Kong DS, Park K. A surgical strategy to prevent delayed epidural hematoma after posterior fossa surgery using lateral suboccipital retrosigmoid approach. J Clin Neurosci. 2018;52:156–8.
7. Matsushima T, Fukui M, Suzuki S, Rhoton AL Jr. The microsurgical anatomy of the infratentorial lateral supracerebellar approach to the trigeminal nerve for tic douloureux. Neurosurgery. 1989;24(6):890–5.
8. Matsushima T, Suzuki SO, Fukui M, Rhoton AL Jr, de Oliveira E, Ono M. Microsurgical anatomy of the tentorial sinuses. J Neurosurg. 1989;71(6):923–8.
9. Masuoka J, Matsushima T, Hikita T, Inoue E. Cerebellar swelling after sacrifice of the superior petrosal vein during microvascular decompression for trigeminal neuralgia. J Clin Neurosci. 2009;16(10):1342–4.
10. Strauss C, Naraghi R, Bischoff B, Huk WJ, Romstöck J. Contralateral hearing loss as an effect of venous congestion at the ipsilateral inferior colliculus after microvascular decompression: report of a case. J Neurol Neurosurg Psychiatry. 2000;69(5):679–82.
11. Koerbel A, Wolf SA, Kiss A. Peduncular hallucinosis after sacrifice of veins of the petrosal venous complex for trigeminal neuralgia. Acta Neurochir. 2007;149(8):831–2. discussion 832–833.
12. Tsukamoto H, Matsushima T, Fujiwara S, Fukui M. Peduncular hallucinosis following microvascular decompression for trigeminal neuralgia: case report. Surg Neurol. 1993;40(1):31–4.
13. Anichini G, Iqbal M, Rafiq NM, Ironside JW, Kamel M. Sacrificing the superior petrosal vein during microvascular decompression. Is it safe? Learning the hard way. Case report and review of literature. Surg Neurol Int. 2016;7(Suppl 14):S415–20.
14. Pathmanaban ON, O'Brien F, Al-Tamimi YZ, Hammerbeck-Ward CL, Rutherford SA, King AT. Safety of superior petrosal vein sacrifice during microvascular decompression of the trigeminal nerve. World Neurosurg. 2017;103:84–7.
15. Choudhari KA. Superior petrosal vein in trigeminal neuralgia. Br J Neurosurg. 2007;21(3):288–92.

Microvascular Decompression for Trigeminal Neuralgia; Transposition Procedure

Jae Meen Lee and Young Hwan Ahn

Since Dr. Jannetta PJ introduced microvascular decompression surgery as a microscopic surgical modality treating patients with trigeminal neuralgia, trigeminal neuralgia became a curable cranial nerve rhizopathy. With MVD, long-term relief of neuralgic pain can be achieved [1]. The practical aims of the MVD surgery are a separation of the causative vessel from the trigeminal REZ and to maintain their separation. The placement of insulating material as a cushion between the causative vessel and trigeminal nerve is commonly carried out for the MVD and is technically easy and safe [2–4]. The pain improvement rate after trigeminal MVD is reported up to 91–97%; however, with a review of large series of report, about 65–70% of patients remained pain-free with no medications during the follow-up for 10 years or more after MVD [2–4]. Most of the surgical failures developed within 2 years after the initial MVD [3]. Annual recurrence after an initial MVD is about 2% and a high recurrence rate after redo surgery, as much as 58% at 10 years postoperatively [1].

J. M. Lee
Department of Neurosurgery, Pusan National University Hospital, Busan, Republic of Korea

Y. H. Ahn (✉)
Department of Neurosurgery, Ajou University School of Medicine, Suwon, Republic of Korea

Department of Biomedical Sciences, Neuroscience Graduate Program, Graduate School of Ajou University, Suwon, Republic of Korea
e-mail: yhahn@ajou.ac.kr

The classic technique of MVD is placing Teflon pieces as an insulating material between the offending vessel and trigeminal REZ. This is so-called interposition technique. Placing surgical sponges between blood vessels and nerves is not the primary goal of MVD [5].

The causes of failure and recurrence after initial MVD for trigeminal neuralgia are not yet clearly determined. Adhesion of insulating materials is one of the most common cause [6]. If any insulating material including surgical sponge was not placed between the causative vessel and the REZ, surgical sponge-associated adhesion between them or related granulomas could be eliminated.

For patients with recurrent trigeminal neuralgia, redo MVD is a possible option to choose. However, initial MVD has to be perfectly carried out as the best therapeutic option aiming cure of TN. In this point of view, transposition of the causative vessel from the trigeminal REZ could be an ideal method for MVD. Since the transposition technique in trigeminal MVD aims to keep the offending vessels away from the REZ of the trigeminal nerve, so called 'off the REZ', instead of 'on' it. When the procedure completed, we can see nothing remained on the trigeminal REZ (Figs. 1 and 2).

A recent report evaluated a recurrence rate with 400 patients with trigeminal neuralgia who underwent MVD and demonstrated that recompression was observed in 15 of 31 recurrent patients who underwent reoperation. That report

K. Park, K. R. Cho (eds.), *Trigeminal Neuralgia*, https://doi.org/10.1007/978-981-19-9171-4_13

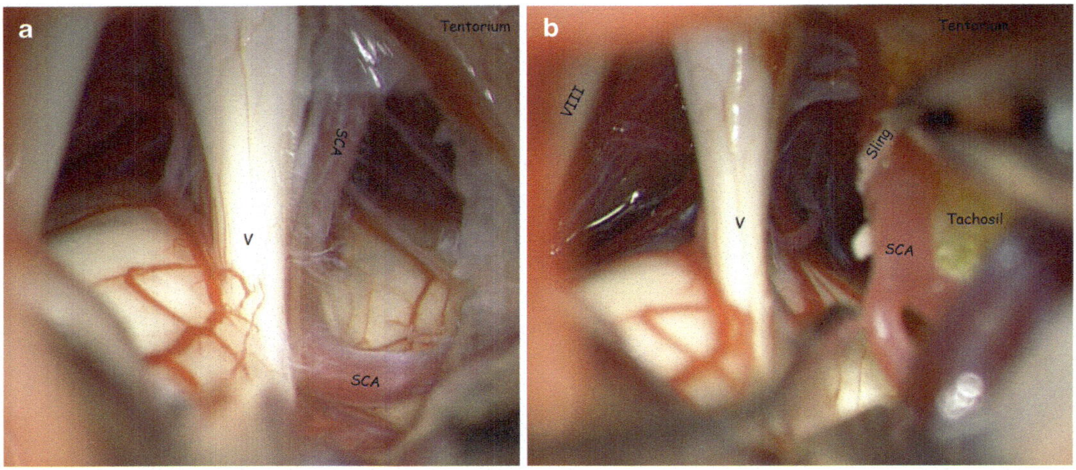

Fig. 1 Sling transposition of SCA using a glue-coated Teflon sling. (**a**) SCA is compressing the REZ (arrow) of the trigeminal nerve and along it. (**b**) The position and trajectory of the SCA is altered by the glue-coated Teflon sling, and the REZ of the trigeminal nerve is freed from the SCA. The trigeminal nerve became straight with no vascular conflict. The SCA was securely fixated with Tachosil pieces and finally "transposition" of the SCA was completed

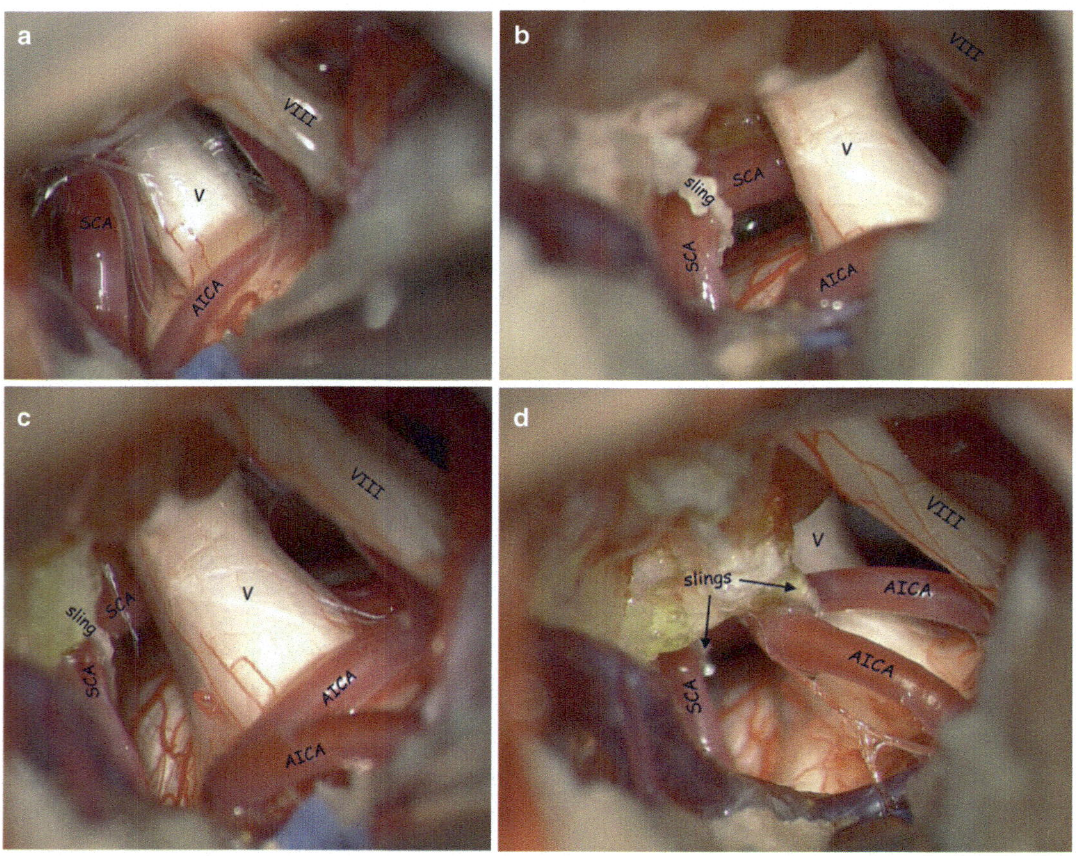

Fig. 2 Sling transposition of SCA and AICA using two glue-coated Teflon slings. (**a**) SCA and AICA contacting trigeminal nerve were shown. (**b**) Transposition of SCA was carried out using a glue-coated Teflon sling. (**c**) AICA is compressing the REZ of the trigeminal nerve. (**d**) A fibrin glue-coated Teflon sling is lifting up AICA to change its position and trajectory off the REZ. These fixations were securely finalized with Tachosil pieces and Tisseel bioglue

pointed out that recompressing causes were artery (7 cases), vein (4 cases), and decompressing material adhesions (4 cases). The report showed that 70.9% (22/31 patients) showed improvement in reoperation pain [7]. The other report summarized that arachnoid adhesions around the previous Teflon felt were also found in 5 cases of 6 who underwent a redo MVD (83.3%) [8]. A report also summarized that 82 patients with trigeminal neuralgia were operated on through microvascular decompression using the technique of interposing Teflon felt between the offending artery and the pons and/or nerve. Recurrence occurred in 14 cases (17.1%) and reoperations were carried out in 6 severe cases. The adhesion of the interposed Teflon felt was found at the trigeminal nerve in all cases and the adhesions were the main cause of recurrence in those 6 patients in whom reoperation was carried out[9]. They suggest that adhesion of the interposed Teflon felt is associated with recurrent trigeminal neuralgia in 70–100% of patients. In some patients, recurred neuralgic pain was so severe that they need to be treated with redo MVD. However, reoperation around the brain stem and cranial nerves is critically dangerous and the cure rate could be lower than initial surgery.

1 Decompressing Materials for MVD Surgery

In MVD surgery, various materials were used as insulating ones. The materials such as neurosurgical sponges have been used for brain protection during arachnoid dissection and brain separation with a metallic retractor to create a surgical corridor [10, 11]. Various materials were recently introduced and some of them were also applied for MVD as a microvascular decompressing material. In the literature, autologous tissue such as muscle, arachnoid membrane, or tentorium, cotton pieces, gel foam, Teflon, Gore-Tex, aneurysmal clips, Fibrin glues, and fibrin sealant patch have been introduced as materials useful in MVD surgery [12]. The characteristics, applicability, merits, effectiveness, and safety of those candidate materials used for MVD were briefly reviewed in the safety point of view.

Cotton is a soft and fluffy natural cellulose fiber that has been used in textiles since prehistoric times. It is familiar material to neurosurgeon as cotton piece or cotton ball which has been used as the most versatile and effective option to maintain a proper unobscured operation view and to clear blood and fluid safely from the operating area [13]. *It is* 20% stronger when it is *wet* because hydrogen bonding in the fiber is enhanced by water and is more adhesive under wet conditions [11]. Adhesions at the cotton-neural tissue interface have been shown to damage when the cotton is removed and the liquid-mediated adhesion mechanism may contribute to the overall stickiness of the cotton sponges, especially within the wet environment typically maintained in a neurosurgical operation field [10, 11]. As neurosurgeon applied cotton balls as a protecting barrier between other surgical tools and the brain, it functions as a spacer to keep away the arteries causing cranial rhizopathies such as trigeminal neuralgia and hemifacial spasm from the REZ of the cranial nerves [14]. However, it leads to cotton gauze foreign-body granuloma after microvascular decompression for trigeminal neuralgia and hemifacial spasm [14]. Therefore, cotton should not be used as a decompressing material during MVD surgery.

Teflon (Dupont, USA), a polytetrafluoroethylene (PTFE), is a synthetic fluoropolymer of tetrafluoroethylene and is considered to be the most slippery material that exists and has been used since 1940s in various fields. It is highly flexible, chemical resistant (highly insoluble in most solvents or chemicals except alkaline metal), thermal resistant (stable range of temperature −270 ~ 250 °C), non-stick with low friction coefficient, resistant to water or oil, and electrically resistant material. When Dr. Jannetta introduced MVD as a curative treatment method, Teflon pieces were used to separate causative vessels from the REZ of trigeminal nerve at the brain stem [15]. Teflon is relatively inert and has therefore advocated its use in MVD procedure [15]. Since then, Teflon is one of the most acceptable material which can act as an implanting graft for the decompression of the causative vessel from the REZ [16].

IVALON®, a unique hydroxylated polyvinyl acetal (PVAc) sponge, which is smooth, soft, highly absorbant, and easily compressible, has been used in medical applications for over 40 years [17, 18]. Dr. Jennetta did not use it and explained that it was a fair hard implant, assuming that it had the effect of transmitting vessel beats to nearby nerves and was highly likely to recur [18]. There are several reports showing surgical results of microvascular decompression surgery [17]. This material has been used less than Teflon™ though it is associated with similar success rates and similar complication rates [17].

Gore-Tex was invented in 1969 for expanding the Teflon polymer [19]. A 100 mm thin expanded PTEF (ePTEF) layer of open structure expanded PTFE film is oriented at right angles to the microstructure of the base tube in order to reinforce the exterior of the tubes [19]. This tube-shaped material invented for vascular graft is kink-resistant, compression-resistant, strongly comfortable, and easy to handle [20], and mainly used in thoracic vascular surgery. This however is so slippery that implanted tube-shaped Gore-Tex might be possible to use as a decompressing material placed between the causative vessel and the REZ. However, biocompatibility with no adhesion is not an ideal property for the transposition surgery since the Gore-Tex holding the causative vessel can be slipped over time when it holds the causative vessel to maintain the separation between the vessel and REZ.

Fibrin glues, known as fibrin sealants or fibrin tissue adhesives, are composed of thrombin, fibrinogen, and sometimes factor XIII and antifibrinolytic agents. Fibrin sealant is the first material approved as a hemostat in the US in 1998 [21]. There are various commercially available types of fibrin glues. Tisseel (Baxter, Westlake Village, CA, USA) is one of them and contain a bovine product therefore has a risk of anaphylactic reaction to bovine proteins or the theoretic risk of bovine spongiform encephalopathy transmission. Crosseal (Evicel in US, Quixil in European Union) is another type of fibrin sealant and does not contain human-derived product, instead of bovine one which is contraindicated for use in neurosurgery because of potential neurotoxicity. This can be ready to apply when assembled in dual syringe applicators with only a brief period of thawing (as little as 5 min). During the MVD surgery, this is used as an adhesive to securely fixate the transposed vessel around the REZ and is also used as a single material for decompression surgery to fix with no additional artificial materials [5]. During the procedure, if the glue gets into blood vessels, it could cause a dangerous situation such as thromboembolism. Fibrin sealant is useful during MVD and this material induces a strong fixation within a minute therefore its topical application has to be carried out at the last step of the procedure. It is not possible to remove the sealant completely even immediately after its application.

Tachosil (Baxter, Westlake Village, CA, USA), a fibrin sealant in sponge form is also useful material during MVD. As this is a material with Human pooled plasma and equine collagen. It is ready-to-use and is possible to be removed even after primary application as adhesives therefore is safer than glue-type material.

2 Decompression Procedure: Transposition

For the retrosigmoid craniotomy, the inferomedial point of the transverse-sigmoid sinus junction was localized as a perforating location for craniotomy using a surgical navigation system with preoperative 3D computed tomography (Fig. 3a). The bone was removed as a flap (Fig. 3b) and the surrounding soft tissues were protected with moisturized gauzes.

Various methods of transposition have been reported. A transposition technique using an adhesive fibrin glue is the simplest one [22]. Adhesive glue such as Tisseel glue is easy to handle, and it is easy to fix the causative vessel during the procedure using it. However, there are several risk factors for whether or not fixation will be well maintained after fixation [23]. The transposition technique using fibrin glue alone

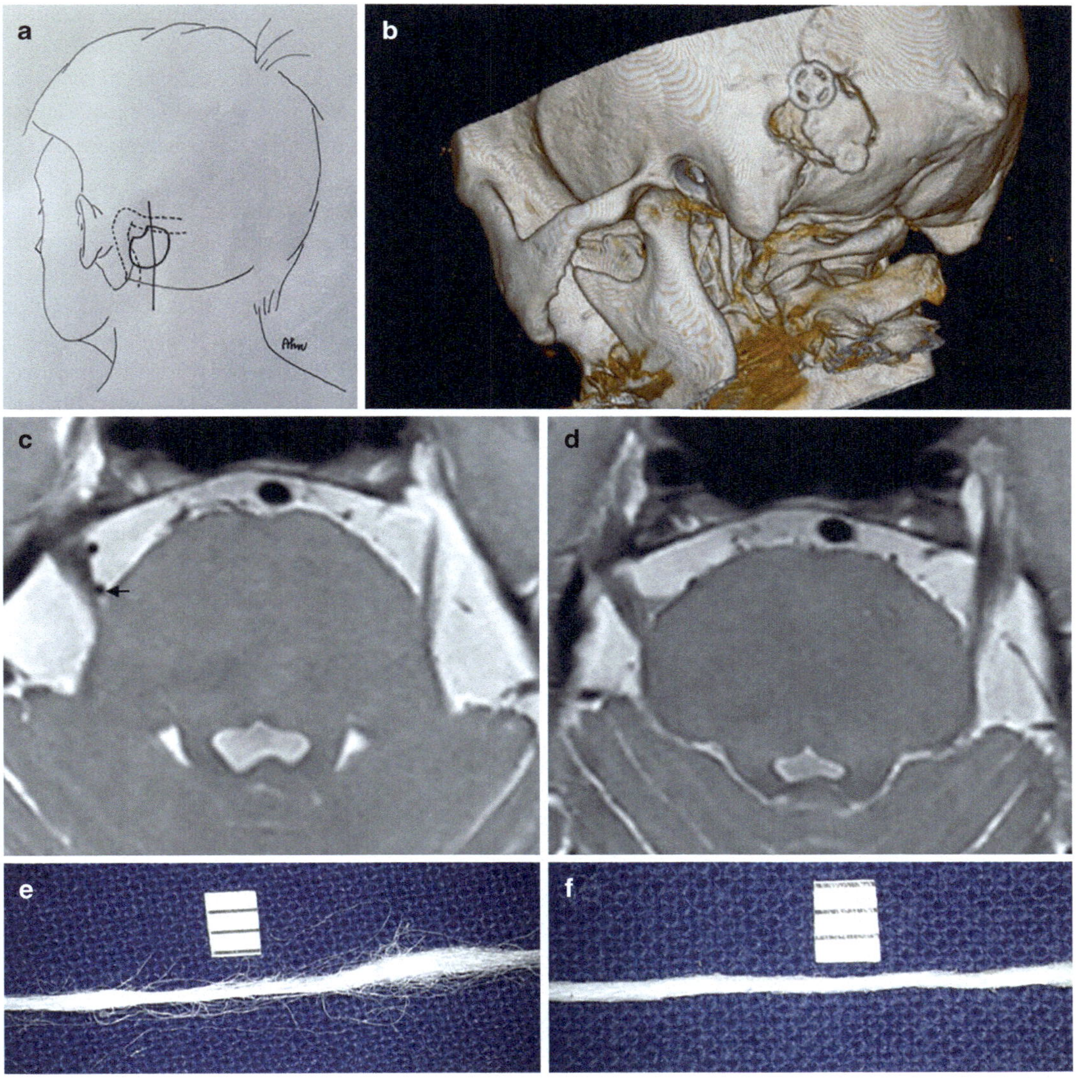

Fig. 3 (**a**) A linear scalp incision was made behind the ear. An outline of the transverse and sigmoid sinuses (dotted line). A craniotomy bone flap (line). (**b**) postoperative 3D CT image showing the size and shape of the suboccipital craniotomy. (**c**) Preoperative MR. The SCA loop is compressing trigeminal nerve and trigeminal REZ (arrows). (**d**) Postoperative MR. The offending artery disappeared in this photo since it was transposed and fixated onto the tentorium. (**e**) Teflon fibers were prepared as a bundle shape before a manual twist with fibrin glue. (**f**) Teflon fiber bundle was manually twisted with Fibrin glue and became a fibrin glue-coated Teflon sling which shows lint-free and sleek

may be enough to avoid some cases of pain recurrence. And removing any compression near the trigeminal nerve root provides long-term pain-free rates for patients with TN [5]. However, additional procedures might be needed to secure long-term maintenance of separation between the offending vessel and trigeminal REZ. A transposition using a sling could be ideal to reduce the risk of recurrence or surgical failure [24]. Teflon fibers or a fibrin glue-coated Teflon sling can be applied for secure fixation of the transposed vessel which was transposed with fibrin glue alone.

As one of the transposition methods, fixation for offending vessels using aneurysm fenestrated-type aneurysmal clip [25]. As aneurysmal clip holding the vessel is so slippery that transposition using aneurysmal clip alone is not safe and can even be dangerous. To avoid this risk, the authors applied a large volume of shredded Teflon felt implants to maintain the vessel position. And they emphasized the placement of the fenestrated clip around the SCA and attachment of it to the lateral tentacles sufficiently to keep it away from the trigeminal nerve [25]. Therefore, transposition using various types of aneurysmal clips is a possible option however additional procedures might be necessary to keep a secure transposition of the causative vessel (Fig. 1). With transposition MVD, the offending artery contacting the trigeminal nerve and trigeminal nerve REZ (arrow) was moved and fixated to the tentorium using a glue-coated Teflon sling (Fig. 1). Post-operative MR showed that the SCA loop, the offending artery (arrow) and become disappeared compared to preoperative MR since it was transposed (Fig. 3c and 3d). A sling transposition procedure was demonstrated (Fig. 1). The SCA contacting the trigeminal REZ and along it was transposed to change the position and trajectory of the SCA with a Tisseel glue-coated Teflon sling. The trigeminal REZ became freed from the SCA. After transposition of offending artery, the trigeminal nerve became straight with no vascular conflict. Thiws procedure can make 'off the trigeminal REZ' as a successful "transposition" procedure (Fig. 1). During transposition MVD, multiple slings can be used to transpose one offending artery away from the trigeminal REZ, and individual slings can be used to transpose multiple arteries (Fig. 2). In this case, two slings were used, one for SCA and the other for AICA (Fig. 2).

To transpose the offending vessel, a tie using Gore-Tex tape was also used [26]. This technique requires the insertion of Gore-Tex tape or thread around the arteries and the suture to the dura mater, requiring adequate work space to operate. Accordingly, they suggest that it is necessary to open the bone flap wide. The Gore-Tex tape can be directly passed around the artery and sutured to the petrous dura. They commented that the great advantage of Gore-Tex is that it does not adhere to surrounding tissues after mplantation. However, it could also be a disadvantage because the vessel can be slipped away which results in a serious neurologic deficit. To keep a secure transposition of the causative vessel, adequate additional procedure for inducing adhesion might be necessary.

Transposition of offending vessels using an autologous fascia strip can be carried out with autologous grafts derived from the patient's occipital fascia [27]. The graft is formed in the shape of a longitudinal band of 15–20 mm long and 4–5 mm wide. A properly prepared myofascial graft passes under the superior cerebellar artery and is twisted around it, forming a loop in which the artery "hanged" from the lateral tentorial surface using sutures. The posterolateral portion of the tentorium was used to suture the graft using 4-0 monofilament absorbable suture. If necessary, additional sutures of the graft were made in the adjacent petrous dura mater [27].

A transposition method using a tentorial flap was introduced [12]. In this method, the dura mater flap was elevated from the tentorium and the fenestrated clip was used to encircle the superior branch of the superior cerebellar artery to secure the clip to the dura mater flap. They emphasized the necessity of checking the blood flow because both were used with the aneurysm clip.

For transposition of offending vessels, a stitched sling method was also tried [28]. For this procedure, the SCA was transposed in the super-intermediate direction to free the compressed trigeminal nerve. The 5-0 thread was stitched through the cerebellar tentorium to transpose the SCA superomedially, then passed it around the SCA, and knotted to make the sling so that the blood vessels would not get twisted. They placed a stitch in the center of the tent and used a long sling to transpose the SCA.

For the safe stitch points on the tentorium, the surgeon needs to care for the tentorial arteries and sinuses that are located near the edge of the tentorium and in the dorsomedial location of the tentorium. The surgeon has to avoid bleeding from the tentorium and perform procedures in a narrow operating field. The arteries were transposed in the caudolateral direction because AICA delivered the caudal to the trigeminal nerve, compressing the nerves from the caudolateral side. A stitch was attached to the petrous dura mater to transpose the AICA inferolaterally. The dura mater of the petrous tubercle is so thin that you should be careful not to tear the dura mater (Fig. 2).

The authors also introduced a transposition method using a glue-coated Teflon sling [29]. For this procedure, a glue-coated sling needs to be crafted. They commented that the great advantage of Gore-Tex is that it does not adhere to surrounding tissues after implantation (Fig. 3e and 3f). For this procedure, Teflon threads were prepared and placed in a shape of a bundle on the table. Fibrin glue was poured over the Teflon threads using a prefilled syringe and the Teflon threads sprinkled with fibrin glue were twisted using fingers to form elongated strands. This fibrin glue-coating procedure changed the elongated threads into a lint-free and smooth-surfaced Teflon sling. This glue-coated Teflon sling therefore became easier to be manipulated safely by surgeons. The tensile strength of the glue-coated sling increased markedly and so it became suitable to use the sling as a secure material for the transposition of the offending artery. Since fibrin glue is used as the coating material for the sling, if the blood vessel is covered with this sling, the blood vessel is properly attached to the sling, so it can be maintained almost permanently in a non-slip state. The length and thickness of the glue-coated sling can be adjusted according to the amount of Teflon thread used. The surgeon can decide the length and thickness of the sling depending on the surgical conditions, and the sling could usually be about 0.1–1 mm thick and about 3–5 cm long. The sling can be easily handcrafted whenever it is needed.

The purpose of sling application is to keep the transposed causative vessels safe, so the sling used for fixation must be permanently fixed. For this purpose, each end of the sling could be fixed with various techniques using a fascia, dura, or a stitch, that was introduced previously [25–28]. Authors usually fix the tip of a Teflon sling coated with adhesive to the deep tentorium or petrosal dura, considering the location of the causative vessel and the flow dynamics of blood flow after transposition. The offending vessel was moved away from the trigeminal REZ carefully by the sling and let it be fixed. In case of SCA, the deep end of the sling is fixed on the deep tentorium and in case of AICA, it is fixed to the petrosal dura. The superficial end of the sling covering the offending vessel is fixed on the tentorium near the petrosal vein or the petrosal dura according to the position of offending vessel. For the fixation of the ends of the sling, stitch is usually unnecessary. If stitch fixation is needed, a stitch onto the Petrosal dura with 5-0 black silk could be enough. Both ends of the sling can be stitch-fixated; however, separate fixation of each end of the sling is recommended to avoid vascular narrowing by sling compression [29].

3 Role of Transposition in Vein as an Offending Vessel

The importance of the vein as a causative vessel of TN was already emphasized by Dr. Jannetta [1]. He commented that a vein contributed to the compression in 68% of 1165 patients with TN and was the only compressing vessel in 12% [1]. Venous compression alone as the cause of TN was reported to be a relatively lower rate of 6–18% [30]. A small unspecified artery or vein was more frequently the only compressing vessel in women than in men. Together with small arteries, veins were the compressing vessels most frequently found in patients with TN undergoing second operations [1]. And vein as a causative vessel was one of the four factors predicting higher rates of recurrence after MVD [1]. Recent publications also commented on the importance of vein as a causative vessel of TN. Coagulation and division of the veins may provide a more satisfactory outcome if the vein is a causative vessel causing TN. However, appropriate management method has not been established yet and still been controversial [9, 31]. There are several veins that can contribute as a causative vessel of TN and transverse pontine vein (TPV) was the most frequently involved vessel [31].

If a vein is considered as a causative vessel of TN, or contributing to the TN, coagulation and division of the vein is the best option to control the neuralgic pain. Veins are usually thin and anchored with the arachnoid membrane, making it difficult to be dissected and separated from the surrounding cranial nerves and brain stem. Coagulation and division of the vein has a risk of disrupted venous drainage followed by cerebellar or brainstem infarction and edema [32]. It is very difficult to determine the sacrifice of the veins.

In a report, the vein of the cerebellopontine fissure (VCPF) was suggested as a reference vein for the decision of sacrifice [31]. They suggested that division of the culprit veins is recommended if the diameter is smaller than the VCPF as it provides a good outcome [31]. However, it is still not yet a definite reference to decide a venous division.

Authors suggest a transposition of vein when the vein is so large and division of the vein is expected to be dangerous. The transposition method for vein is similar to that of artery. If the vein was transposed, the flow could be restored as was not divided (Fig. 4). When the vein was transposed with a glue-coated Teflon sling, the vein might look collapsed however is not been divided yet. The venous flow will be completely restored if the venous drainage using the transposed vein is critical. As we do not know whether the offending venous flow is critical or not, we have to save venous flow.

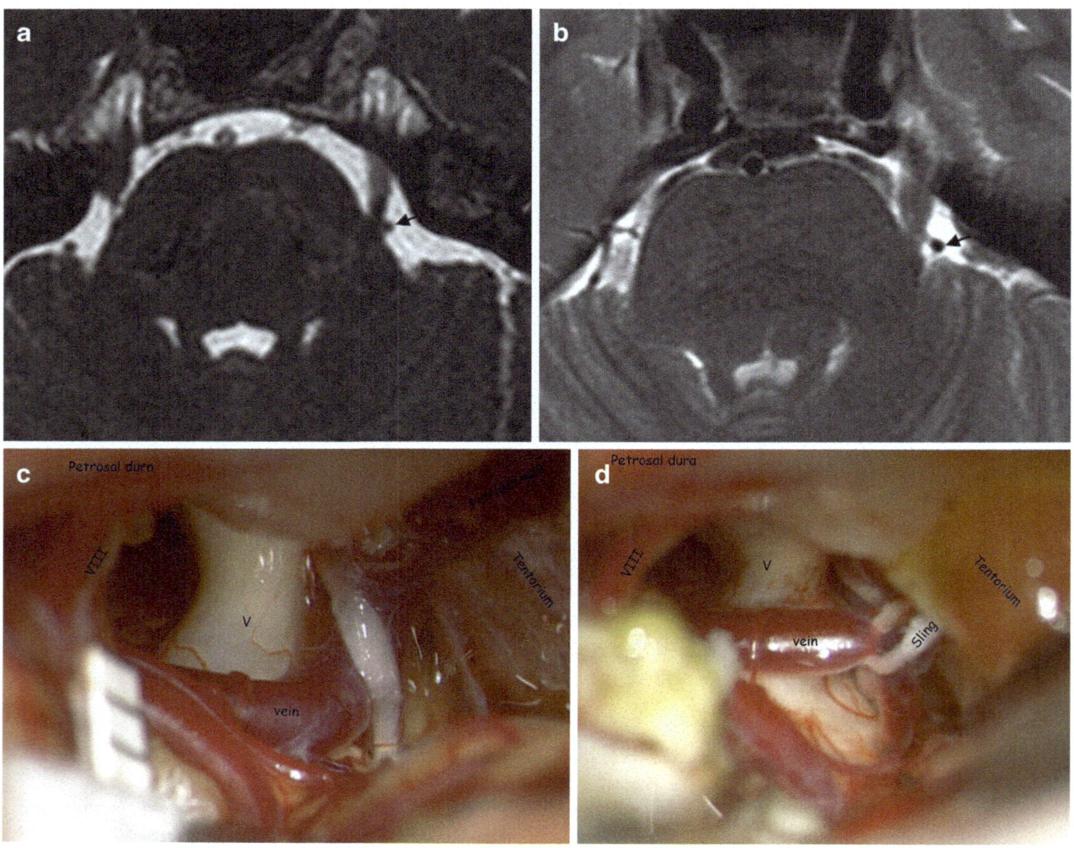

Fig. 4 (**a**) Preoperative MR. A large vein is contacting the REZ of the trigeminal nerve. (**b**) Postoperative MR. The offending vein was transposed and venous flow was well preserved. (**c**) A large petrosal vein is contacting the REZ of the trigeminal nerve and passes along the nerve between the main trunk and the motor branch of the nerve. (**d**) The vein was carefully dissected out from the REZ of the trigeminal nerve and pons. A fibrin glue-coated Teflon sling was used to lift up the petrosal vein and the position of the offending vein was changed therefore compressing force onto the REZ conveyed from the large vein was removed as the flow dynamic trajectory was off from the REZ. In the surgical view, the vein looked partially collapsed, but the venous flow was maintained

References

1. Barker FG 2nd, Jannetta PJ, Bissonette DJ, Larkins MV, Jho HD. The long-term outcome of microvascular decompression for trigeminal neuralgia. N Engl J Med. 1996;334(17):1077–83. https://doi.org/10.1056/NEJM199604253341701.
2. Sarsam Z, Garcia-Finana M, Nurmikko TJ, Varma TR, Eldridge P. The long-term outcome of microvascular decompression for trigeminal neuralgia. Br J Neurosurg. 2010;24(1):18–25. https://doi.org/10.3109/02688690903370289.
3. Pollock BE. Surgical management of medically refractory trigeminal neuralgia. Curr Neurol Neurosci Rep. 2012;12(2):125–31. https://doi.org/10.1007/s11910-011-0242-7.
4. Sindou M, Leston J, Decullier E, Chapuis F. Microvascular decompression for primary trigeminal neuralgia: long-term effectiveness and prognostic factors in a series of 362 consecutive patients with clear-cut neurovascular conflicts who underwent pure decompression. J Neurosurg. 2007;107(6):1144–53. https://doi.org/10.3171/JNS-07/12/1144.
5. Pines AR, Butterfield RJ, Turcotte EL, Garcia JO, De Lucia N, Algier EJ, et al. Microvascular transposition without Teflon: a single Institution's 17-year experience treating trigeminal neuralgia. Oper Neurosurg (Hagerstown). 2021;20(4):397–405. https://doi.org/10.1093/ons/opaa413.
6. Amador N, Pollock BE. Repeat posterior fossa exploration for patients with persistent or recurrent idiopathic trigeminal neuralgia. J Neurosurg. 2008;108(5):916–20. https://doi.org/10.3171/JNS/2008/108/5/0916.
7. Cho DY, Chang CG, Wang YC, Wang FH, Shen CC, Yang DY. Repeat operations in failed microvascular decompression for trigeminal neuralgia. Neurosurgery. 1994;35(4):665–9. ; discussion 9-70. https://doi.org/10.1227/00006123-199410000-00012.
8. Ugwuanyi UC, Kitchen ND. The operative findings in re-do microvascular decompression for recurrent trigeminal neuralgia. Br J Neurosurg. 2010;24(1):26–30. https://doi.org/10.3109/02688690903507489.
9. Matsushima T, Yamaguchi T, Inoue TK, Matsukado K, Fukui M. Recurrent trigeminal neuralgia after microvascular decompression using an interposing technique. Teflon felt adhesion and the sling retraction technique. Acta Neurochir. 2000;142(5):557–61. https://doi.org/10.1007/s007010050469.
10. Menovsky T, De Ridder D, de Vries J. Neurosurgical patties and their intraoperative interaction with neural tissue. Surg Neurol. 2009;71(3):326–9. https://doi.org/10.1016/j.surneu.2007.12.018; discussion 9.
11. Stratton-Powell AA, Anderson IA, Timothy J, Kapur N, Culmer P. Neurosurgical patties: adhesion and damage mitigation. J Neurosurg. 2015;123(1):153–60. https://doi.org/10.3171/2014.12.JNS14917.
12. Gonzalez-Quarante LH, Ruiz-Juretschke F, Agarwal V, Garcia-Leal R. Microvascular decompression for trigeminal neuralgia using a novel fenestrated clip and tentorial flap technique. World Neurosurg. 2017;106:775–84. https://doi.org/10.1016/j.wneu.2017.07.110.
13. Bechtold R, Garlow B, Liu R, Tandon A, Szewc A, Zhu W, et al. Minimizing cotton ball retention in neurological procedures. Des Med Devices Conf (2020). 2020;2020:V001T06A006. https://doi.org/10.1115/dmd2020-9042.
14. Parmar DN, Sharr MM. Cotton gauze foreign body granuloma following microvascular decompression. Br J Neurosurg. 1999;13(1):87–9. https://doi.org/10.1080/02688699944294.
15. Ammar A, Lagenaur C, Jannetta P. Neural tissue compatibility of Teflon as an implant material for microvascular decompression. Neurosurg Rev. 1990;13(4):299–303. https://doi.org/10.1007/BF00346368.
16. Premsagar IC, Moss T, Coakham HB. Teflon-induced granuloma following treatment of trigeminal neuralgia by microvascular decompression. Report of two cases. J Neurosurg. 1997;87(3):454–7. https://doi.org/10.3171/jns.1997.87.3.0454.
17. Pressman E, Jha RT, Zavadskiy G, Kumar JI, van Loveren H, van Gompel JJ, et al. Teflon or Ivalon(R): a scoping review of implants used in microvascular decompression for trigeminal neuralgia. Neurosurg Rev. 2020;43(1):79–86. https://doi.org/10.1007/s10143-019-01187-0.
18. Jannetta PJ, Bissonette DJ. Management of the failed patient with trigeminal neuralgia. Clin Neurosurg. 1985;32:334–47.
19. Jorgensen CS, Paaske WP. Physical and mechanical properties of ePTFE stretch vascular grafts determined by time-resolved scanning acoustic microscopy. Eur J Vasc Endovasc Surg. 1998;15(5):416–22. https://doi.org/10.1016/s1078-5884(98)80203-7.
20. Zaidi HA, Awad AW, Chowdhry SA, Fusco D, Nakaji P, Spetzler RF. Microvascular decompression for hemifacial spasm secondary to vertebrobasilar dolichoectasia: surgical strategies, technical nuances and clinical outcomes. J Clin Neurosci. 2015;22(1):62–8. https://doi.org/10.1016/j.jocn.2014.09.008.
21. Spotnitz WD. Fibrin sealant: the only approved hemostat, sealant, and adhesive-a laboratory and clinical perspective. ISRN Surg. 2014;2014:203943. https://doi.org/10.1155/2014/203943.
22. Ryu H, Yamamoto S. A simple technique for neurovascular decompression of the cranial nerves. Br J Neurosurg. 2000;14(2):132–4. https://doi.org/10.1080/02688690050004561.
23. Ohta M, Komatsu F, Abe H, Sakamoto S, Tsugu H, Oshiro S, et al. Complication caused by use of fibrin glue in vessel transposition for trigeminal neuralgia. Neurol Med Chir (Tokyo). 2008;48(1):30–2. https://doi.org/10.2176/nmc.48.30.
24. Fukushima T. Posterior cranial fossa neurovascular decompression (Jannetta method) for trigeminal neuralgia and facial spasm. No Shinkei Geka. 1982;10(12):1257–61. Epub 1982/12/01

25. Attabib N, Kaufmann AM. Use of fenestrated aneurysm clips in microvascular decompression surgery. Technical note and case series. J Neurosurg. 2007;106(5):929–31. https://doi.org/10.3171/jns.2007.106.5.929.
26. Shigeno T, Kumai J, Endo M, Oya S, Hotta S. Snare technique of vascular transposition for microvascular decompression–technical note. Neurol Med Chir (Tokyo). 2002;42(4):184–9. https://doi.org/10.2176/nmc.42.184; discussion 90.
27. Mitsos AP, Georgakoulias N, Lafazanos SA, Konstantinou EA. The "hanging technique" of vascular transposition in microvascular decompression for trigeminal neuralgia: technical report of four cases. Neurosurg Rev. 2008;31(3):327–30. https://doi.org/10.1007/s10143-008-0144-6.
28. Masuoka J, Matsushima T, Kawashima M, Nakahara Y, Funaki T, Mineta T. Stitched sling retraction technique for microvascular decompression: procedures and techniques based on an anatomical viewpoint. Neurosurg Rev. 2011;34(3):373–9. https://doi.org/10.1007/s10143-011-0310-0; discussion 9-80.
29. Lee SH, Park JS, Ahn YH. Bioglue-coated teflon sling technique in microvascular decompression for hemifacial spasm involving the vertebral artery. J Korean Neurosurg Soc. 2016;59(5):505–11. https://doi.org/10.3340/jkns.2016.59.5.505.
30. Oishi M, Fukuda M, Noto Y, Kawaguchi T, Hiraishi T, Fujii Y. Trigeminal neuralgia associated with the specific bridging pattern of transverse pontine vein: diagnostic value of three-dimensional multifusion volumetric imaging. Stereotact Funct Neurosurg. 2011;89(4):226–33. https://doi.org/10.1159/000326778.
31. Inoue T, Hirai H, Shima A, Suzuki F, Fukushima T, Matsuda M. Diagnosis and management for trigeminal neuralgia caused solely by venous compression. Acta Neurochir. 2017;159(4):681–8. https://doi.org/10.1007/s00701-017-3085-4.
32. Anichini G, Iqbal M, Rafiq NM, Ironside JW, Kamel M. Sacrificing the superior petrosal vein during microvascular decompression. Is it safe? Learning the hard way. Case report and review of literature. Surg Neurol Int. 2016;7(Suppl 14):S415–20. https://doi.org/10.4103/2152-7806.183520.

Postoperative Cerebrospinal Fluid Leakage and Closing Technique for Microvascular Decompression

Hyun Seok Lee and Kwan Park

1 Postoperative CSF Leakage

Cerebrospinal fluid (CSF) leakage is one of the most common complication in the neurosurgical procedure including microvascular decompression (MVD) surgery [1].

So far, various techniques were proposed to prevent and manage CSF leakage. Although CSF leakage has decreased compared to the past, it is still a major cause of morbidity following MVD surgery [2].

In addition to pseudomeningocele, CSF leakage can cause complications such as meningitis, encephalitis, and brain abscess, which can be potentially fatal [1]. These complications increase hospital costs and prolong the length of hospital stay [3, 4].

Hospital costs for patients with postoperative CSF leakage increase by about 141% more than those without [5].

Therefore, it is important to understand and prevent postoperative CSF leakage.

H. S. Lee · K. Park (✉)
Department of Neurosurgery, Konkuk University Medical Center, Konkuk University School of Medicine, Seoul, Republic of Korea
e-mail: 20220205@kuh.ac.kr; kwanpark@skku.edu

2 Incidence

The rate of postoperative CSF leakage according to many neurosurgical approaches has been reported variously in previous literatures. The rate of postoperative CSF leakage in the practice of neurosurgery has been reported to be ranging from 5 to 30% [1]. The incidence rate of CSF leakage after surgery in the infratentorial approach is known to be about six times higher than in the supratentorial approach [5]. The incidence of CSF leakage after retro-sigmoid approach for multiple pathologies such as hemifacial spasm, trigeminal neuralgia, tumor, and cavernous malformation has been reported to range from 0 to 22% [6, 7]. Among them, the incidence rate following MVD surgery has been reported to range from 0.9 to 12.5% in the previous review of literatures [8, 9].

3 Factors Affecting Postoperative CSF Leakage

CSF leakage is caused by connection between the subarachnoid space and the external environment. This connection can be made by several causes and many factors are thought to affect CSF leakage.

The fragile dura mater and strong attachment between the dura mater and skull especially in elderly patients can cause dural tear during

K. Park, K. R. Cho (eds.), *Trigeminal Neuralgia*, https://doi.org/10.1007/978-981-19-9171-4_14

craniotomy or craniectomy. The dura overlying the cerebellum is quite thin and friable, which is also one of the factors that make dura tear more likely.

Pinholes on the dura mater created by needle used during dura suture may also cause CSF leakage.

Retracting the dural flap with stay sutures during surgery can lead to dehydration and contraction of the dura mater. This progresses further as the operation time increases. These factors make dura closure difficult.

The mastoid air cells may be opened while drilling the margin of the sigmoid sinus. If the mastoid air cell is not sufficiently sealed during surgery, fluid may flow through it. For this reason, the leaked CSF enters the middle ear cavity and flows through the Eustachian tube into the nasopharynx, resulting in paradoxical rhinorrhea and fills the tympanic membrane, resulting in ear fullness and CSF otorrhea [8].

Well-pneumatized petrous bone and well-developed mastoid air cells may predispose to open the mastoid air cell during craniectomy and are associated with a higher risk of CSF leakage.

If the opening site of mastoid air cell is small, it might not be noticed and packed during surgery [9].

Through a temporal bone computed tomography (CT) scan, the extent of mastoid air cells can be checked before surgery, and the possibility of opening can be predicted in advance [10]. If mastoid air cells are exposed, they should be sealed with bone wax during bone drilling and sealing again prior to final dura closure.

In addition, other factors affecting CSF leakage and poor wound healing include diabetes, malnutrition, and steroid use [11, 12]. These factors should also be checked prior to surgery. Especially, obese patients need particular attention to CSF leakage because BMI greater than 25 kg/m^2 is also associated with higher rate of CSF leakage after posterior fossa surgery [11, 12].

4 Clinical Symptoms

CSF leakage may occur as form of a surgical site leak, otorrhea, or rhinorrhea [4, 13, 14].

Wound leak is diagnosed if the clear fluid was drained through the skin incision site or if CSF fluid is collected in the subcutaneous layer as pseudomeningocele [13, 14].

CSF otorrhea was defined as a clear fluid which was observed through the ear ipsilateral to the surgical site and CSF rhinorrhea was diagnosed when a clear fluid was leaking through the ipsilateral or bilateral nostril [13]. Wound leak may occur through a defect of the dural incision site, and otorrhea or rhinorrhea may occur through the middle ear and Eustachian tube because of communication between the intradural space of posterior fossa and mastoid air cells.

Patients with CSF rhinorrhea may complain of intermittent watery discharge into the nasopharynx, ear fullness, and conductive hearing loss [15]. CSF rhinorrhea was induced by Valsalva maneuver, jugular venous compression, or position change with neck flexion [13].

Pseudo-CSF rhinorrhea, due to irrigation water entering the opened mastoid air cell during surgery, not from active CSF leakage, is difficult to differentiate from true rhinorrhea. This temporary rhinorrhea usually occurs after immediate surgery and is easier to control with conservative management than true paradoxical CSF rhinorrhea.

"Reservoir sign" which would show large volume of fluid flowing out of the nose following a change in head position may be seen in patients with CSF rhinorrhea. This is when leaked CSF that has been accumulating in the sphenoid sinus is discharged due to a change in posture.

In the cases of bloody CSF rhinorrhea, the "Ring sign" or "Halo sign" which refers to the formation of pattern by differential diffusion of CSF and blood on a filter paper or dry gauze can also be used as a clinical evidence of CSF rhinorrhea.

It is also necessary to differentiate CSF rhinorrhea from other diseases that may cause rhinorrhea symptoms, such as allergic or vasomotor rhinitis [15].

5 Diagnosis

Accurate and rapid identification of postoperative CSF leakage is important to determine appropriate management and to reduce the comorbidity.

5.1 Biochemical Diagnosis

If patient has symptoms of a CSF leak, it is important to determine whether it is CSF or not. In these cases, biochemical methods can help.

5.1.1 Glucose Oxidase Test

Glucose oxidase test is the most commonly used easy method for screening CSF leakage. However, due to high false-positive and negative rates, it is not recommended as a confirmatory test [16]. The test shows positive result if the concentration of glucose in the sample is more than 20 mg/day [15]. Since the glucose concentration in nasal secretions without CSF is usually about 10 mg/dL, it is possible to simply rule out whether CSF is mixed or not [15]. However, it has poor diagnostic sensitivity and specificity because the results can be easily affected by the patient's medical conditions. False-positive results may be obtained in patients with diabetes mellitus or nasal epithelial inflammation and false-negative results can be obtained in patients with bacterial meningitis [16]. Therefore, the results should be interpreted in combination with the patient's clinical symptoms.

5.1.2 Beta-2 Transferrin Test (β-2 TRF)

Beta-2 transferrin is produced by neuraminidase within the brain and is only detected in CSF, vitreous humor, and perilymph. This test has a high sensitivity (99%) and specificity (97%) [17]. However, this test is expensive and takes longer time for the results and is not available in some hospitals [16].

5.1.3 Beta-Trace Protein Test (β-TP)

Beta-trace protein (β-TP) test is also useful for detecting CSF leaks. β-TP is the second most common protein in the CSF, produced by the epithelial cell lining of the leptomeninges and by the choroid plexus [17]. This test can confirm CSF leak because the concentration of β-TP in CSF is more than 30 times higher than in serum (14.6 ± 4.6 mg/L in CSF and 0.4 6 ± 0.13 mg/L in serum) [16]. Although this test is less expensive and less time-consuming than the β-2 TRF test, it is not yet commonly used clinically [16].

5.2 Radiologic Diagnosis

Imaging methods for diagnosing CSF leakage after MVD surgery are differ from those of traumatic CSF leakage. Because postoperative CSF leakage occurs dura defect at the surgical site, it is no need to perform all of the tests used to find the CSF leakage site in the case of traumatic CSF leakage. It is difficult to distinguish whether the CSF is continuously leaking because the mastoid air cell is open, or whether the irrigation water during surgery is stagnant even when the mastoid air cell is well-clogged.

5.2.1 Temporal Bone Computed Tomography (TBCT)

Temporal bone CT is not only suitable for predicting the size of mastoid air cells before surgery but is also useful for confirming the presence of water in mastoid air cells in patients with symptoms of CSF leakage after surgery. If the open site of the mastoid air cell was not seen in the surgical field, it may be a good examination to find it. And also the test that can be used quickly and easily to compare before and after the management of CSF leakage patients.

However, this test can only check for the presence of effusion in mastoid air cells, and it is difficult to prove the leak itself or to locate the site of the dural defect.

5.2.2 Magnetic Resonance Imaging (MRI)

Through T2-weighted MR images (T2WI), CSF leakage seen as high-signal intensity in mastoid air cells can be demonstrated. In patients with CSF otorhinorrhea, the route of CSF within the mastoid air cell, middle ear cavity, eustachian tube, and nasal cavity can be identified [18].

However, compared with TBCT, the main disadvantages are high cost and limited access [16].

5.3 Endoscopic Ear Examination

Endoscopic examination of the ipsilateral ear may be helpful for the diagnosis of CSF leakage. Accumulated clear fluid on the tympanic membrane may be seen in patients with CSF leakage. In some cases, for example, in a patient who has a persistent feeling of ear fullness but does not have active rhinorrhea, puncture of the tympanic membrane and draining this fluid may be helpful in diagnosis and rule out CSF leakage.

6 Management

CSF leakage increases the risk of infection such as meningitis and brain abscess that can proceed to fatal. Therefore, early diagnosis and treatment are important. Although the management of CSF leak has been proposed by many studies, it still remains a difficult problem.

There are three main steps for the management of postoperative CSF leakage that consists of conservative management, lumbar drainage, and surgical management.

6.1 Conservative Management

If a patient has symptoms of CSF leakage following MVD surgery, conservative treatment can be the first step. The conservative treatment includes bed rest, 30–45° head elevation, pressure dressings, and using drugs to reduce CSF production [13]. Preventing the patient from sneezing, coughing, or stringing. Careful monitoring is necessary for the development of CSF infection, which may include fever, neurological deterioration, leukocytosis, and increase in erythrocyte sedimentation rate (ESR) and C-reactive protein (CRP).

Oral administration of 250 mg acetazolamide (carbonic anhydrase inhibitor) twice a day for 3 days helps to lower intracranial pressure (ICP) by reducing CSF secretion via its action on the choroid plexus [13]. Maintain conservative treatment for at least 3 days and check for patient's response.

6.2 Lumbar Drainage

If CSF leakage persists despite at least 3 days of conservative treatment in a patient, more invasive treatment should be considered. Continuous CSF diversion via lumbar drainage catheter is relatively simple and efficient to manage postoperative CSF leakage. A catheter placed in the vertebral intrathecal space to drain the CSF to lower the pressure gradient and CSF diversion helps to seal the CSF fistula of the operation site by granulation tissue [13]. In some cases, the insertion of a lumbar drainage catheter is simultaneous with conservative treatment [5]. CSF diversion is performed at the rate of 10–15 mL/h increasing the rate as necessary and is continued for a minimal of 5 days to a maximum of 10 days [13, 19]. The lumbar CSF drainage is maintained until the dry and compressed surgical wound is obtained or rhinorrhea (or otorrhea) symptoms are relieved. The CSF should be examined to detect infection early [4, 10]. Minor complications including headache, nausea, vomiting and pneumocephalus may occur following lumbar drainage placement. More severe complications such as meningitis, intracranial hemorrhage, or brain herniation due to excessive CSF drainage have been reported. Careful hourly monitoring of the amount and rate of

CSF drainage is important to prevent over-drainage of CSF. Mechanical complications relating to catheters such as catheter blockage and catheter dislodging from the subarachnoid space because of patient movement also have been reported [13]. Caution should be exercised when inserting and managing a lumbar drainage catheter.

If the CSF leakage persists up to 7~10 days after lumbar drainage, further invasive management is required.

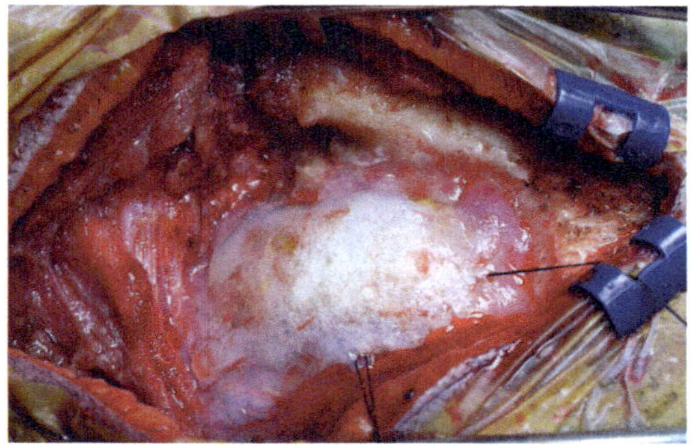

Fig. 1 After (a) to (c) procedures, sealing with Tisseel over the Duragen and Tachosils layers

6.3 Surgical Management

Persistent CSF leakage that does not respond to conservative management and lumbar drainage is likely to require revision surgery. The surgical wound should be reexplored and repaired surgically [13]. Careful identification of CSF leakage point and extent of the dural defect is needed. Perform direct dural repairment if possible, otherwise close dural defect using muscle graft, artificial dural substitute material, and fibrin glue. Check for the presence of any opened mastoid air cells and seal them securely.

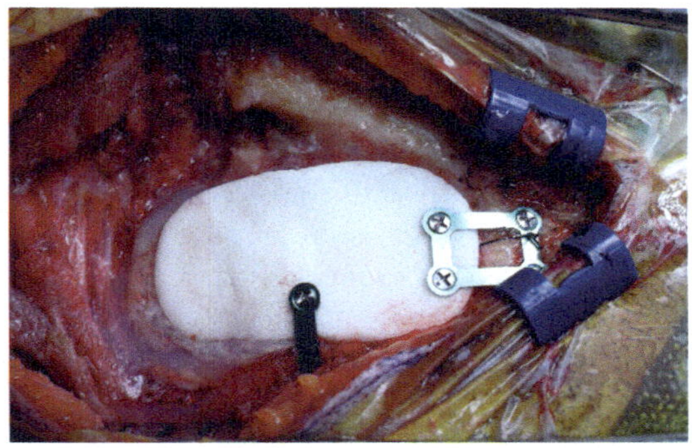

Fig. 2 Polymethyl methacrylate (PMMC) bone cement flap fixation

7 Dural Closure Technique

Watertight dural closure and complete sealing of the opened mastoid air cells is the most important thing to prevent postoperative CSF leakage. Numerous attempts have been made and various dural closing techniques have been proposed using different materials to reduce CSF leakage rate.

We introduce triple layer reinforced dural repair technique using: (a) primary watertight dural repair, (b) Collagen matrix (Duragen, Integralife) (c) Fibrin sealant patch (TachoSil, Nycomed), (d) surgical adhesive (Tisseel, Baxter or Greenplast, Green cross CO) (Fig. 1), (e) polymethyl methacrylate bone cement (Fig. 2), (f) layered soft tissue closure. Triple layer means collagen matrix, fibrin sealant patch, and polymethyl methacrylate bone cement.

7.1 Triple Layer Reinforced Dural Repair Technique: Durogen, Tachosil, Artificial Bone Cement

Following decompression of nerve, fill the posterior fossa space with warm saline. Check that there is any opened mastoid air cell and that it is securely sealed with bone wax. If opened mastoid air cells are visualized, make sure to pack them completely with bone wax. After removing the stay suture, dural flaps are gathered in its place. Three to four stitches are made on dural incision site at similar intervals using 4-0 vicryl. Two slits are made at each side of Duragen. Duragens are placed over the dura between previously stitched knots. Then, Duragens are sutured with dura mater below it with 4-0 vicryl. Duragens are used to close the gaps between the dural flaps and pinholes on the dura mater created by needle used during dural suture. Two surgical knots are made on dura at upper and posterior margin of skull defect. Fibrin sealant patches are placed over the epidural space and thrombin glue sealant is sprayed over the fibrin sealant patches. Bone flap using polymethyl methacrylate bone cement is placed over the entire skull defect and is fixed by plates and screws tagging with previously made two surgical knots. While the Duragen, Tachosils, and bone cement apply pressure to press the dura inward, the tagged surgical knots force the dura to lift outward. This eliminates the dead space between the cranioplasty site and the duroplasty site, helping the CSF not to accumulate. Bone dusts are removed through massive saline irrigation. Layered closure of muscle and subcutaneous layer is performed with 2-0 and 3-0 vicryl (Ethicon), respectively and superficial skin layer suture is done using skin stapler of 3-0 nylon suture. The closed wound is washed with a saline-soaked gauze and dressed sterilely.

Previously used technique named "muscle plugging technique" [20] was designed to prevent CSF leakage after retro-sigmoid craniotomy [21]. Dumbbell-shaped muscle pieces were plugged inside and outside dura incision to prevent outward flow of CSF. However, it seems that the muscle fragments attached to the inside of the dura mater act as foreign body and cause postoperative infection. Therefore, triple layer reinforced closure technique was designed to accomplish watertight closure of the dura mater and avoid putting foreign material that can cause infection and inflammation into the dura mater.

We performed over 4000 cases of MVD surgery and used this closing technique. At the latest follow-up, the incidence of CSF leakage was 1.1%. This technique seems to be effective and ready to lower the incidence of CSF leakage following MVD surgery.

References

1. Abuzayed B, Kafadar AM, Oguzoglu SA, Canbaz B, Kaynar MY. Duraplasty using autologous fascia lata reinforced by on-site pedicled muscle flap: technical note. J Craniofac Surg. 2009;20(2):435–8.
2. Stoker MA, Forbes JA, Hanif R, Cooper C, Nian H, Konrad PE, et al. Decreased rate of CSF leakage associated with complete reconstruction of suboccipital cranial defects. J Neurol Surg B Skull Base. 2012;73(4):281–6.
3. Sherif C, Di Ieva A, Gibson D, Pakrah-Bodingbauer B, Widhalm G, Krusche-Mandl I, et al. A management algorithm for cerebrospinal fluid leak associated with anterior skull base fractures: detailed clinical and radiological follow-up. Neurosurg Rev. 2012;35(2):227–37. discussion 37–8.
4. Arlt F, Trantakis C, Krupp W, Renner C, Winkler D, Strauss G, et al. Cerebrospinal fluid leak after microsurgical surgery in vestibular schwannomas via retrosigmoidal craniotomy. Neurol Res. 2011;33(9):947–52.
5. Altaf I, Vohra AH, Shams S. Management of cerebrospinal fluid leak following posterior cranial fossa surgery. Pak J Med Sci. 2016;32(6):1439–43.
6. Khan SA, Laulloo A, Vats A, Nath F. Microvascular decompression: incidence and prevention of postoperative CSF leakage in a consecutive series of 134 patients. Br J Neurosurg. 2020;34(4):416–8.
7. Venable GT, Roberts ML, Lee RP, Michael LM 2nd. Primary dural closure for retrosigmoid approaches. J Neurol Surg B Skull Base. 2018;79(4):330–4.
8. Li N, Zhao WG, Pu CH, Shen JK. Clinical application of artificial dura mater to avoid cerebrospinal fluid leaks after microvascular decompression surgery. Minim Invasive Neurosurg. 2005;48(6):369–72.
9. Yanagawa T, Hatayama T, Harada Y, Sato E, Yamashita K, Tanaka M, et al. Preoperative risk assessment for predicting the opening of mastoid air cells in lateral suboccipital craniotomy for microvascular decompression. Clin Neurol Neurosurg. 2020;189:105624.
10. Bani A, Gilsbach JM. Incidence of cerebrospinal fluid leak after microsurgical removal of vestibular schwannomas. Acta Neurochir. 2002;144(10):979–82. discussion 82.
11. Eseonu CI, Goodwin CR, Zhou X, Theodros D, Bender MT, Mathios D, et al. Reduced CSF leak in complete calvarial reconstructions of microvascular decompression craniectomies using calcium phosphate cement. J Neurosurg. 2015;123(6):1476–9.
12. Tang R, Mao S, Li D, Ye H, Zhang W. Treatment and outcomes of iatrogenic cerebrospinal fluid leak caused by different surgical procedures. World Neurosurg. 2020;143:e667–e75.
13. Allen KP, Isaacson B, Purcell P, Kutz JW Jr, Roland PS. Lumbar subarachnoid drainage in cerebrospinal fluid leaks after lateral skull base surgery. Otol Neurotol. 2011;32(9):1522–4.
14. Mangus BD, Rivas A, Yoo MJ, Alvarez J, Wanna GB, Haynes DS, et al. Management of cerebrospinal fluid leaks after vestibular schwannoma surgery. Otol Neurotol. 2011;32(9):1525–9.
15. Oh JW, Kim SH, Whang K. Traumatic cerebrospinal fluid leak: diagnosis and management. Korean J Neurotrauma. 2017;13(2):63–7.
16. Mantur M, Lukaszewicz-Zajac M, Mroczko B, Kulakowska A, Ganslandt O, Kemona H, et al. Cerebrospinal fluid leakage–reliable diagnostic methods. Clin Chim Acta. 2011;412(11–12):837–40.

17. Phang SY, Whitehouse K, Lee L, Khalil H, McArdle P, Whitfield PC. Management of CSF leak in base of skull fractures in adults. Br J Neurosurg. 2016;30(6):596–604.
18. Kabuto M, Kubota T, Kobayashi H, Handa Y, Tuchida A, Takeuchi H. MR imaging of cerebrospinal fluid rhinorrhea following the suboccipital approach to the cerebellopontine angle and the internal auditory canal: report of the two cases. Surg Neurol. 1996;45(4):336–40.
19. Krishnan SS, Nigam P, Manuel A, Vasudevan MC. Bone sandwich closure technique for posterior fossa craniectomy. J Neurol Surg B Skull Base. 2020;81(1):8–14.
20. Park JS, Kong DS, Lee JA, Park K. Intraoperative management to prevent cerebrospinal fluid leakage after microvascular decompression: dural closure with a "plugging muscle" method. Neurosurg Rev. 2007;30(2):139–42. discussion 42.
21. Lee MH, Jee TK, Lee JA, Park K. Postoperative complications of microvascular decompression for hemifacial spasm: lessons from experience of 2040 cases. Neurosurg Rev. 2016;39(1):151–8. discussion 8.

Operative Complications of Microvascular Decompression for Trigeminal Neuralgia

Min Ho Lee

1 Introduction

Since Jannetta performed the first procedure 50 years ago, microvascular decompression (MVD) remains an effective and safe treatment for trigeminal neuralgia (TN) [1]. Surgical techniques of MVD have been modified and improved by many pioneers over the past 50 years [2–8]. Nevertheless, minor and serious postoperative complications continue to be reported in the literature. Because TN is not a life-threatening disease and MVD is a functional treatment, many efforts are needed to achieve the lowest complication rate.

This chapter will review various complications that may occur after MVD in TN patients and their frequency of occurrence, and I would discuss how to reduce these complications. In addition to the common operative complications, specific vascular complications will be described separately in another chapter, so I wound not discuss them in this chapter.

2 Methods

A search of the PubMed/MEDLINE and Ovid databases was conducted for studies published from database inception from 2018 to 2021. The search terms used included, "microvascular decompression" and "trigeminal neuralgia." Relevant references from the chosen articles were also included.

Inclusion criteria for studies in this article were established as follows: adult patients, clinical studies with more than ten patients, utilization MVD to treat TN, Retro-mastoid suboccipital craniotomy with retro-auricular incision, English-language studies, and articles that listed specific complications. Exclusion criteria for the analysis were as follows: clinical studies involving other procedures (e.g., radiosurgery, balloon compression, glycerol rhizolysis, or percutaneous radiofrequency lesioning), pediatric, animal, basic science, and cadaver studies, commentary articles, operation with endoscope, and related with other pathologies (e.g., neoplasm or multiple sclerosis). First, the selection was made using abstract. Secondarily, the full text was reviewed to determine whether it was a suitable article.

M. H. Lee (✉)
Department of Neurosurgery, Uijeongbu St. Mary's Hospital, The Catholic University of Korea, Seoul, Republic of Korea
e-mail: minho919.lee@catholic.ac.kr

K. Park, K. R. Cho (eds.), *Trigeminal Neuralgia*, https://doi.org/10.1007/978-981-19-9171-4_15

3 Results

According to the criteria mentioned above, 15 articles were selected and reviewed. In recent papers, many cases using endoscopic surgery were excluded, and among them, cases where conventional microscopic surgery could be separately analyzed were included. (Table 1) Not all articles are mentioned in detail about all complications. Also, there were several papers that mentioned hearing loss and facial palsy without distinguishing between permanent and transient complications. Therefore, all complications were determined and arranged as permanent complications. Meanwhile, through searched review papers, the results of previous studies date before 2018 were also checked and each complication was summarized.

3.1 Operative Complications

1. Facial nerve—Facial nerve palsy

   Facial palsy is perhaps the biggest concern for neurosurgeons performing MVD surgery. It is a complication that is highly likely to occur in MVD surgery, along with hearing loss, which will be mentioned below. Although the incidence is lower than that of hemifacial spasm, when proceeding to the retro-sigmoid approach, the facial nerve is a structure that must be paid attention to. Previous studies have reported less than 1%. However, through a systemic review of more than 6000 patients, it was reported that up to 2.9% of the occurrence of facial palsy could occur [23]. These results are thought to be attributed to the difference in operator. However, the incidence did not decrease significantly in recent studies [10, 11, 16, 20, 22].

2. Cochlear-vestibular nerve—Hearing loss, tinnitus, vertigo

   Hearing loss is likewise a very critical complication. In previous papers, 1–2% were reported. As the cochlear nerve lies parallel to the facial nerve, there is a risk of such symptoms. Hearing loss may occur immediately after surgery, but in some cases, it may also occur due to delayed onset. Lee et al. reported delayed hearing loss 22 days (range 10–45 days) after MVD surgery. Although the results were based on hemifacial spasm patients, it is not expected to be significantly different in TN patients. Herta et al. [11] reported postoperative complications, 1.20% of tinnitus and 1.80% of vertigo. This may be a rather minor symptom compared to other complications, so it is often overlooked and

Table 1 The literature reviews of operative complications after microvascular decompression for trigeminal neuralgia

Author	Year	Number of patients	Wound infection	Facial palsy	Facial numbness	Hearing difficulty	Tinnitus	Vertigo	CSF leak
Wang [9]	2021	42	0.60			1.80	1.20	1.80	2.30
Singh [10]	2021	106		0.34	9.60	11.80			
Herta [11]	2021	165		1.80	6.00	2.40			
Pressman [12]	2021	291			2.85	1.84			1.96
Mizobuchi [13]	2021	166			23.00	3.84			
Inoue [14]	2020	26			6.30				4.50
Tomasello [15]	2020	72		9.52		4.76			2.38
Li [16]	2020	111	0.94	1.89	4.72	1.89			2.83
Lee [5]	2019	222				1.40			1.40
Bick [17]	2019	29			37.93	6.89			10.34
Mastronardi [18]	2019	66							1.51
Zhao [19]	2018	34	1.56		6.25	1.56			
Wu [20]	2018	64	2.70	0.00	12.60	4.50			
Xiang [21]	2018	111	2.12		4.47	0.94			0.47
Wei [22]	2018	425	1.35	0.90		0.90			4.48

not reported in several other papers. In general, these symptoms (tinnitus and vertigo) are self-limited, and most can be improved by appropriate management of the symptoms.

3. Trigeminal nerve—Facial numbness

   In addition to the improvement of pain after MVD surgery in TN patients, the incidence of numbness, i.e., hypesthesia, is also a problem. However, since this symptom is also related to the outcome of the surgery, and there is a very high possibility that there was already hypesthesia before surgery due to neurovascular conflict, the results reported in previous papers (incidence of 2.28~37.93%) should not be accepted as they are [10, 11, 13, 16, 17]. Rather, I think it would be better to view this problem as one of the outcomes of surgery. The problem of pain exacerbation also will be dealt with in another chapter.

4. Wound problem

   Cerebrospinal fluid (CSF) leak remains a significant source of morbidity in neurosurgery, particularly after posterior fossa surgery. It is six times more likely to occur in the infratentorial procedures than in the supratentorial procedures [24–26]. In many studies, CSF leakage has been reported from 1.4 to 10.3% [5, 9, 16, 17]. This, in turn, has a high risk of leading to wound infection, and wound infection rates ranged from 0.6 to 2.7% [9, 20, 22].

3.2 Tricks to Overcome Complications

There have been many efforts by neurosurgeons to reduce the complications mentioned above. As MVD is functional surgery unlike other skull base surgery, it is important to improve patient satisfaction, and for this purpose it is moving towards minimally invasive surgery. And, the smaller the skin incision wound or craniotomy area, the narrower the surgical corridor. Therefore, the optimal position is very important. By setting the perfect position, unnecessary exposure and nerve manipulation can be reduced. If the correct corridor surgical is established, retraction can be reduced. Cerebellar retraction can cause hearing loss when performing a retro-sigmoid approach [27]. Recently, to find such an optimal position, augmented reality or virtual reality is used [28–31].

3.2.1 Paresthesia and Skin Incision

Paresthesia of the postauricular region is one of the most common complaints of patients after MVD surgery. Although it may feel less important compared to other complications mentioned above, it is another important complication that affects the quality of pain from the patient's point of view. In order to avoid damage to the greater auricular nerve and to the lesser occipital nerve, it may be beneficial to insert the incision parallel to the nerve's direction. Also, avoiding unnecessarily long incisions is a way to reduce these complications.

3.2.2 Optimal Position

The patient is placed in the park-bench position. The operator is placed behind the patient. The patient's ipsilateral shoulder is allowed to fall forward and is mobilized caudally away from the incision, to provide additional space within the surgical field. The patient's head should be put in a proper position to facilitate cerebellar detaching from the petrous bone with its gravity and without the use of retractors. Since the operation should be performed with a supralateral cerebellar approach, the craniotomy should be opened close to the transverse-sigmoid sinus junction. Through this, the shortest surgical trajectory can be obtained.

3.2.3 Intradural Procedure

During the supralateral cerebellar approach, it is inevitable to encounter the petrosal vein, even though there are many variations. Petrosal veins should be saved as much as possible. There is an opinion that there is no problem with the sacrifice of the petrosal vein, but there have been reports of cerebellar infarction or hemorrhage after petrosal vein damage.

The cranial nerves of the skull base travel through the arachnoid cistern, and the opening of this cistern is crucial. The root entry zone of the trigeminal nerve should be approached after microdissection of the arachnoid and slow suction of the CSF. Opening cerebellar fissures allows the root entry zone to be seen more directly. Careful dissection of the surrounding arachnoid membrane can reduce nerve manipulation and reduce damage. To reduce CSF leakage and postoperative infection, the surgical field should be irrigated thoroughly, before dural closure and the dura must be sutured in a watertight fashion.

Previous studies have shown that MVD is associated with low mortality and morbidity rates. However, this is mostly a result of specialized centers, and many MVD procedures are performed outside such centers. Morbidity rates are significantly lower at high-volume hospitals and with high-volume surgeons [32]. Recently, efforts are being made to further reduce complications by using a wide variety of modalities such as endoscopic surgery or augmented reality. In the future, it is expected that MVD surgery will be further developed and will go in the direction of upward leveling.

4 Conclusion

After Jannetta's procedure was introduced, the current MVD surgery was developed through various changes by many pioneers. However, even now, after MVD surgery in TN patients, various complications can occur. We have to be aware of this and always be careful. Neurosurgeons need to refine the standard procedure in order to lower the complications.

References

1. Jannetta PJ, Rand RW. Transtentorial retrogasserian rhizotomy in trigeminal neuralgia by microneurosurgical technique. Bull Los Angel Neurol Soc. 1966;31(3):93–9.
2. Jannetta PJ. Arterial compression of the trigeminal nerve at the pons in patients with trigeminal neuralgia. J Neurosurg. 1967;26(1):Suppl: 159–62.
3. McLaughlin MR, et al. Microvascular decompression of cranial nerves: lessons learned after 4400 operations. J Neurosurg. 1999;90(1):1–8.
4. Jannetta PJ, McLaughlin MR, Casey KF. Technique of microvascular decompression. Technical note. Neurosurg Focus. 2005;18(5):E5.
5. Lee MH, Lee JA, Park K. Different roles of microvascular decompression in Hemifacial spasm and trigeminal neuralgia. J Neurol Surg B Skull Base. 2019;80(5):511–7.
6. Sindou M, et al. Treatment of trigeminal neuralgia with microvascular decompression. Neurochirurgie. 2009;55(2):185–96.
7. Sindou M, et al. Microvascular decompression for primary trigeminal neuralgia: long-term effectiveness and prognostic factors in a series of 362 consecutive patients with clear-cut neurovascular conflicts who underwent pure decompression. J Neurosurg. 2007;107(6):1144–53.
8. Cohen-Gadol AA. Microvascular decompression surgery for trigeminal neuralgia and hemifacial spasm: naunces of the technique based on experiences with 100 patients and review of the literature. Clin Neurol Neurosurg. 2011;113(10):844–53.
9. Wang P, et al. Complete neuroendoscopic versus microscopical trigeminal neuralgia microvascular decompression (MVD) in primary trigeminal neuralgia (PTN). Am J Transl Res. 2021;13(11):12905–12.
10. Singh D, et al. Microvascular decompression for trigeminal neuralgia: experience of a tertiary Care Center in India and a brief review of literature. Neurol India. 2021;69(Supplement):S206–s212.
11. Herta J, et al. Microvascular decompression in trigeminal neuralgia: predictors of pain relief, complication avoidance, and lessons learned. Acta Neurochir. 2021;163(12):3321–36.
12. Pressman E, et al. Teflon versus Ivalon in microvascular decompression for trigeminal neuralgia: a 2-center 10-year comparison. World Neurosurg. 2021;146:e822–8.
13. Mizobuchi Y, et al. Microvascular decompression for trigeminal neuralgia: a prospective, Multicenter Study. Neurosurgery. 2021;89(4):557–64.
14. Inoue T, et al. Microvascular decompression for trigeminal neuralgia attributable to the vertebrobasilar artery: decompression technique and significance of separation from the nerve root. Acta Neurochir. 2021;163(4):1037–43.
15. Tomasello F, et al. A novel technical refinement of microvascular decompression: pain relief and complication rate in a consecutive series of patients with trigeminal neuralgia. Oper Neurosurg (Hagerstown). 2020;19(3):226–33.
16. Li L, et al. Microvascular decompression versus stereotactic radiosurgery for trigeminal neuralgia: a single-institution experience. World Neurosurg. 2020;143:e400–8.
17. Bick SK, et al. Older patients have better pain outcomes following microvascular decompression for trigeminal neuralgia. Neurosurgery. 2019;84(1):116–22.
18. Mastronardi L, et al. Typical trigeminal neuralgia: comparison of results between patients older and younger than 65 years operated on with microvascular

decompression by Retrosigmoid approach. J Neurol Surg A Cent Eur Neurosurg. 2020;81(1):28–32.
19. Zhao Y, et al. Microvascular decompression for trigeminal neuralgia due to venous compression alone. J Craniofac Surg. 2018;29(1):178–81.
20. Wu M, et al. Microvascular decompression for classical trigeminal neuralgia caused by venous compression: novel anatomic classifications and surgical strategy. World Neurosurg. 2018;113:e707–13.
21. Xiang H, et al. Prospective study of Neuroendoscopy versus microscopy: 213 cases of microvascular decompression for trigeminal neuralgia performed by one neurosurgeon. World Neurosurg. 2018;111:e335–9.
22. Wei Y, et al. Long-term therapeutic effect of microvascular decompression for trigeminal neuralgia: Kaplan-Meier analysis in a consecutive series of 425 patients. Turk Neurosurg. 2018:28(1):88–93.
23. Xia L, et al. Effectiveness and safety of microvascular decompression surgery for treatment of trigeminal neuralgia: a systematic review. J Craniofac Surg. 2014;25(4):1413–7.
24. Schiariti M, et al. Two alternative dural sealing techniques in posterior fossa surgery: (Polylactide-co-glycolide) self-adhesive resorbable membrane versus polyethylene glycol hydrogel. Surg Neurol Int. 2014;5:171.
25. Jito J, Nitta N, Nozaki K. Delayed cerebrospinal fluid leak after watertight dural closure with a polyethylene glycol hydrogel dural sealant in posterior fossa surgery: case report. Neurol Med Chir (Tokyo). 2014;54(8):634–9.
26. Park JS, et al. Intraoperative management to prevent cerebrospinal fluid leakage after microvascular decompression: dural closure with a "plugging muscle" method. Neurosurg Rev. 2007;30(2):139–42; discussion 142.
27. Lee MH, et al. Cerebellar retraction and hearing loss after microvascular decompression for hemifacial spasm. Acta Neurochir. 2015;157(2):337–43.
28. Panesar SS, et al. Patient-specific 3-dimensionally printed models for neurosurgical planning and education. Neurosurg Focus. 2019;47(6):E12.
29. Christiano LD, et al. Microvascular decompression for trigeminal neuralgia: visualization of results in a 3D stereoscopic virtual reality environment. Minim Invasive Neurosurg. 2011;54(1):12–5.
30. Yao S, et al. Multimodal image-based virtual reality Presurgical simulation and evaluation for trigeminal neuralgia and Hemifacial spasm. World Neurosurg. 2018;113:e499–507.
31. Zawy Alsofy S, et al. Virtual reality-based evaluation of neurovascular conflict for the surgical planning of microvascular decompression in trigeminal neuralgia patients. Neurosurg Rev. 2021;44(6):3309–21.
32. Kalkanis SN, et al. Microvascular decompression surgery in the United States, 1996 to 2000: mortality rates, morbidity rates, and the effects of hospital and surgeon volumes. Neurosurgery. 2003;52(6):1251–61; discussion 1261–2.

Postoperative Prognosis After Microvascular Decompression for Trigeminal Neuralgia

Jeong-A Lee and Kwan Park

Trigeminal neuralgia (TN) is a disorder characterized by severe episodes of lancinating pain in the distribution of the branches of the trigeminal nerve. The most common factor associated with the etiology of TN is vascular compression of the trigeminal nerve. For patients with refractory pain to medication, microvascular decompression (MVD) is the gold standard. In addition, stereotactic radiosurgery (SRS) and percutaneous procedures such as glycerol rhizotomy, radiofrequency rhizotomy (RF), and balloon compression are available [1, 2]. This chapter aims to investigate clinical outcomes and predictors of outcomes after MVD in patients with TN, and to compare the outcomes with other treatments through a literature review. And we introduce a study to compare the prognosis of primary MVD with that of subsequent MVD and to provide the prognosis of redo MVD in TN patients.

J.-A. Lee
Department of Neurosurgery, Samsung Medical Center, Sungkyunkwan University School of Medicine, Seoul, Republic of Korea
e-mail: jalee@skku.edu

K. Park (✉)
Department of Neurosurgery, Konkuk University Medical Center, Konkuk University School of Medicine, Seoul, Republic of Korea
e-mail: 20200454@kuh.ac.kr

1 Pain Outcomes After Microvascular Decompression

A systematic review of 26 papers with 6847 patients indexed on PubMed between 2000 and 2013 found that 83.5% (79.6–89.1) of patients were completely pain-free postoperatively. The average follow-up period was 35.8 months (26.2–56.6) [3]. In a prospective, multicenter study of 166 patients enrolled from 2012 to 2015, complete pain relief at 7 days and 3 years after surgery was 78.9% and 80.0%, respectively. Of patients, 155 patients (93.4%) completed a 3-year follow-up [4]. In our unpublished data, all 317 consecutive TN patients underwent MVD from February 1998 to October 2016. The patients were followed up for a mean 62.3 months (median 48.2, range 0.4–273.5). At the last follow-up, the rate of complete pain-free without medication (Barrow Neurological Institute (BNI) pain intensity score of I) was 66.6%. Although MVD for TN is an effective treatment, MVD-treated TN had a risk of recurrence. Of the 181 TN patients treated with MVD, 43 had a BNI score worse than III and 12 were worsened to a BNI score of IV [5].

In addition to pain relief, MVD for TN significantly improved depression and anxiety and relieved the patient's burdens related to working ability and use of health resources [6, 7]. However, in a study using the Patient's Subjective Assessment of Treatment Effectiveness Scale

K. Park, K. R. Cho (eds.), *Trigeminal Neuralgia*, https://doi.org/10.1007/978-981-19-9171-4_16

(PSATES), pain relief was completed in most TN patients, but none of the patients rated the MVD as "excellent," with only 16.1% of the patients rated it as "good." Thus, regardless of the pain outcome after MVD, time and psychological support are needed for social adjustment due to changes in social status [8].

2 Prognostic Factors for Outcome of Microvascular Decompression

Our previous study included 141 patients with a mean follow-up 26.3 months (6 months-10 years). A high degree of intraoperative neurovascular conflict, single arterial offending vessel during surgery, and positive findings on preoperative magnetic resonance imaging (MRI) were good prognostic factor for MVD in TN [9]. In a retrospective case series including 124 patients with an average follow-up period of 42.4 months, older age, male, and preoperative drug responsiveness were correlated with low long-term pain scores, and V2 branch involvement with high long-term pain scores [10]. A prospective, systematic study of 59 patients who completed 1-year follow-up found that neurovascular contact with morphological changes on preoperative 3.0 Tesla MRI and male were better prognostic factors for MVD outcome [11]. In the data analyzed for 3897 patients from 46 studies, the predictors of pain-free were less than 5 years of disease duration, arterial compression, superior cerebellar artery (SCA) involvement, and type 1 Burchiel classification [12].

For further investigation, prognostic factors for the outcome of MVD in TN were randomly grouped into three factors: patient-related factors, disease-related factors, and surgery-related factors (Fig. 1).

2.1 Patient-Related Factors

2.1.1 Age

Pain relief rates after MVD were similar between older (≥70 years) and younger (<70 years) TN patients. Despite the high prevalence of comorbidities in older patients, MVD-related complications did not differ from those in younger patients [13]. Clinical outcomes in young-onset TN patients <30 years of age were similar to those in older patients [14].

2.1.2 Brain Structure

In TN patients who underwent MVD surgery, trigeminal nerve, hippocampal volume, and thalamic structure on preoperative MRI were associated with surgical response [15, 16]. The thalamus is an essential element of the trigeminal sensory pathway. In addition to the structure of the thalamus, metabolic changes after surgery in the thalamus had an effect on postoperative pain relief [16].

2.2 Disease-Related Factors

2.2.1 Coexistence with Ipsilateral HFS or Contralateral TN

Tic convulsif (TC) is characterized by the coexistence of TN and ipsilateral hemifacial spasm

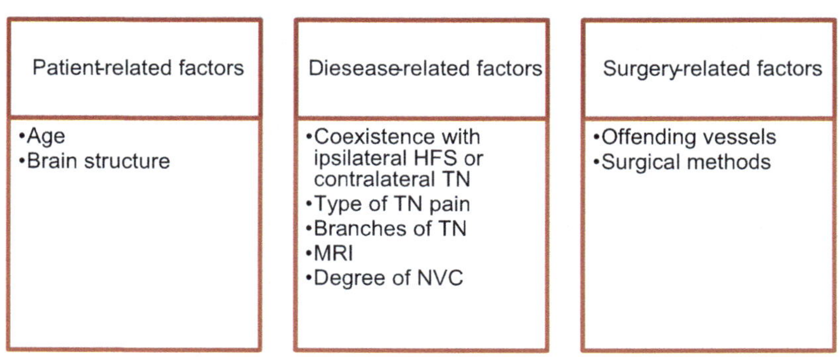

Fig. 1 Prognostic factors. *HFS* hemifacial spasm; *MRI* magnetic resonance imaging; *NVC* neurovascular compression; *TN* trigeminal neuralgia

(HFS) and is rare. In an analysis of 192 patients with TC, the cure rate for MVD was >80%. The involvement of anterior inferior cerebellar artery (AICA) or posterior inferior cerebellar artery and older age predicted successful prognosis and recurrence after surgery, respectively [17]. Bilateral TN is also rare. Of the 13 bilateral TN patients treated with MVD, 11 and 2 patients showed postoperative excellent and good outcomes on the operated side, respectively. In 3 patients, the contralateral symptom also improved, and out of 10 patients who did not improve, 9 patients who underwent MVD on the opposite side improved [18].

2.2.2 Type of TN Pain

The presence of mechanical allodynia (MA; trigger point) and the type of TN pain (shock-like or constant) were significant predictors of outcome after MVD for TN. MA was not only an independent predictor of surgical outcome but also a significant predictor of the presence of neurovascular compression (NVC) and low recurrence rates after surgery [19].

2.2.3 Branches of TN

On a comparative analysis of remission rates at 1 day and 3 years after MVD according to branches of TN, the results were as follows: V1 division, 100% and 100%; V1–2 division, 93.5% and 67.7%; V1–3 division, 91.7% and 66.7%; V2 division, 88.4% and 69.8%; V2–3 division, 90.2% and 75.6%; and V3 division, 100% and 92.9%. Postoperative prognosis for TN without V2 branch (V1 and V3) was better than that with V2 branch (V2, V1–2, V2–3, and V1–3) [20].

2.2.4 Magnetic Resonance Imaging (MRI)

Studies on the following preoperative imaging tools in TN have reported that they improved post-MVD outcome prediction performance: T2 VISTA and FLAIR VISTA fusion imaging, trigeminal nerve diffusion tensor imaging (DTI), contrast-enhanced CISS imaging, three-dimensional high-resolution MRI with DRIVE sequences, and balanced Steady State Free Precession (b-SSFP) sequences and the newly developed Fast-Spin-Echo (FSE)-sequences in combination with Time-of-Flight (TOF) angiography [21–25]. The changes in DTI revealed microstructural alteration of the trigeminal nerve in TN without NVC and showed a correlation with the prognosis of patients after internal neurolysis [26]. On the other hand, since the efficacy of MVD on TN cannot be perfectly predicted by MRI yet, some suggested that the decision to MVD should be based on the typical symptoms of TN rather than the evidence of vascular compression by preoperative MRI [27, 28].

2.2.5 Degree of Neurovascular Compression

NVC on preoperative MRI prior to MVD for TN was graded according to its presence and severity. Patients with severe NVC on preoperative MRI were more than six times more likely to be pain-free without medication after MVD compared to those without severe NVC [29].

2.3 Surgery-Related Factors

2.3.1 Offending Vessels

The usual offending vessels in TN are SCA or AICA. Studies have been focused on rare offending vessels such as vertebrobasilar artery (VBA) or venous compression. In a case series review, 19 of 23 (83%) patients with VBA-compressed TN treated with MVD were pain-free after surgery. An additional 3 patients (13%) were pain-free within 3 months and the success rate was 96%. Three patients (13%) experienced pain recurrence [30]. In a systematic review and meta-analysis of 9 studies, the overall proportion of VBA-compressed TN among MVD was 3.4%. Of these, 96% were pain-free immediately after surgery, and 93% experienced pain relief with BNI pain intensity score of I–II at the last follow-up [31]. MVD in TN due to VBA compression showed good results, but further studies on long-term outcomes are needed. MVD surgery of TN by vertebrobasilar dolichoectasia, which is the elongation and dilatation of the vertebral and basilar arteries, also showed excellent surgical outcomes [32].

On the other hand, among 121 patients with MVD for TN, venous compression alone and arterial and venous compression were reported in 4% and 22%, respectively. The surgical cure rates of venous compression alone and arterial and venous compression were 60% and 92%, respectively and the recurrence rates were 20% and 12%, respectively. Venous compression was correlated with a bad prognosis [33]. In a systematic review and meta-analysis of 24 studies with 330 patients with purely venous compression, 76% of patients were pain-free with an average follow-up of 38 months after MVD and 23% of patients recurred at an average follow-up of 51.4 months. Pain control rates after MVD in patients with purely venous compression were similar to those with arterial compression, but recurrence rates were higher [34]. Both short-term and long-term outcomes were worse in venous compression compared with arterial compression and the delayed cure rate was higher in venous compression [35].

When NVC is absent, internal neurolysis (nerve combing), which is a surgical technique to separate the fascicles of the trigeminal nerve, can be used. The postoperative outcomes showed a BNI pain intensity score of I for 50% with a mean follow-up of 20 months (range 3–40). Six patients (19%) experienced pain recurrence [36].

2.3.2 Surgical Methods

Endoscopic surgery, which has revolutionized the ventral skull base, was adopted for use in the cerebellopontine angle. Pain outcomes and complication rates between the endoscopic MVD (E-MVD) and microscopic MVD (M-MVD) for TN were similar, but the rate of headaches 1 month after the E-MVD was significantly lower [37]. In a systematic review and comparative meta-analysis, pain relief was also similar between E-MVD and M-MVD for TN. However, the incidence of complications such as facial palsy and hearing loss were lower in E-MVD. Although the advantages of E-MVD should be exploited, the authors recommended caution in interpreting these data [38].

Tentorial sling technique for MVD in patients with TN was introduced as an alternative method for traditional MVD. The technique uses a sling to transpose the compressive vessel away from the nerve without the use of foreign material. Although the clinical outcomes were similar to the historical outcomes, additional data are needed to evaluate the long-term durability of this method [39].

For patients who are not suitable to undergo pure MVD, MVD combined with partial sensory rhizotomy (MVD + PSR) can be used as an alternative for TN. If MVD + PSR was performed, 1/3–2/3 of the trigeminal sensory root was cut. There was no significant difference in long-term outcomes between the pure MVD and MVD + PSR groups [40].

In MVD for TN, a conventional lateral supracerebellar approach can be difficult to expose and decompress the entire trigeminal nerve due to blockage of the superior petrosal vein complex, cerebellum, and vestibulocochlear nerve. Suprafloccular approach via the petrosal fissure and venous corridors for MVD was used as a substitute for the conventional route used to treat TN. This approach reported a high cure rate and a low complication rate [41].

2.4 Models

A predictive pain-free scoring system was constructed based on preoperative clinical and radiographic factors (Table 1). Patients with type 1 Burchiel classification and severe NVC had the best long-term pain-free outcome [42]. Another preoperative TN scoring system to predict long-term pain relief following MVD was as follows (Table 2). Classical TN type, positive response to ox/carbamazepine, and presence and nature of NVC on MRI predicted pain-free status [43]. A prognostic nomogram for MVD-

Table 1 Predictive pain-free scoring system

Characteristics		Points
TN type	TN2	0
	TN1	1
Offending vessel	No	0
	Vein or artery	1
Compression severity[a]	No vessel or grade I	0
	Grade II or III	1
Total score		0–3

TN trigeminal neuralgia
Higher scores predicted better pain relief than lower scores
[a]Grade I, vessel not touching the nerve; grade II, compression; grade III, distortion TN2, Type 2 Burchiel classification; TN1, Type 1 Burchiel classification

treated TN was established based on a retrospective cohort study of 1054 patients with TN. This nomogram was developed to predict a 3-year overall remission rate after MVD treatment of TN (Fig. 2) [44].

Clinical factors correspond to specific points by drawing a straight line upward to the 'points' axis. After the sum of the points is located on the 'total points' axis, the sum represents the probabilityof a 3-year remission rate by drawing straight downward to the 'remission rate at 3 years' axis.

Table 2 TN scoring system to predict pain relief

Characteristics		Points
TN type[a]	All other forms	0
	Classical TN	1
Response to ox/carbamazepine	No response	0
	Complete or partial resolution	1
Neurovascular contact	Venous contact or absent NVC	1
	Arterial contact; the vessel touching but not indenting the surface of the nerve	2
	Arterial deformity; any indentation/deformity of the surface of the trigeminal nerve	3
Total score		1–5

NVC neurovascular compression, *TN* trigeminal neuralgia
Higher scores predicted long-term pain-free status without medications following MVD
[a]Criteria established by the International Headache Society, the International Association for the Study of Pain, and the European Academy of Neurology

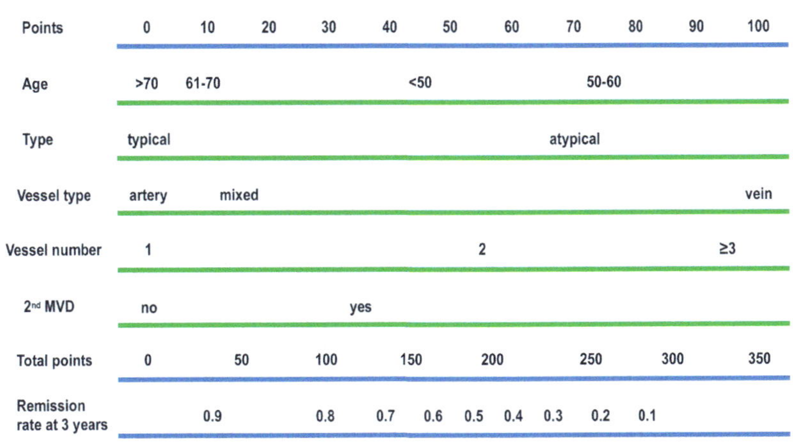

Fig. 2 Prognostic nomogram. *MVD* microvascular decompression

3 Microvascular Decompression Versus Other Treatments

3.1 Versus Radiofrequency Rhizotomy

Nine studies involving 2163 patients in patients with TN were reviewed. Compared to RF group, MVD group had a lower risk of requiring a secondary procedure and postoperative facial numbness, although there was no significant difference in postoperative drug use. The total cost of MVD was higher than that of RF. The authors suggested that RF could be considered in patients who are not suitable for MVD or refused invasive treatment [48].

3.2 Versus Stereotactic Radiosurgery

A prospective comparison of long-term pain relief rates after MVD and SRS for TN was studied. The mean follow-up periods for MVD and SRS groups were 59 ± 35 months and 59 ± 45 months, respectively and approximately 38% of patients who underwent MVD or SRS had >5 years of follow-up. Compared to those who underwent SRS, patients who received MVD were younger. The rates of pain-free at <3 months, 1, 5, and 10 years after MVD were 96%, 83%, 61%, and 44%, and the corresponding rates after SRS were 75%, 71%, 47%, and 27%, respectively. The median time to pain recurrence was 94 months for MVD and 53 months for SRS. The authors proposed that these results can help physicians counsel patients with TN on treatment selection, although surgical decision-making depends upon many factors [49]. In another study, patients who received MVD had a longer duration of pain-free than those who received SRS but adverse events were fewer after SRS. The researchers also proposed that treatment selection can be tailored to the patients' condition and wishes [50].

3.3 Versus Percutaneous Balloon Compression

One study evaluated the surgical outcomes of percutaneous balloon compression (PBC) and MVD in the treatment of elderly patients with TN. The pain relief rate was 90% and 87% after PBC and MVD, respectively ($P > 0.05$). The recurrence rates were also similar between the groups. The postoperative complication rates related to masticatory muscle weakness and facial numbness in the PBC group were higher than MVD group ($P < 0.05$) [51].

3.4 Versus Percutaneous Thermocoagulation

The study compared the surgical outcomes of patients with percutaneous thermocoagulation (PT) with those with MVD. Compared to the MVD group, the mean age of patients was older and comorbidity was higher in the PT group. Neurovascular conflict was identified in 78 (98.7%) MVD and 17 (43.6%) PT patients on preoperative MRI. The BNI pain intensity score at the last follow-up was higher and the mean pain-free survival was shorter after PT than MVD. The facial hypesthesia rate was higher in the PT group [52].

4 Primary Microvascular Decompression Versus Subsequent Microvascular Decompression

Researchers compared the surgical outcomes of patients receiving MVD as an initial intervention (primary MVD) with those receiving MVD as an intervention following other surgeries (subsequent MVD). Patients who underwent subsequent MVD had older age and longer duration of symptoms than patients who underwent primary MVD. Patients who underwent subsequent MVD experienced less pain relief and a higher incidence of facial numbness despite rates of complications similar to patients who underwent primary MVD [45].

In a meta-analysis, patients who received MVD after failed gamma knife surgery (GKS) showed better complete pain relief at 1 year, despite similar adequate pain relief at 1 year, postoperative facial numbness, and retreatment rates compared to repeat GKS [46]. A prospective comparison study had ≥1 year of follow-up. Patients who received MVD after failed GKS also had a longer duration of favorable outcome compared to those who received repeat GKS, although the risk of facial numbness was higher in patients with prior GKS than in patients without prior GKS [47].

5 Redo Microvascular Decompression

For recurrent TN patients, redo MVD can achieve good outcomes. For redo MVD in patients with recurrent TN, the postoperative follow-up period was 63–167 months. Of 127 patients, the postoperative BNI pain intensity score was excellent for 69 patients (53%) and good for 46 patients (36%). During the follow-up, no recurrence was noted. All complications were improved [53]. Reasons for 63 cases with redo MVD were divided into arterial compression (13 patients, 21%), venous compression (11 patients, 17%), prosthesis-related (25 patients, 40%), and adhesion or negative exploration (14 patients, 22%) [54]. Significant factors for surgical success were older age and direct absence of pain after redo MVD [55]. Negative finding at exploration during reoperation and no postoperative pain relief after the initial surgery influenced success rates negatively after redo MVD [56].

References

1. Bick SKB, Eskandar EN. Surgical treatment of trigeminal neuralgia. Neurosurg Clin N Am. 2017;28(3):429–38.
2. Jones MR, Urits I, Ehrhardt KP, Cefalu JN, Kendrick JB, Park DJ, Cornett EM, Kaye AD, Viswanath O. A comprehensive review of trigeminal neuralgia. Curr Pain Headache Rep. 2019;23(10):74.
3. Xia L, Zhong J, Zhu J, Wang YN, Dou NN, Liu MX, Visocchi M, Li ST. Effectiveness and safety of microvascular decompression surgery for treatment of trigeminal neuralgia: a systematic review. J Craniofac Surg. 2014;25(4):1413–7.
4. Mizobuchi Y, et al. Microvascular decompression for trigeminal neuralgia: a prospective, multicenter study. Neurosurgery. 2021;89(4):557–64.
5. Lee MH, Lee JA, Park K. Different roles of microvascular decompression in hemifacial spasm and trigeminal neuralgia. J Neurol Surg B Skull Base. 2019;80(5):511–7.
6. Cheng J, Long J, Hui X, Lei D, Zhang H. Effects of microvascular decompression on depression and anxiety in trigeminal neuralgia: a prospective cohort study focused on risk factors and prognosis. Clin Neurol Neurosurg. 2017;161:59–64.
7. Obermueller K, Shiban E, Obermueller T, Meyer B, Lehmberg J. Working ability and use of healthcare resources for patients with trigeminal neuralgia treated via microvascular decompression. Acta Neurochir. 2018;160(12):2521–7.
8. Moisak GI, Amelina EV, Zubok NA, Rzaev JA. Psychological status before and after surgery in patients with trigeminal neuralgia. Clin Neurol Neurosurg. 2021;203:106578.
9. Jo KW, Kong DS, Hong KS, Lee JA, Park K. Long-term prognostic factors for microvascular decompression for trigeminal neuralgia. J Clin Neurosci. 2013;20(3):440–5.
10. Bick SK, Huie D, Sneh G, Eskandar EN. Older patients have better pain outcomes following microvascular decompression for trigeminal neuralgia. Neurosurgery. 2019;84(1):116–22.
11. Heinskou TB, Rochat P, Maarbjerg S, Wolfram F, Brennum J, Olesen J, Bendtsen L. Prognostic factors for outcome of microvascular decompression in trigeminal neuralgia: a prospective systematic study using independent assessors. Cephalalgia. 2019;39(2):197–208.
12. Holste K, Chan AY, Rolston JD, Englot DJ. Pain outcomes following microvascular decompression for drug-resistant trigeminal neuralgia: a systematic review and meta-analysis. Neurosurgery. 2020;86(2):182–90.
13. Greve T, Tonn JC, Mehrkens JH. Microvascular decompression for trigeminal neuralgia in the elderly: efficacy and safety. J Neurol. 2021;268(2):532–40.
14. Yu F, Yin J. Young-onset trigeminal neuralgia: a clinical study and literature review. Acta Neurochir. 2021;163(6):1617–21.
15. Danyluk H, Lee EK, Wong S, Sajida S, Broad R, Wheatley M, Elliott C, Sankar T. Hippocampal and trigeminal nerve volume predict outcome of surgical treatment for trigeminal neuralgia. Cephalalgia. 2020;40(6):586–96.
16. Danyluk H, Andrews J, Kesarwani R, Seres P, Broad R, Wheatley BM, Sankar T. The thalamus in trigemi-

nal neuralgia: structural and metabolic abnormalities, and influence on surgical response. BMC Neurol. 2021;21(1):290.
17. Yin Z, Liu Y, Bai Y, Zhang H, Yao W, Yu F, Zhang J, Liu R, Yang A. The epidemiology, cause, and prognosis of painful tic convulsif syndrome: an individual patient data analysis of 192 cases. World Neurosurg. 2021;147:e130–47.
18. Zhao H, Wang XH, Zhang Y, Zhang X, Tang YD, Zhou P, Zhu J, Li ST. Management of primary bilateral trigeminal neuralgia with microvascular decompression: 13-case series. World Neurosurg. 2018;109:e724–30.
19. Liao C, Zhang W, Yang M, Zhong W, Liu P, Li S. Microvascular decompression for trigeminal neuralgia: the role of mechanical allodynia. World Neurosurg. 2016;91:468–72.
20. Zhang WB, Min LZ, Tao BB, Sun QY, Li ST, Wang XQ. Prognosis comparison of different branches of trigeminal neuralgia. World Neurosurg. 2020;133:e1–5.
21. Hung PSP, Chen DQ, Davis KD, Zhong J, Hodaie M. Predicting pain relief: use of pre-surgical trigeminal nerve diffusion metrics in trigeminal neuralgia. Neuroimage Clin. 2017;15:710–8.
22. Blitz AM, Northcutt B, Shin J, Aygun N, Herzka DA, Theodros D, Goodwin CR, Lim M, Seeburg DP. Contrast-enhanced CISS imaging for evaluation of neurovascular compression in trigeminal neuralgia: improved correlation with symptoms and prediction of surgical outcomes. Am J Neuroradiol. 2018;39(9):1724–32.
23. Cha J, Kim ST, Kim HJ, Choi JW, Kim HJ, Jeon P, Kim KH, Byun HS, Park K. Trigeminal neuralgia: assessment with T2 VISTA and FLAIR VISTA fusion imaging. Eur Radiol. 2011;21(12):2633–9.
24. Ruiz-Juretschke F, Guzmán-de-Villoria JG, García-Leal R, Sañudo JR. Predictive value of magnetic resonance for identifying neurovascular compressions in trigeminal neuralgia. Neurologia (Engl Ed). 2019;34(8):510–9.
25. Müller S, Khadhraoui E, Khanafer A, Psychogios M, Rohde V, Tanrikulu L. Differentiation of arterial and venous neurovascular conflicts estimates the clinical outcome after microvascular decompression in trigeminal neuralgia. BMC Neurol. 2020;20(1):279.
26. Wu M, Qiu J, Jiang X, Li M, Wang SD, Dong Q, Fu X, Niu C. Diffusion tensor imaging reveals microstructural alteration of the trigeminal nerve root in classical trigeminal neuralgia without neurovascular compression and correlation with outcome after internal neurolysis. Magn Reson Imaging. 2020;71:37–44.
27. Wei SC, Yu R, Meng Q, Qu C. Efficacy of microvascular decompression in patients with trigeminal neuralgia with negative neurovascular relationship shown by magnetic resonance tomography. Clin Neurol Neurosurg. 2020;197:106063.
28. Mooney J, Erickson N, Pittman B, Agee BS, Guthrie BL. The use of MRI in preoperative decision-making for trigeminal neuralgia: a single-center study. World Neurosurg. 2021;146:e651–7.
29. Hughes MA, Jani RH, Fakhran S, Chang YF, Branstetter BF, Thirumala PD, Sekula RF. Significance of degree of neurovascular compression in surgery for trigeminal neuralgia. J Neurosurg. 2019:1–6.
30. Wang X, Wang H, Chen S, Liang H, Wang H, Xu M, Xu L. The long-term clinical outcomes of microvascular decompression for treatment of trigeminal neuralgia compressed by the vertebra-basilar artery: a case series review. BMC Neurol. 2019;19(1):217.
31. Carlo DTD, Benedetto N, Marani W, Montemurro N, Perrini P. Microvascular decompression for trigeminal neuralgia due to vertebrobasilar artery compression: a systematic review and meta-analysis. Neurosurg Rev. 2021;45:285. https://doi.org/10.1007/s10143-021-01606-1.
32. Sun S, Jiang W, Wang J, Gao P, Zhang X, Jiao L, Liu W, Shu K, Lei T. Clinical analysis and surgical treatment of trigeminal neuralgia caused by vertebrobasilar dolichoectasia: a retrospective study. Int J Surg. 2017;41:183–9.
33. Toda H, Iwasaki K, Yoshimoto N, Miki Y, Hashikata H, Goto M, Nishida N. Bridging veins and veins of the brainstem in microvascular decompression surgery for trigeminal neuralgia and hemifacial spasm. Neurosurg Focus. 2018;45(1):E2.
34. Soni P, Potter T, Soni PP, Estemalik E, Recinos PF, Kshettry VR. Outcomes of microvascular decompression for trigeminal neuralgia with purely venous compression: a systematic review and meta-analysis. Clin Neurol Neurosurg. 2020;198:106230.
35. Wang J, Niu H, Zhao K, Shu K, Lei T. Comparative analysis of trigeminal neuralgia caused by sole arterial and venous compression: clinical features and surgical outcomes from 222 cases. Front Neurol. 2021;12:634945.
36. Sabourin V, Mazza J, Garzon T, Head J, Ye D, Stefanelli A, Saiegh FA, Lavergne P, Evans J. Internal neurolysis with and without microvascular decompression for trigeminal neuralgia: case series. World Neurosurg. 2020;143:e70–7.
37. Lee JYK, Pierce JT, Sandhu SK, Petrov D, Yang AI. Endoscopic versus microscopic microvascular decompression for trigeminal neuralgia: equivalent pain outcomes with possibly decreased postoperative headache after endoscopic surgery. J Neurosurg. 2017;126(5):1676–84.
38. Zagzoog N, Attar A, Takroni R, Alotaibi MB, Reddy K. Endoscopic versus open microvascular decompression for trigeminal neuralgia: a systematic review and comparative meta-analysis. J Neurosurg. 2018:1–9.
39. Steinberg JA, Sack J, Wilson B, Weingarten D, Carter B, Khalessi A, Ben-Haim S, Alksne J. Tentorial sling for microvascular decompression in patients with trigeminal neuralgia: a description of operative technique and clinical outcomes. J Neurosurg. 2018:1–6.
40. Liu R, Deng Z, Zhang L, Liu Y, Wang Z, Yu Y. The long-term outcomes and predictors of microvascular decompression with or without partial sensory rhizotomy for trigeminal neuralgia. J Pain Res. 2020;13:301–12.

41. Wang H, Ying X, Yu WH, Zhu Q, Dong XQ, Sheng YF, Wang D. Suprafloccular approach via the petrosal fissure and venous corridors for microvascular decompression of the trigeminal nerve: technique notes and clinical outcomes. J Neurosurg. 2018;129(2):324–33.
42. Hardaway FA, Gustafsson HC, Holste K, Burchiel KJ, Raslan AM. A novel scoring system as a preoperative predictor for pain-free survival after microsurgery for trigeminal neuralgia. J Neurosurg. 2019:1–8.
43. Panczykowski DM, Jani RH, Hughes MA, Sekula RF. Development and evaluation of a preoperative trigeminal neuralgia scoring system to predict long-term outcome following microvascular decompression. Neurosurgery. 2020;87(1):71–9.
44. Zhang WB, Zeng YY, Chang BW, Min LZ, Sun QY, Li B, Tao BB, Wang XQ. Prognostic nomogram for microvascular decompression-treated trigeminal neuralgia. Neurosurg Rev. 2021;44(1):571–7.
45. Theodros D, et al. Efficacy of primary microvascular decompression versus subsequent microvascular decompression for trigeminal neuralgia. J Neurosurg. 2017;126(5):1691–7.
46. Patra DP, Savardekar AR, Dossani RH, Narayan V, Mohammed N, Nanda A. Repeat gamma knife radiosurgery versus microvascular decompression following failure of GKRS in trigeminal neuralgia: a systematic review and meta-analysis. J Neurosurg. 2018:1–10.
47. Raygor KP, Wang DD, Ward MM, Barbaro NM, Chang EF. Long-term pain outcomes for recurrent idiopathic trigeminal neuralgia after stereotactic radiosurgery: a prospective comparison of first-time microvascular decompression and repeat stereotactic radiosurgery. J Neurosurg. 2018:1–9.
48. Li Y, Yang L, Ni J, Dou Z. Microvascular decompression and radiofrequency for the treatment of trigeminal neuralgia: a meta-analysis. J Pain Res. 2019;12:1937–45.
49. Wang DD, Raygor KP, Cage TA, Ward MM, Westcott S, Barbaro NM, Chang EF. Prospective comparison of long-term pain relief rates after first-time microvascular decompression and stereotactic radiosurgery for trigeminal neuralgia. J Neurosurg. 2018;128(1):68–77.
50. Raygor KP, Lee AT, Nichols N, Wang DD, Ward MM, Barbaro NM, Chang EF. Long-term pain outcomes in elderly patients with trigeminal neuralgia: comparison of first-time microvascular decompression and stereotactic radiosurgery. Neurosurg Focus. 2020;49(4):E23.
51. Ni H, Wang Y, Chen X, Gu W. Outcomes of treatment for elderly patients with trigeminal neuralgia: percutaneous balloon compression versus microvascular decompression. J Craniofac Surg. 2020;31(7):e685–8.
52. Keric N, Kalasauskas D, Kreth SL, Glaser MB, Krenzlin H, Kantelhardt SR, Ringel F. An age-dependent outcome analysis of microvascular decompression and percutaneous thermocoagulation in trigeminal neuralgia. BMC Neurol. 2021;21(1):182.
53. Liu J, Wu G, Xiang H, Liu R, Li F, Hei B, Qian W, Song H, Liu Z. Long-term retrospective analysis of microvascular decompression in patients with recurrent trigeminal neuralgia. Front Neurol. 2020;11:584224.
54. Inoue T, Shitara S, Goto Y, Prasetya M, Radcliffe L, Fukushima T. Redo surgery for trigeminal neuralgia: reasons for re-exploration and long-term outcomes. Acta Neurochir. 2021;163(9):2407–16.
55. Bakker NA, Van Dijk JM, Immenga S, Wagemakers M, Metzemaekers JD. Repeat microvascular decompression for recurrent idiopathic trigeminal neuralgia. J Neurosurg. 2014;121(4):936–9.
56. Cheng J, Meng J, Lei D, Hui X. Repeat microvascular decompression for patients with persistent or recurrent trigeminal neuralgia: prognostic factors and long-term outcomes. Medicine (Baltimore). 2019;98(18):e15167.

Redo Surgery for Failed MVD

Sang Hoon Lee, Yeon Soo Choo, and Sang Wook Joo

Trigeminal neuralgia often results in severe pain on one side of the face.

Typical case of trigeminal neuralgia shows distinct characteristic of unbearable and repetitive pain on one side of the facial trigeminal branches.

The aspect of pain is often described as electric shock and/or piercing by a sharp gimlet or knife. As time passes, the frequency of severe pain increases without silence and patients suffer in pain as long as they are awake. Daily life activities become difficult as the pain results from everyday actions such as washing face, doing makeup, brushing teeth, and eating. Most patients show teeth or oral pain thus they visit neurology or neurosurgery clinics even after their visit to a dentist. In most cases, a latent period of weeks or months or even many years may exist since the first attack of pain after that period, the pain is more severe and frequent. Because the pain is so severe, patients visit pain clinics, acupuncturists, or herbal medical clinics.

Trigeminal neuralgia is classified into two kinds.

S. H. Lee (✉) · Y. S. Choo
Department of Neurosurgery, Dongrae Bongseng Hospital, Busan, Republic of Korea

S. W. Joo
Department of Neurosurgery, Inje University School of Medicine, Pusan Paik Hospital, Busan, Republic of Korea

The first kind is classic, primary, or idiopathic. The second kind is symptomatic or secondary. In this case, intrinsic brain stem lesions (i.e., tumor, vascular lesion) are shown in the trigeminal nucleus or trigeminal tract. Most trigeminal neuralgia patients (>85%) are typical trigeminal neuralgia patients or it is imperative to differentiate from other illness with similar clinical symptoms.

Postsurgery persistent pain and recurrent pain have different definitions; however, both cases fall into failed surgery category. Recurrent pain is defined as recurrance of severe pain as like presurgery while no symptoms were shown postsurgery for a certain period of time or pain was under control with minimal medication. Persistent pain is defined as no improvement is shown or pain is worsened postsurgery. The patient loses hope and severe fear and horror may lead to panic and in severe cases, depression or suicidal impulse may occur.

Successful surgery shows No symptoms, No recurrence, and No complications after surgery. One hundred percent postsurgery results all the time is impossible thus thorough preparation and perfect surgery skill are needed. In 1985, P.J. Jannetta says "Neurosurgeons would like to be perfect and like all physicians, want our patients to do well. A failed patient is a signal that we are not perfect and that the forces of nature have again outwitted us. We can not hide these failure, avoid them or ignore them, Rather, we

K. Park, K. R. Cho (eds.), *Trigeminal Neuralgia*, https://doi.org/10.1007/978-981-19-9171-4_17

can learn from them and, frequently, can make the patients feel better or even cure them." [1].

Reasons of Failed MVD are suspected as follows [2].

1. Incomplete decompression or omission of offenders

   Often times are shown in unexperienced surgeon. It is imperative to decompress in order to find the causing blood vessel after complete dissection around the trigeminal nerve area. However, lack of experience may cause missing an offender or insufficient decompression which may cause recurrence or persistence of the symptoms.
2. Progressive elongation of vessels can cause additional vascular insult

   In this case of the aging process, offender is elongated and other parts of the nerve are compressed or in case the vein is the offender, new veins are developed and compressed again.
3. Interpositer displacement

   In this case of recurrent after short-term postsurgery, already inserted interpositer may slip due to the sudden head movement.
4. Teflon adhesion or granuloma

   It is the most often cause of recurrent pain. It is the foreign body reaction of interposition Teflon. As the adhesion fibrosis granuloma occurs between the nerve and offender, fibrotic adhesion rotates the axis of the nerve or distorts which symptoms occur due to the persistent compression.
5. Negative (Intrinsic factor)

   In this case, there is no causing blood vessel in the surgery site. There is no adherence or the axis of the nerve is normal. In this case, it is explained by the intrinsic factor of the inside of the nerve, trigeminal nerve's chronic vascular compression causes focal demyelination thus the development of ectopic neuronal pacemaker and segmental inhibitory interneuron dysfunction.

In case of recurrence or persistent pain after the surgery, medication is started again in the initial stage. Categories of drug are shown in the following table. (Table 1).

However, in most cases, drug medication shows no efficacy or side effect of the drug leading to surgical treatment.

Redosurgery is decided after the consideration of patient's age, health status, complications of the first surgery, etc. We can choose many kinds of surgery in failed cases. For resurgery, surgical methods are such as Glycerol rhizotomy, RFR, percutaneous balloon compression, gamma-knife radiosurgery, and MVD revision (Fig. 1).

MVD revision is considered preferentially because of the possibility of complete healing other than the case of old age or danger of general anesthesia, danger from other physical illness, and also patient's strong refusal.

It may be difficult to choose redosurgery because MVD revision is technically more difficult than other surgical methods and will be fatal when complications occur. Despite the difficulties, an experienced surgeon brings sufficiently satisfying results. When possible, a detailed review of the first surgery video and imaging examination such as MRI, MRA CISII, and TOF is crucial, and then carrying out the surgery is preferred.

Table 1 Medications used for trigeminal neuralgia

Drug	Level of evidence	Effect	Adverse effect	Suggested dose	Comment
Carbamazepine (the only first-line agent)	Systematic review of four randomized Controlled trials ($n = 160$)	NNT for pain relief is 19; 72 (72% of patients or 72 patients) of patient had an excellent or good response	Drowsiness, ataxia, nausea, constipation (minor); NNT3	100 mg twice a day; Increase if necessary by 50~100 mg every 3–4 days; target range 400 ~ 1000 mg/day	Dose may need to be adjusted after 3 weeks because of enzyme induction
Baclofen	One controlled trial Compared Baclofen with placebo ($n = 10$)	Seven of 10 patients improved With baclofen; 0 of 10 improved withplacebo ($P = 0.05$)	Drowsiness, hypotonia; avoid abrupt withdrawal	10 mg three times daily; increase as necessary by 10 mg/day; target dose 50–60 mg daily	May be useful in patients with multiple sclerosis when its antispasticity effects can be hamessed
Gabapentin	Five uncontrolled Studie ($n = 123$)	Good to excellent pain relief in 40% any pain relief in 53%	Drowsiness, ataxia, diarrhea (min or) NNT 2.5	300 mg once daily; increase as necessary by 300 mg every 3 days in divided doses (three times daily); target Dose 900–2400 mg daily	Widely used for trigeminal neuralgia although evidence is weak; evidence based on other types of neuropathic pains much stronger
Lamotrigine	One randomized controlled trial with lamotrigine as add on to carbamazepine or phenytoin ($n = 14$)	10 of 13 patients improved on lamotrigine; 8 of 14 improved on placebo; (NS)	Drowsiness, dizziness, constipation, nausea (no different from placebo)	300 mg twice daily; increase by 600 mg weekly; target dose 600–2400 mg daily	Evidence weak; structurally similar to carbamazepine although probably better tolerated
Oxcarbazepine	Two uncontrolled studies ($n = 21$)	Pain relief in all 21 patients	Dizziness, fatigue, rash, hyponatremia	300 mg twice daily; increase by 600 mg weekly; target dose 600–2400 mg daily	Evidence weak; structurally similar to carbamazepine although probably better tolerated
Phenytoin	Three uncontrolled studies ($n = 30$)	About 77% of patients reported some pain relief	Drowsiness, ataxia, dizziness, gum hypertrophy	300 mg a day; dose altered to achieve therapeutic plasma concentration	First drug used in the successful management of trigeminal neuralgia; little evidence but rapid dose titration and once-daily dosing are advantages

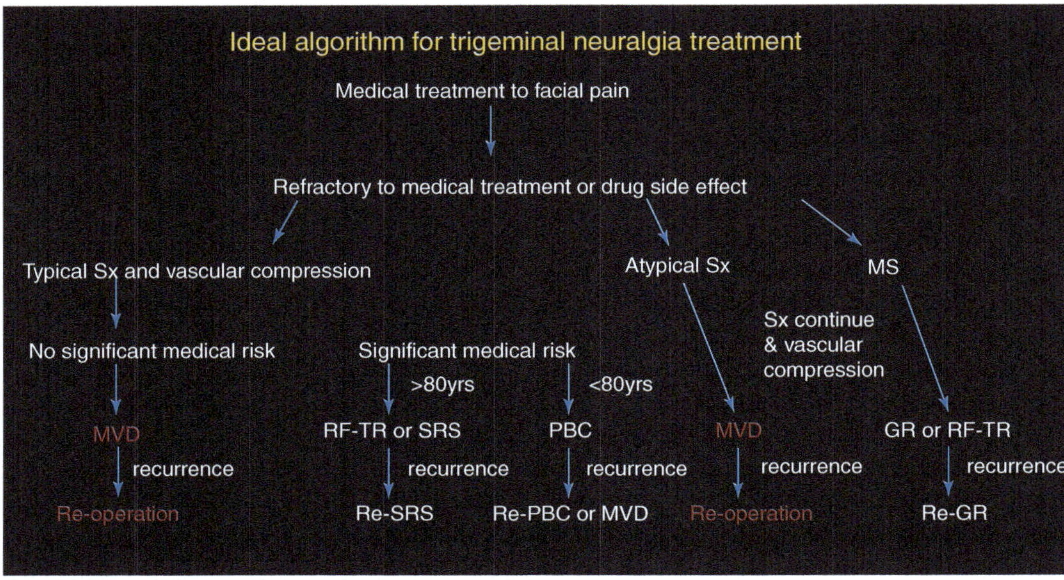

Fig. 1 Ideal algorithm, for trigeminal neuralgia treatment

1 Operative Technique

During operation, standard neuroanesthetic techniques are required, with chemically paralyzed and controlled ventilation to avoid any minimal motion in the field and prevent the patient from developing gasp reflex. IF gasp reflex occurs, massive air embolism may occur even with a small air entrainment. To detect air embolization, a Doppler precordial detector and an end-tidal carbon dioxide monitor are used because they can detect even minute amounts of air. This air embolism usually occurs frequently in sitting position but does not occur frequently in lateral decubitus position. However, this monitoring is essential to observe a small air embolism. In addition, for all neuroanesthesia, it is important to perform endotracheal intubation as smoothly as possible and not to burden the patient even after anesthesia is terminated.

Preoperative brainstem auditory evoked potentials proved baseline information for the neurophysiology team members so that they can warn the surgeon of any deviations observed during intraoperative monitoring. Deviation, such as delays or shifts in interpeak latencies of more than 1.5–2 ms, can signify potential stretch-induced injury to the eighth nerve [3]. But we keep in mind that in many patients, it may be difficult to obtain adequate responses, it may take a significant period of time to obtain a meaningful average, and there is the problem of false-negative and false-positive responses.

As in any microvascular decompression for trigeminal neuralgia, patient positioning is essential for surgical success. The patient can be positioned in the prone position, lateral decubitus position (Park-bench position), and supine position with head turned to the affected side, as well as in the sitting position. Lateral decubitus position is our preference because this position is familiar and skilled to us.

The patient is placed on the operating table such that his or her armpit is located outside the bed. This ensures the surgeon's most optimal working room during microscopic control. A three-point head fixation device is applied, and the patient is placed in the lateral decubitus position. Fix the back, chest, and pelvis with a soft pad or chest roll to minimize movement, an axillary roll is applied under armpit, and the padding is placed on other pressing points. The head is rotated slightly from the affected side and flexed, maintaining two or more finger breaths between

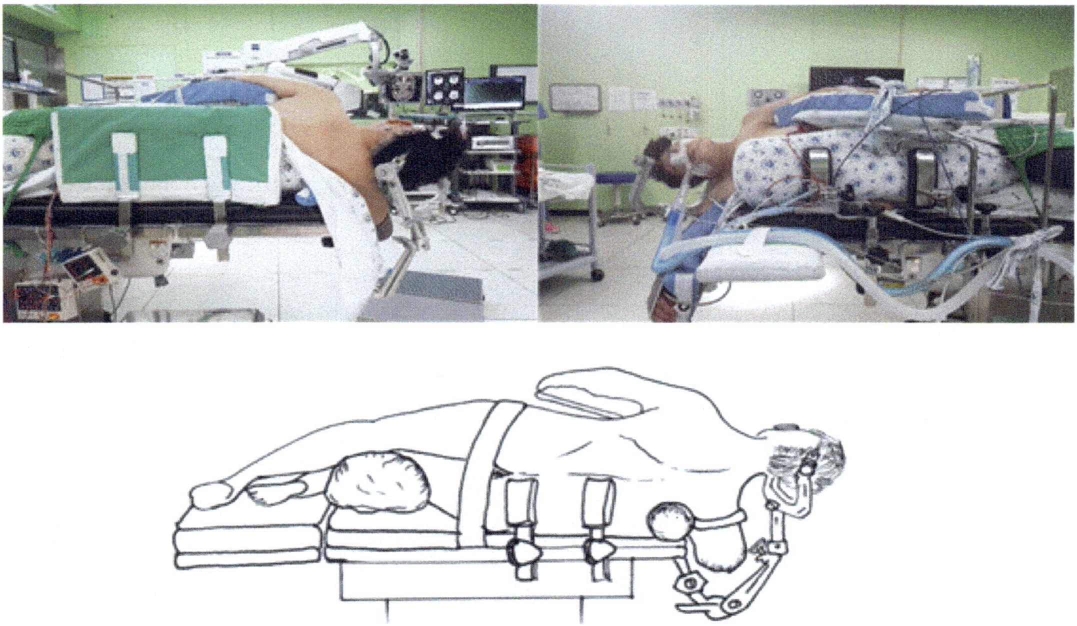

Fig. 2 The patient is placed on the operating table such that his or her armpit is located outside the bed. A three-point head fixation device is applied, and the patient is placed in the lateral decubitus position. Fix the back, chest, and pelvis with a soft pad or chest roll to minimize movement, an axillary roll applied under armpit, and the padding is placed on other pressing points. The head is rotated slightly from the affected side and flexed, maintaining two or more finger breaths between the patient's chin and sternum. Always the vertex of the head is positioned parallel to the floor, placing the seventh-eighth nerve complex at a more inferior position relative to the trigeminal nerve. The head fixation device is fastened into position and the patient's shoulder is taped caudally for maximal operating field

the patient's chin and sternum. (Depending on the case, the head can be flexed, extended, or still neutral). Always the vertex of the head is positioned parallel to the floor, placing the seventh-eighth nerve complex at a more inferior position relative to the trigeminal nerve [4]. The head fixation device is fastened into position and the patient's shoulder is taped caudally for maximal operating field (Fig. 2).

Before positioning, lumbar drain is performed if severe adhesion between cerebellar cortex and dura is expected in preoperative magnetic resonance images, or if the cerebral spinal drain is expected to be difficult in the surgical field due to lack of cistern or no brain atrophy from previous surgery.

Our standard procedure is to set up the operating microscope and the surgical assistant being located on the other side of the surgeon. The scrub nurse is positioned on the surgeon's right for left side MVD and left for right side MVD. It is to ensure that the operating team (surgeons, nurses, and assistants) is standardized in performing surgery and produce optimal results.

Bony landmarks allow us to guess the transverse sinus and sigmoid sinus, and these landmarks have mastoid eminence, digastric groove, and inion. The line connecting inion to external auditory meatus identifies the transverse sinus, and the sigmoid sinus runs along the digastric groove posterior to the mastoid eminence. The hair is shaved only from the retromastoid area on the affected side, and the head is sterilized and draped in the usual fashion. In order to reduce scalp bleeding, lidocaine with epinephrine is injected into the scalp. A linear skin incision runs longitudinally 5 mm medial to the hairline and extends about 5–7 cm, with one-quarter above

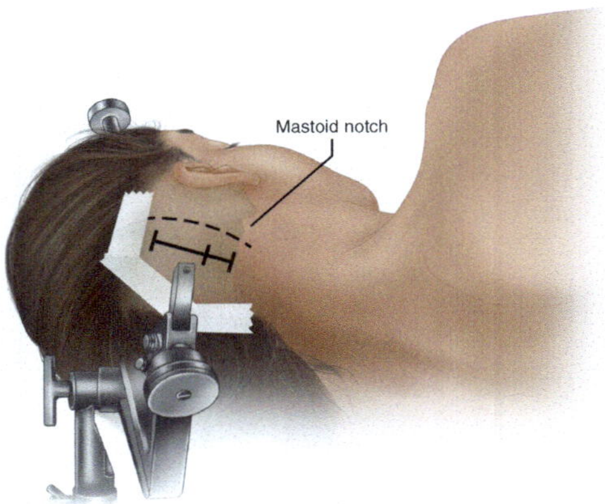

Fig. 3 A linear skin incision runs longitudinally 5 mm medial to the hairline and extends about 5–7 cm, with one-quarter above the iniomeatal line and three-quarters below. (or two-thirds above and one-third below the mastoid notch is utilized)

iniomeatal line and three-quarters below. (or two-thirds above and one-third below the mastoid notch is utilized) (Fig. 3). If it is not much different from our standard skin incision during redo MVD, we use the incision line from the previous surgery as it is. Monopolar electrocautery is used to divide the muscle and soft tissue down to the occipital bone until the digastric groove is seen. The occipital artery and emissary vein are often encountered in this exposure and coagulated. Lateral bony exposure is extended to the curving part of the suboccipital bone. In the case of reoperation, there is relatively less bleeding during muscular dissection and lateral extension of muscle and soft tissue is restricted because of hardened tissue due to the previous surgery. The wound is secured with a self-retaining retractor (cerebellar retractor).

Retromastoid craniectomy is performed using a high-speed air drill and Kerrison punches about longitudinally oval shaped 2 × 3 cm sized. This craniectomy continues until exposure of transverse sinus cranially and sigmoid sinus laterally. Dura nearby such sinuses is very thin, so we have to be especially careful during craniectomy. If small injuries to the sinus have happened, avoid electrical cauterization as much as possible, and cover it with surgical glue-soaked Gelfoam or tack-up suture. The mastoid air cells will be visible at the lateral margin of bony exposure and are then waxed thoroughly. Meticulous bleeding control is obtained to prevent blood from running over the subarachnoid space. During redo surgery, the bone flap or the metal mesh is removed during previous operation, and if the craniectomy is sufficient, only the adhesive connective tissue is removed, and if not enough, additional craniectomy is performed carefully. Care should be taken because there may be a lot of bleeding and the dura may tear when removing the adhesive connective tissue until the dura is exposed.

The linear dura incision is made 5 mm parallel to the sigmoid sinus. The dura is then secured with tack-up sutures laterally to retract the sigmoid sinus and the major portion of the dura is not retracted over the cerebellum to protect the cerebellar surface. Even during redo surgery, it is performed in the same way regardless of the dura incision in the previous operation. At this point, there may be an adhesion between the brain cortex and dura, so careful dissection is needed.

After dura opening, we retract carefully the petrosal surface of the cerebellum with a cottonoid under microscope, cerebrospinal fluid is drawn from the cerebellomedullary cistern to let the cerebellum relax further. If the cerebellum is not relaxed enough, drain about 20–30 cc of cerebrospinal fluid through the lumbar drain performed before surgery.

Many surgeons generally use a self-retaining brain retractor for cerebellar retraction, but we avoid using a self-retaining brain retractor as much as possible, place cottonoids on the cerebellar surface, and gently retract the brain using a suction tip. When we enter further using suction and bipolar, the petrosal vein complex is encountered, which usually has a Y- or V-shaped. In order to prevent venous infarction that may occur due to electrical cauterization of petrosal veins, we should preserve these vessels. During reoperation, there are times when there is severe adhesion with the surrounding arachnoid or no vein complex. In this situation, more attention should be paid to dissect from other structures.

By advancing over the superior surface of the cerebellum, the surgeon can avoid the seventh and eighth nerves. The arachnoid around these

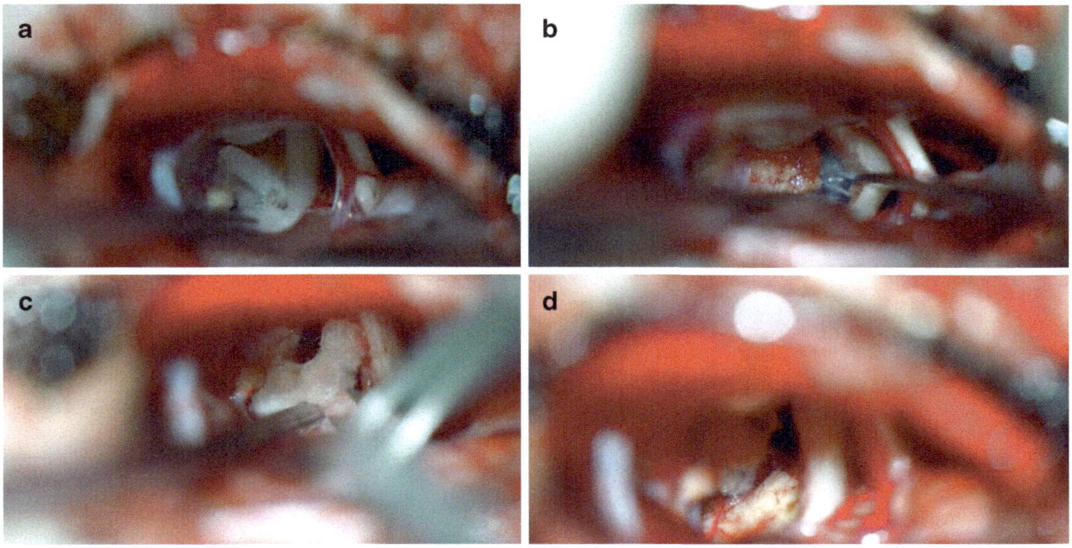

Fig. 4 (**a**) Teflon, which was previously inserted during the first MVD, is severely adhered to the trigeminal nerve and brainstem, forming Teflon granuloma. (**b**) Careful dissection between Teflon granuloma and trigeminal nerve using microscopic blunt dissector. (**c**) We remove the remaining lumped Teflon granuloma with microscissors. At this time, must be careful not to damage the surrounding blood vessels or brainstem. (**d**) This picture shows the complete removal of Teflon granuloma, and there are no offending vessels

nerves does not need to be opened, and this helps to prevent stretch-induced nerve injury as much as possible due to the retraction of the cerebellum. If the surgical field around the fifth nerve is narrow due to adhesion caused by previous operation, the arachnoid around seventh and eighth nerves is removed to secure the sufficient operative field.

Penetration of the trigeminal cistern and sharp dissection of the arachnoid allow complete inspection of the fifth nerve. In the first surgery, the arachnoid is thin and translucent, it is relatively easy to be dissected. But during reoperation, the arachnoid is generally thick and opaque in many cases, so care should be taken to avoid injury to the trigeminal nerve, the trochlear nerve, or small vascular branches in subarachnoid space.

It is necessary to closely analyze brain MRI performed by preoperative evaluation of recurrent trigeminal neuralgia patients to determine whether it is the new vascular compression or Teflon granuloma. If fibrotic adhesion is induced by Teflon felt, microsurgical sharp dissection, preserving the trigeminal nerve and corresponding vessel, with complete removal of the Teflon granuloma is performed. At this time, if Teflon felt adhesion is severe, bleeding may occur during dissection, so meticulous bleeding control is required at the same time, and when pulling adhesive Teflon felt, stretch-induced injury may occur to fifth nerve or brainstem, so much caution is required (Fig. 4).

After the complete removal of Teflon granuloma, we do not insert the Teflon felt between the offending vessel and the trigeminal nerve in case new fibrotic adhesion was induced by previous foreign materials. Teflon felt has been thought to be an ideal material because of its tissue acceptance, little dislocation, and lack of resorption [5]. However, it also has some complications, the major one is inflammatory foreign body reaction, which may cause severe adhesion, fibrotic change, or even granulomatous formation around the trigeminal nerve and lead to the recurrence of trigeminal neuralgia [6] (Fig. 5). As a matter of fact, using any kind of implant in the interposing techniques would cause compression and may produce adhesions to the trigeminal nerve, which may be reasons for recurrence. Thus, an ideal technique should only push the vessels off the tri-

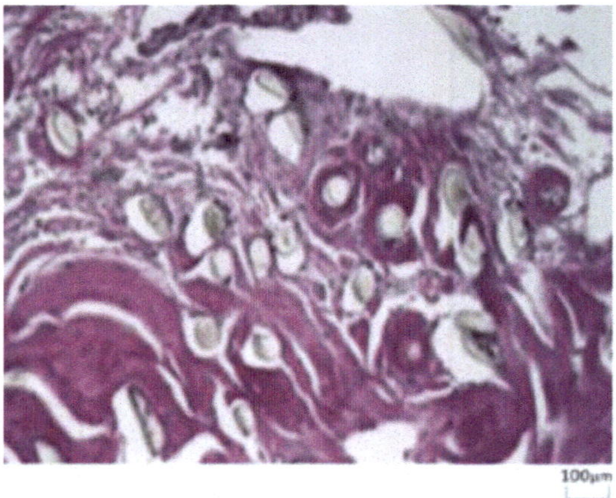

Fig. 5 Teflon granuloma in redo MVD (hematoxylin and eosin staining, ×100). (Adapted from Jiayu Liu, Guangyong Wu, Hui Xiang et al. Long-term retrospective analysis of microvascular decompression in patients with recurrent trigeminal neuralgia. *Front. Neurol.* 2020;11:1–11)

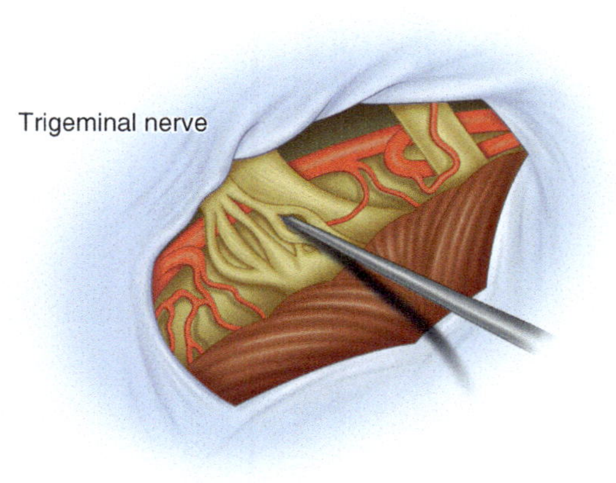

Fig. 6 The trigeminal nerve and root entry zone are carefully examined for neurovascular compression by an artery or vein. When none is found, the trigeminal nerve itself is then longitudinally divided along its fibers, using a straight blunt-tip bayonet probe, into 5–10 bundles from the root entry zone to the petrous bone

geminal nerve and avoid any contact with the nerve itself [7–9]. After the trigeminal nerve is completely freed, a piece of Teflon felt is shaped as a sling measuring 10–20 mm in length and 2–3 mm in width. This sling wrapping around offending vessel is fixed to the inferior surface of the tentorium or petrous dura using surgical glue. To make a strong attachment, Tachosil (fibrin sealant patch) is applied additionally. If the offending vessel is large and does not work this method, a thin and long Gore-Tex can be used to wind the offending vessel and tie it to the surrounding dura. The vessels that are displaced should be carefully inspected. If there is any tendency toward kinking, they need to be positioned in a gentle arc. Some pieces of Gelfoam placed at the center of the curvature help conform these vessels to a gentle arc and avoid kinking. If any spasm occurs due to manipulation, the spasm is lysed immediately when the cottonoid soaked in papaverine is placed in affected vessels. Transposition techniques require high proficiency and wide operative fields, but in recurrent cases, the cerebellar cortex may be relatively atrophic due to previous operation, making it easy to use transposition techniques.

After transposition, it is important to completely inspect around the trigeminal nerve. In some cases, micromirror or endoscope can be used to see the ventral side of the fifth nerve. If the vein is the cause of compressing the nerve, sharply dissect the vein as much as possible, otherwise perform electrical coagulation to divide it. If only electrical coagulation is performed and not divided, it may be recanalized, so much care must be required.

The trigeminal nerve and root entry zone are carefully examined for neurovascular compression by an artery or vein. When none is found, the trigeminal nerve itself is then longitudinally divided along its fibers, using a straight blunt-tip bayonet probe, into 5–10 bundles from the root entry zone to the petrous bone (Fig. 6). We include both the portio minor and portio major in the neurolysis, as the portio minor has been shown to carry unmyelinated fibers implicated in pathological facial pain, and neural anastomoses exist between these components of the trigeminal nerve [10–11].

The operative field is liberally irrigated, cottonoids covered over the cerebellum are removed, and Valsalva maneuver is performed by anesthesiologist to ensure there is no bleeding. We placed a piece of Durafoam over the cerebellar surface beneath the dura prior to closure, to prevent adhesion between the cerebellar cortex and the dura.

The dura is closed with continuous or interrupted No.4-0 braided nylon sutures in a near water-tight fashion. If a water-tight closure cannot be obtained, muscle graft is used to patch the leak and surgical glue (fibrin sealant) is applied over it. A piece of Durafoam is placed over the dura, and cranioplasty with wire mesh is performed. Wound closure is done in layers, using 2-0 vicryl sutures for the deep layers, 3-0 vicryl for the more superficial layers, and skin suture is done by stapler.

After the surgery, the patient is carefully observed overnight in the intensive care unit. Systolic blood pressure can be adjusted to 160 mmHg or less, analgesics are administered when complaining of headache, and antiemetics are administered if there is nausea. If there is a severe headache that is not controlled by analgesics or neurological changes, brain computed tomographic scan is done immediately to check for intracranial hemorrhage. On the first operative day, the computed tomographic scan is taken and if there are no specific abnormalities, the patient moves to a general ward, and diet and activity are gradually increased. Dressing of the surgical wound is performed once every 2 days, and the removal of the stapler is performed on the 7th day after surgery, and discharged the next day. Daily life activity after discharge is possible without restrictions, and almost all patients return to normal life activity within a month after surgery.

Complications after MVD usually do not occur, but various complications can occur. The most common type of complication is cranial nerve palsy. Facial hypesthesia or numbness accounts for about 30%. Most of these recover on their own about 2–3 months after surgery. Double vision due to fourth nerve palsy is relatively common but usually has subsided over a few weeks to several months. Facial nerve palsies generally have been self-limited but may remain a permanent disability in some cases. Hearing loss can occur after MVD. Hearing loss caused by fluid filling in mastoid air cells can be recovered naturally after several weeks, but hearing loss due to brain stem injury due to excessive cerebellar retraction or microvascular damage is permanent. Care must be taken to prevent cranial nerve injuries by gentle retraction, careful manipulation, and treatment of any vasospasms that occur. CSF rhinorrhea is caused by leakage of CSF through the dural opening into mastoid air cells, that occurs more often with redo surgery, and can be prevented by meticulous waxing of the mastoid air cell and water-tight dura closure with surgical glue. When the lumbar drain is applied for 2–3 days, most CSF rhinorrhea usually stops. Cerebellar hemorrhagic infarction may occur from venous injury, so it is important to preserve the vein complex as much as possible. Wound infection presents as swelling of operative wound, fever, or discharge of pus, and in this case, requires reoperation to remove all sources of infection and intravenous antibiotics for 2–4 weeks.

2 Our Results

From 1984 to June 2021, a total of 3771 microvascular decompression (MVD) cases were performed, of which 2937 cases were hemifacial spasm (HFS) and 490 cases were TN. Among them, HFS recurrence occurred in 76 cases and TN recurrence occurred in 51(10.4%) cases.

The 51 patients who underwent redo surgery for recurrent or persistent TN included 12 males (23.5%) and 39 females (76.5%) with a mean age of 64.08 (range, 31–92) at the time of revision. The right side was affected in 33 patients (64.7%) and the left in 18 patients (35.3%). The mean duration of pain at the time of initial MVD surgery for TN was 5.6 years. Pain distribution was V2 area in 7 patients (13.7%), V3 area in 3 patients (5.8%), V1 + V2 area in 7 patients (13.7%), V2 + V3 area in 20 patients (39.2%), and V1 + V2 + V3 in 14 patients (27.5%) (Table 2). Among the reoperation patients, there were a total of 4 patients who underwent early revision within 2 months of the first MVD surgery, and all of them were due to missed offenders. Three patients underwent 2 redo surgeries, and one patient underwent 3 redo surgeries.

The cause of reoperation was Teflon adhesion with granuloma in 31 cases (60.7%), new vessel

Table 2 Patients characteristics

Characteristics	Number of patients
Male:Female	12:39
Age (years)	64.08 (31–92)
Right:Left	33:18
Pain distribution	
V2	7
V3	3
V1 + V2	7
V2 + V3	20
V1 + V2 + V3	14

Table 3 Cause of TN recurrence in our hospital

Cause		Number of patients
Teflon adhesion and granuloma		31 (60.7%)
New vessel compression	Vein (5)	10 (19.6%)
	Small artery (5)	
Missed offender		5 (9.8%)
Negative		5 (9.8%)

Table 4 Prognosis after redo surgery of TN

Prognosis	Number of patients
Excellent	30 (58.8%)
Good	12 (23.5%)
Fair	5 (9.8%)
Poor	4 (7.8%)

Excellent: No pain without medication
Good: No pain with medication
Fair: Remain pain with medication, but tolerable
Poor: No difference compared preoperative condition

Table 5 Complications after redo surgery of TN

Complications	Number of patients
Mortality	0
Wound infection	0
CSF leakage	0
Ischemia (brain stem, cerebellar)	0
Facial paresthesia	12 (23.5%)
Transient hearing loss	2 (3.9%)
Transient facial palsy	1 (1.9%)

compression 10 (vein 5, small artery 5) (19.6%), missed offender 5 (9.8%), and negative 5 (9.8%). In all negative cases, internal neurolysis was performed (Table 3). The prognosis after redo surgery for recurrent or persistent TN was Excellent in 30 patients (58.8%) and Good in 12 patients (23.5%). However, in 9 patients, unsatisfactory or preoperative pain persisted (Table 4). Complications were facial paresthesia in 12 cases (23.5%), transient facial nerve palsy in 1 case (1.9%), and transient hearing loss in 2 cases (3.9). There was no mortality, CSF leakage, or wound infection (Table 5).

In conclusion, successful first surgery is most important.

For successful result, it is good to choose the patient for MVD and treatment of causing illness after patient's symptoms or imaging results, and a thorough review of prerecord to differentiate distinguished illness. If secondary trigeminal neuralgia is caused by tumor, AVM, or aneurysm, we have to plan to remove the causative lesion and then also MVD surgery.

To minimize the complications before/after or during the surgery, it is crucial to be well informed about the precautions stated in the operative technic. As possible, transposition is better than interposition as Teflon may cause complications and recurrence.

We have to develop a new prosthesis instead of Teflon for no foreign body reaction and fibrosis.

After the first surgery, if symptoms are persistent or recurrent, active reoperation is needed after considering the patient's many conditions. If the patient's condition is not appropriate, other surgical methods may be chosen.

References

1. Jannetta PJ, Bissonette DJ. Management of the failed patient with trigeminal neuralgia. Clin Neurosurg. 1985;32:334–47.
2. Liao JJ, Cheng WC, Chang CN, Yong JT, Wei KC, Hsu YH, Lin TK. Reoperation for recurrent trigeminal neuralgia after MVD. Surg Neurol. 1997;47:562–70.
3. Moller AR, Jannetta PJ. Monitoring auditory functions during cranial nerve microvascular decompression operations by direct recording from the eighth nerve. J Neurosurg. 1983;59:493–9.
4. McLaughlin MR, Jannetta PJ, Clyde BL, et al. Microvascular decompression of cranial nerves: lessons learned after 4400 operations. J Neurosurg. 1999;90:1–8.

5. Capelle HH, Brandis A, Tschan CA, et al. Treatment of recurrent trigeminal neuralgia due to Teflon granuloma. J Headache Pain. 2010;11:339–44.
6. Cheng J, Meng J, et al. Repeat microvascular decompression for patients with persistent or recurrent trigeminal neuralgia. Medicine. 2019;98:1–6.
7. Masuoka J, Matsushima T, Kawashima M, et al. Stitched sling retraction technique for microvascular decompression: procedures and techniques based on an anatomical viewpoint. Neurosurg Rev. 2011;34:373–9.
8. Khoo HM, Yoshimine T, Taki T. A "sling swing transposition" technique with pedicled dural flap for microvascular decompression in hemifacial spasm. Neurosurgery. 2012;71:25–30.
9. Sindou M, Leston JM, Decullier E, et al. Microvascular decompression for trigeminal neuralgia: the importance of a noncompressive technique–Kaplan-Meier analysis in a consecutive series of 330 patients. Neurosurgery. 2008;63:341–50.
10. RS T, Griessenauer CJ, Hogan E, Louskas M, Cohen-Gadol AA. Neural interconnections between portio minor and portio major at the Porus trigeminus: application to failed surgical treatment of trigeminal neuralgia. Clin Anat. 2010;27:160–7.
11. Ko AL, Ozpinar A, Lee A, et al. Long-term efficacy and safety of internal neurolysis for trigeminal neuralgia without neurovascular compression. J Neurosurg. 2015;122:1048–57.

Part III

Ablative Treatment and Related Issues

Nerve Block, Pulsed RF Treatment, and Percutaneous Neurolysis for Trigeminal Neuralgia

Jae Hun Kim

Trigeminal nerve block is performed for diagnostic and therapeutic purposes in trigeminal neuralgia. Trigeminal nerve block can be performed for trigeminal neuralgia as well as trigeminal nerve disorders such as postherpetic neuralgia of the trigeminal nerve and trigeminal nerve injury, anesthesia for facial surgery, and postoperative analgesia of the face. There are three major branches of the trigeminal nerve: the ophthalmic nerve (V1), maxillary nerve (V2), and mandibular nerve (V3). These three major branches are divided into several small branches. Although there are many peripheral branches of the trigeminal nerve, the most commonly performed peripheral nerve blocks are the supraorbital, infraorbital, and mental nerve blocks. Recently, these three peripheral nerve blocks have been performed using ultrasound guidance.

Trigeminal neurolysis is performed for therapeutic purposes in trigeminal neuralgia. Peripheral neurolysis is most commonly performed for the supraorbital, infraorbital, and mental nerves. These three peripheral nerve neurolytic blocks have been performed using ultrasound guidance.

J. H. Kim (✉)
Department of Anesthesiology and Pain Medicine, Konkuk University Medical Center, Konkuk University School of Medicine, Seoul, Republic of Korea
e-mail: painfree@kuh.ac.kr

1 Peripheral Branch Block of the Trigeminal Nerve and Percutaneous Neurolysis for Peripheral Branch of Trigeminal Nerve

There are several branches of the trigeminal nerve. In these branches, the supraorbital, infraorbital, and mental nerves exit through the foramen or notch. These foramina or notches can be anatomical landmarks for nerve blocks or peripheral neurolysis.

1.1 Supraorbital Nerve Block and Pulsed Radiofrequency (RF) Treatment [1, 2]

1.1.1 Anatomy

The supraorbital nerve is a branch of the frontal nerve, which is a branch of the ophthalmic nerve. The ophthalmic nerve is purely sensory. The supraorbital and supratrochlear nerves are the two branches of the frontal nerve. The supraorbital nerve exits through the supraorbital notch (Fig. 1A) or foramen in the superior margin of the orbit and divides into the medial and lateral branches. These branches head toward the head. The supraorbital foramen is a landmark of the supraorbital nerve. According to a study of multidetector computed tomography, 76.5% (right) and 77.7% (left) patients had a single foramen or

K. Park, K. R. Cho (eds.), *Trigeminal Neuralgia*, https://doi.org/10.1007/978-981-19-9171-4_18

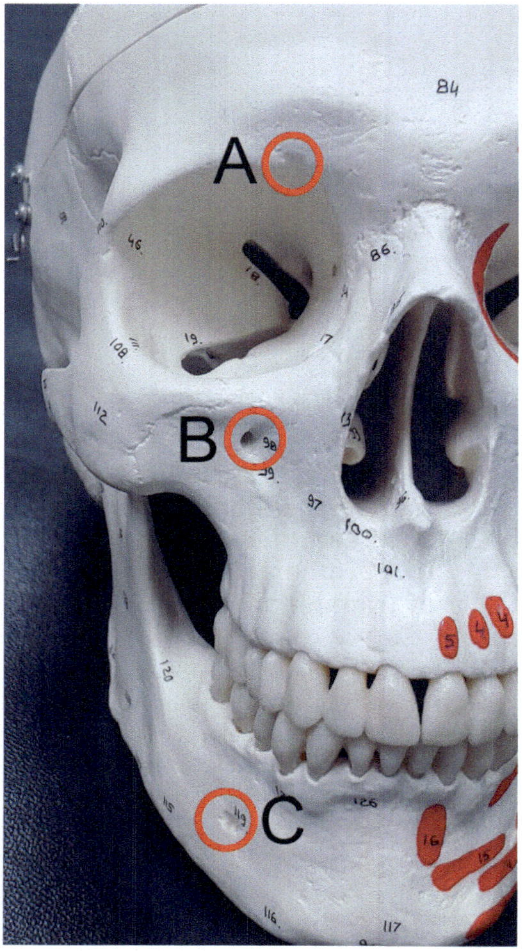

Fig. 1 The position of supraorbital notch (A), infraorbital foramen (B), and mental foramen (C)

notch, 13.7% (right) and 10.6% (left) patients had double foramina or notches, 6.3% (right) and 5.1% (left) patients had co-existence of the foramen and notch, and 9/9% (right) and 11.7% (left) had no foramen or notch [3].

The supraorbital nerve provides sensory innervation to the skin, scalp, and periosteum of the frontal head.

1.1.2 Indications

Trigeminal neuralgia, pain of herpes zoster, postherpetic neuralgia, cancer pain, trigeminal nerve injury, surgery of the upper eyelid or frontal area.

1.1.3 Methods

Blind Technique

The patient is placed in the supine position. The supraorbital nerve block can be performed by palpation of the supraorbital notch or foramen. The upper part of the eye is disinfected where the procedure is performed. The physician palpates the patient's superior margin of orbit and should detect the supraorbital notch or foramen [4]. After identification of the supraorbital notch or foramen, a 25-gauge needle is inserted in the medial and cephalad directions into the inferior edge of the supraorbital ridge approximately 0.5 cm below the supraorbital notch or foramen. After assessing no blood aspiration, 0.5–2 mL of local anesthetics with/without steroids is injected. To prevent hematoma or edema of the superior aspect of the eyelid, physicians should instruct the patient to press on the injection site with gauze for at least 5 min.

Ultrasound Guidance Technique

Recently, ultrasound guidance blocks have been commonly used. Thus, this procedure can be performed more accurately and safely. A linear probe or a hockey stick probe can be used. The physician places the probe on the patient's forehead and moves down to the superior margin of the orbit [5]. The supraorbital notch or foramen can be found on the orbital margin (Fig. 2a). To detect the supraorbital artery, a physician can use color Doppler imaging (Fig. 2b). After assessing the artery position, a 25-gauge needle in-plane technique is inserted into the supraorbital notch or foramen. Sometimes, the supraorbital nerve can be identified by ultrasound. After placing the needle near the nerve or supraorbital notch/foramen, 0.5–2 mL of local anesthetics with/without steroids is injected. The needle insertion out-of-plane technique can be used. However, we did not recommend the technique for supraorbital nerve block owing to the risk of orbital trauma.

Pulsed RF Treatment

If the effect of the nerve block is short, pulsed RF treatment can be performed. It can be performed using a blind technique or ultrasound guidance

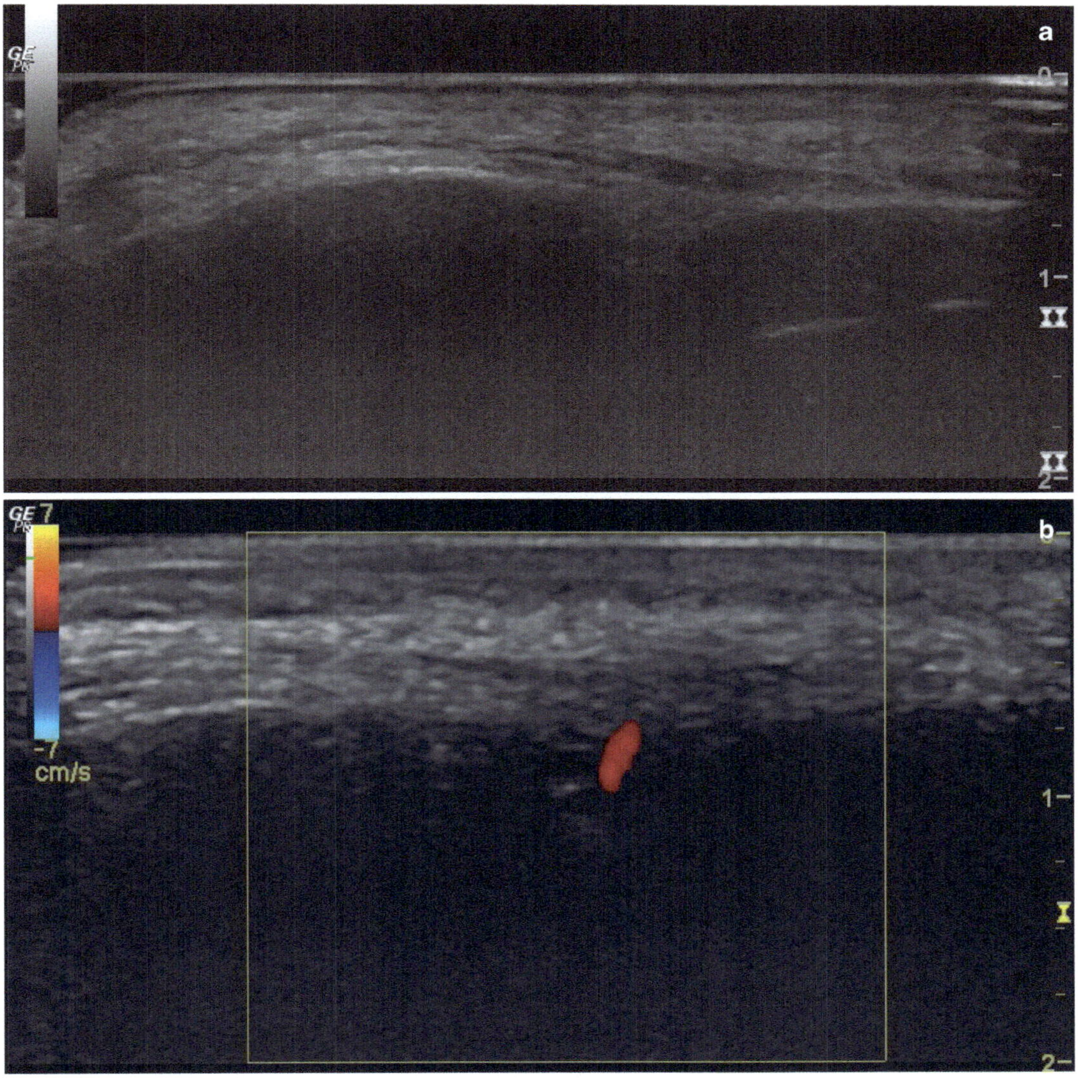

Fig. 2 Ultrasound images of supraorbital notch, (**a**) supraorbital, (**b**) notch supraorbital artery in color Doppler image

technique. Although the RF needle is larger than the block needle, the insertion technique is the same as aforementioned, the RF needle with a 0.2–0.5 cm active tip is positioned near the supraorbital nerve, the physician initiates 50 Hz and 1 V sensory stimulation and detects stimulation of the supraorbital nerve. Then, the needle is moved gradually until the nerve is detected with a stimulation of 0.3–0.5 V. Stimulation below 0.5 V indicates that the needle is in close proximity to or in contact with the nerve. Pulsed RF treatment can be performed for 10 min.

Conventional RF Thermocoagulation

If the effect of the nerve block is short, conventional RF thermocoagulation can be performed. It can be performed using a blind technique or ultrasound guidance technique. The insertion technique is the same as the pulsed RF treatment described above. An RF needle with 0.5–1 cm active tip is positioned near the supraorbital nerve, the physician initiates 50 Hz and 1 V sensory stimulation and detects stimulation of the supraorbital nerve. Then, the needle is moved gradually until the nerve is detected with a stimulation of 0.3–0.5 V. Stimulation below 0.5 V indicates that the needle is in close proximity or in contact with the nerve. After injecting local anesthetics, conventional RF thermocoagulation at 60–80 °C can be performed for 2 min several times. In general, the procedure begins at a low temperature and gradually increases with temperature. Finally, 1–2 mL of local anesthetics with steroids can be injected.

1.1.4 Effects

In patients with supraorbital neuralgia, after single pulsed RF treatment, the effectiveness rates at 6 months, 1 year, and 2 years were 73%, 64%, and 50%, respectively [6]. In the 53 patients with supraorbital neuralgia, the cumulative proportion of recurrence-free survival (RFS) after conventional RF thermocoagulation was 96.2% at 12 months, 88.4% at 24 months, 82.7% at 36 months, 70.0% at 48 months, 66.3% at 60 months, and 49.7% at 97 months [7].

After the second or third RF lesion, recurrent pain was completely relieved, except in one patient. In 54 patients with V1 trigeminal neuralgia, conventional RF lesioning, the effective rate of patients with supraorbital foramen at 0.5, 1, and 2 years was 92%, 80%, and 76%, respectively [8]. The effective rate of patients with supraorbital foramen at 0.5, 1, and 2 years was 82.6%, 65.5%, and 48.2%, respectively, and at 2 years after treatment, the effective rate in the patients with foramen was higher than that in those with notch.

1.1.5 Complications

The possible side effects may be pain at the injection site, edema, hematoma, dizziness, and infection. To prevent edema or hematoma, compression of the injection site for over 5 min is mandatory. After pulsed RF treatment, 23% of patients experienced mild upper eyelid ecchymosis that gradually disappeared after 2 weeks, and no severe complications were observed [6]. After conventional RF treatment, no patients reported anesthesia dolorosa, and there were no serious side effects [7]. In other study on conventional RF thermocoagulation, all patients had numbness of the supraorbital nerve dermatome. Moreover, the degree at 2 years after treatment was lower than 1 day after treatment [8] there were no other serious complications.

1.2 Supraorbital Nerve Neurolysis

1.2.1 Indications

Trigeminal neuralgia, cancer pain, cluster headache, or atypical facial pain [9].

1.2.2 Methods

Blind Technique

The patient is placed in the supine position. The supraorbital nerve neurolysis can be performed by palpation of the supraorbital notch or foramen. The upper part of the eye is disinfected where the procedure is performed. The physician palpates the patient's superior margin of orbit and should detect the supraorbital notch or foramen [4]. After identification of the supraorbital notch or foramen, a 25-gauge needle is inserted in the medial and cephalad directions into the inferior edge of the supraorbital ridge approximately 0.5 cm below the supraorbital notch or foramen. After assessing no blood aspiration, 0.5–1 mL of local anesthetics is injected. After 15–20 min, block efficacy is confirmed, and 0.2–0.5 mL of a neurolytic agent (phenol, alcohol, or glycerol) is injected [10]. To prevent hematoma or edema of the superior aspect of the eyelid, physicians should instruct the patient to press on the injection site with gauze for at least 5 min.

Ultrasound Guidance Technique

Recently, ultrasound guidance blocks have been commonly used. Thus, this procedure can be performed more accurately and safely. A linear probe or a hockey stick probe can be used. The physician places the probe on the patient's forehead and moves down to the superior margin of the orbit [5]. The supraorbital notch or foramen can be found on the orbital margin (Fig. 2a). To detect the supraorbital artery, a physician can use color Doppler imaging (Fig. 2b). After assessing the artery position, a 25-gauge needle in-plane technique is inserted into the supraorbital notch or foramen. Sometimes, the supraorbital nerve can be identified by ultrasound. After placing the needle near the nerve or supraorbital notch/foramen, 0.5–1 mL of local anesthetics is injected. After 15–20 min, block efficacy is confirmed, and 0.2–0.5 mL of a neurolytic agent (phenol, alcohol, or glycerol) is injected. The needle insertion out-of-plane technique can be used. However, we did not recommend the technique for supraorbital nerve block owing to the risk of orbital trauma.

1.2.3 Effects

There are few reports of supraorbital nerve neurolysis. Wakasugi [11] reported a mean effect duration of 19 months, and Wilkins [12] reported a mean effect duration of 8.5 months.

1.2.4 Complications

The possible side effects may be pain at the injection site, anesthesia dolorosa, edema, hematoma, dizziness, and infection. To prevent edema or hematoma, compression of the injection site for over 5 min is mandatory. An accidental intravascular injection of phenol may cause tinnitus and flushing [13]. Partial nerve destruction may cause neuritis of a somatic nerve with subsequent regeneration and dysesthesia or hyperesthesia [13].

1.3 Infraorbital Nerve Block and Pulsed RF Treatment [1, 2]

1.3.1 Anatomy

The infraorbital nerve is a branch of the maxillary nerve. It exits on the face through the infraorbital foramen (Fig. 1B) and provides sensory innervation to the skin of the middle face, lateral nose, and upper lip. The infraorbital foramen is a landmark of the infraorbital nerve. It is located on the midline of the pupil and 0.5–1 cm below the inferior margin of the orbit. The foramen is open from the center to the inside at approximately 20°.

1.3.2 Indications

Trigeminal neuralgia, pain of herpes zoster, postherpetic neuralgia, cancer pain, trigeminal nerve injury, surgery of the lower eyelid, upper lip, or median cheek.

1.3.3 Methods

Blind Technique

The patient is placed in the supine position. An infraorbital nerve block can be administered by palpation of the infraorbital foramen. The cheek should be disinfected below the orbital rim, where the procedure is performed. The physician palpates the patient's cheek at the intersection of a vertical line drawn caudally through the center of the pupil and should find the infraorbital foramen. After identification of the infraorbital foramen, the physician's second or third finger should be placed and maintained over the infraorbital foramen. A 25-gauge needle is slowly inserted into the infraorbital foramen. After assessing no blood aspiration, 0.5–2 mL of local anesthetics with/without steroids are injected. To prevent hematoma or edema, physicians should instruct the patient to press on the injection site with gauze for at least 5 min.

Ultrasound Guidance Technique

Recently, ultrasound guidance blocks have been commonly used. Thus, this procedure can be performed more accurately and safely. A linear probe or a hockey stick probe can be used. The physician places the probe on the patient's cheek (the infraorbital foramen is located on the midline of the pupil and 0.5–1 cm below the inferior margin of the orbit) and detects the infraorbital foramen (Fig. 3a). To detect the infraorbital artery, a physician can use color Doppler imaging (Fig. 3b) [5]. After assessing the artery position, a 25-gauge needle in-plane technique is inserted into the infraorbital foramen. Sometimes, the infraorbital nerve can be identified using ultrasound. After placing the needle near the nerve or infraorbital foramen, 0.5–2 mL of local anesthetics with/without steroids are injected. The needle insertion out-of-plane technique can also be used.

Pulsed RF Treatment

If the effect of the nerve block is short, pulsed RF treatment can be performed. It can be performed using a blind technique or ultrasound guidance

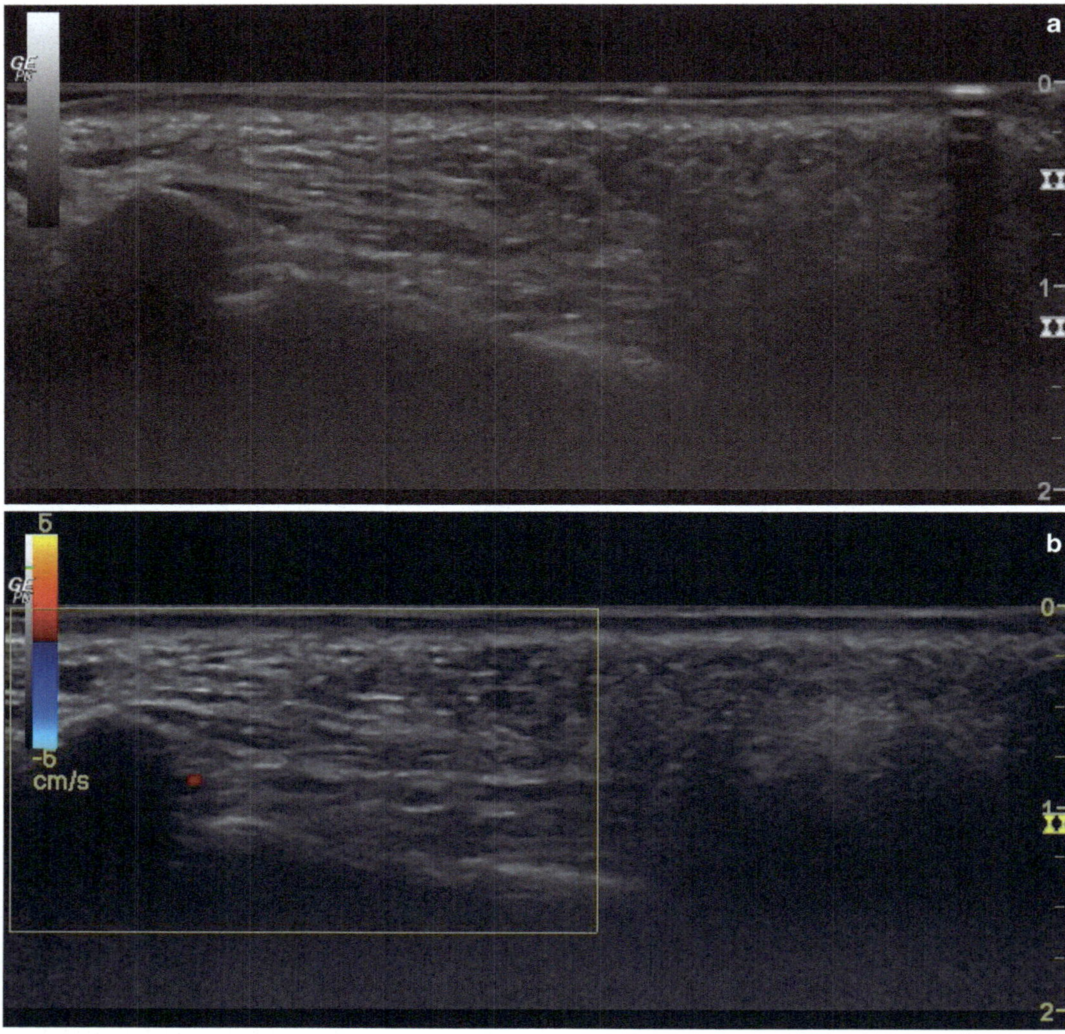

Fig. 3 Ultrasound images of infraorbital foramen, (**a**) infraorbital foramen, (**b**) infraorbital artery in color Doppler image

technique. Although the RF needle is larger than the block needle, the insertion technique is the same as aforementioned. The RF needle with a 0.2–0.5 cm active tip is positioned near the infraorbital nerve, and the physician starts 50 Hz and 1 V sensory stimulation and finds stimulation of the infraorbital nerve. Then, move the needle little by little until the nerve is found with a stimulation of 0.3–0.5 V. Stimulation below 0.5 V means that the needle is quite close to or in contact with the nerve. Pulsed RF treatment was performed for 10 min.

Conventional RF Thermocoagulation
If the effect of the nerve block is short, conventional RF thermocoagulation can be performed. It can be performed using a blind technique or ultrasound guidance technique. The insertion technique is the same as the pulsed RF treatment described above. An RF needle with 0.5–1 cm active tip is positioned near the infraorbital nerve, and the physician starts 50 Hz and 1 V sensory stimulation and detects stimulation of the infraorbital nerve. Then, the needle is gradually moved until the nerve is detected with a stimulation of

0.3–0.5 V. Stimulation below 0.5 V means that the needle is quite close to or in contact with the nerve. After injection of local anesthetics, conventional RF thermocoagulation at 60–80 °C was performed for 2 min several times. In general, the procedure starts at a low temperature and gradually increases with temperature. Finally, 1–2 mL of local anesthetics with steroids can be injected.

1.3.4 Effects

In the patients with infraorbital neuralgia following ineffective conservative therapy, after single pulsed RF treatment, the effectiveness rates at 6 months, 1 year, and 2 years were 64%, 50%, and 50%, respectively [14]. In another investigation, pulsed RF treatment with 270 s of 60 °C conventional RF lesioning was performed for refractory infraorbital neuralgia. The effective rates at 6 months, 1 year, 18 months, and 2 years were 81.8%, 72.7%, 72.7%, and 72.7%, respectively [15]. In comparison with standard voltage pulsed RF treatment and high-voltage pulsed RF treatment, high-voltage pulsed RF treatment was more effective and safe for patients with refractory infraorbital neuralgia [16]. There are some reports on the effectiveness and safety of conventional RF thermocoagulation [17]. However, further investigation of conventional RF thermocoagulation of the infraorbital nerve is needed.

1.3.5 Complications

Pain at the injection site, edema, hematoma, dizziness, and infection can be possible side effects. To prevent edema or hematoma, compression of the injection site for over 5 min is mandatory. After pulsed RF treatment, 25% of patients experienced mild numbness, and the symptoms disappeared in approximately 1 month [14]. There was no serious side effects.

1.4 Infraorbital Nerve Neurolysis

1.4.1 Indications

Trigeminal neuralgia, cancer pain, cluster headache, or atypical facial pain [2].

1.4.2 Methods

Blind Technique

The patient is placed in the supine position. An infraorbital nerve block can be administered by palpation of the infraorbital foramen. The cheek should be disinfected below the orbital rim, where the procedure is performed. The physician palpates the patient's cheek at the intersection of a vertical line drawn caudally through the center of the pupil and should find the infraorbital foramen. After identification of the infraorbital foramen, the physician's second or third finger should be placed and maintained over the infraorbital foramen. A 25-gauge needle is slowly inserted into the infraorbital foramen. After assessing no blood aspiration, 0.5–1 mL of local anesthetics is injected. After 15–20 min, block efficacy is confirmed, and 0.2–0.5 mL of a neurolytic agent (phenol, alcohol, or glycerol) is injected. To prevent hematoma or edema, physicians should instruct the patient to press on the injection site with gauze for at least 5 min.

Ultrasound Guidance Technique

Recently, ultrasound guidance blocks have been commonly used. Thus, this procedure can be performed more accurately and safely. A linear probe or a hockey stick probe can be used. The physician places the probe on the patient's cheek (the infraorbital foramen is located on the midline of the pupil and 0.5–1 cm below the inferior margin of the orbit) and detects the infraorbital foramen (Fig. 3a). To detect the infraorbital artery, a physician can use color Doppler imaging (Fig. 3b) [5]. After assessing the artery position, a 25-gauge needle in-plane technique is inserted into the infraorbital foramen. Sometimes, the infraorbital nerve can be identified using ultrasound. After placing the needle near the nerve or infraorbital foramen, 0.5–1 mL of local anesthetics is injected. After 15–20 min, block efficacy is confirmed, and 0.2–0.5 mL of a neurolytic agent (phenol, alcohol, or glycerol) is injected. The needle insertion out-of-plane technique can also be used.

1.4.3 Effects

With regard to alcohol neurolysis of the infraorbital nerve, Wakasugi [6], Wilkins [7], Kim et al. [9], and Fardy et al. [10] reported mean effect durations of 16 months, 12 months, 15.2 months, and 13 months, respectively. Moreover, Fardy et al. reported that with regard to peripheral neurolysis, alcohol (13 months) had a longer effect than glycerol (7 months) [10].

1.4.4 Complications

Pain at the injection site, anesthesia dolorosa, edema, hematoma, dizziness, and infection can be possible side effects. To prevent edema or hematoma, compression of the injection site for over 5 min is mandatory.

1.5 Mental Nerve Block and Pulsed RF Treatment [1, 2]

1.5.1 Anatomy

The mental nerve is a branch of the inferior alveolar nerve, which is a branch of the mandibular nerve. It exits on the face through the mental foramen (Fig. 1C). The mental foramen is a landmark of the mental nerve. It was located approximately 1 cm below the second premolar. It faces outward and upward. The mental nerve is a sensory nerve that provides the lower lip, gum, lower anterior teeth, and front of the chin.

1.5.2 Indications

Trigeminal neuralgia, pain of herpes zoster, postherpetic neuralgia, cancer pain, trigeminal nerve injury, and surgery of the lower lip or chin.

1.5.3 Methods

Blind Technique

The patient is placed in the supine position. A mental nerve block can be administered by palpation of the mental foramen. The chin is disinfected below the second premolar where the procedure will be performed. The physician palpates the patient's chin below the second premolar and should detect the mental foramen. After identification of the mental foramen, the physician's second or third finger should be placed and maintained over the mental foramen. Then, a 25-gauge needle is inserted slowly into the mental foramen. After assessing no aspiration of blood, 0.5–2 mL of local anesthetics with/without steroids are injected. To prevent hematoma or edema, physicians should instruct the patient to press on the injection site with gauze for at least 5 min.

Ultrasound Guidance Technique

Recently, ultrasound guidance blocks have been commonly used. Thus, this procedure can be performed more accurately and safely. A linear probe or a hockey stick probe was used. The physician places the probe on the patient's chin (the mental foramen is located below the second premolar) and detects the mental foramen (Fig. 4). To determine the mental branch of the inferior alveolar artery, a physician can use color Doppler imaging [18]. After checking the artery position, a 25-gauge needle in-plane technique was inserted into the mental foramen. Sometimes, the mental nerve can be identified using ultrasound. After placing the needle near the nerve or mental foramen, inject 0.5–2 mL of local anesthetics with/without steroids. The needle insertion out-of-plane technique can also be used.

Pulsed RF Treatment

If the effect of the nerve block is short, pulsed RF treatment can be performed. It can be performed using a blind technique or ultrasound guidance technique. Although the RF needle is larger than the block needle, the insertion technique is the same as above. The RF needle with a 0.2–0.5 cm active tip is positioned near the mental nerve, the physician initiates 50 Hz and 1 V sensory stimulation and detects stimulation of the mental nerve. Then, the needle is moved gradually until the nerve is detected with a stimulation of 0.3–0.5 V. Stimulation below 0.5 V indicates that the needle is in close approximation or in contact with the nerve. Pulsed RF treatment can be performed for 10 min.

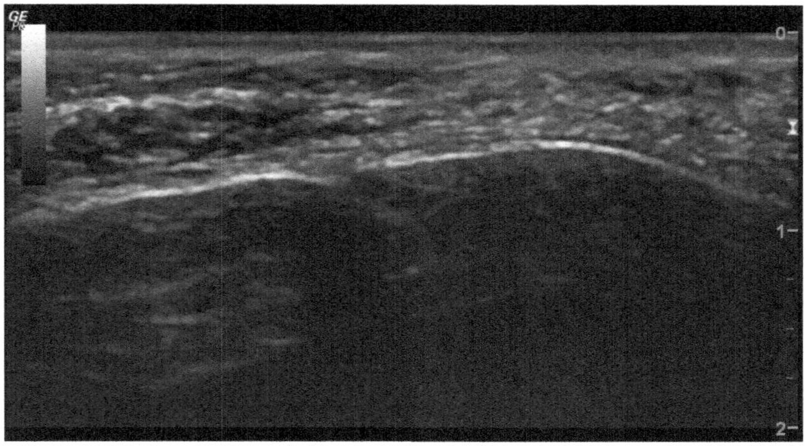

Fig. 4 Ultrasound image of mental foramen

Conventional RF Thermocoagulation

If the effect of the nerve block is short, conventional RF thermocoagulation can be performed. It can be performed using a blind technique or ultrasound guidance technique. The insertion technique is the same as the pulsed RF treatment described above. An RF needle with 0.5–1 cm active tip is positioned near the mental nerve, the physician initiates 50 Hz and 1 V sensory stimulation and detects stimulation of the mental nerve. Then, the needle is gradually moved until the nerve is detected with a stimulation of 0.3–0.5 V. Stimulation below 0.5 V means that the needle is quite close to or in contact with the nerve. After injection of local anesthetics, conventional RF thermocoagulation at 60–80 °C can be performed for 2 min several times. In general, the procedure begins at a low temperature and gradually increases with temperature. Finally, 1–2 mL of local anesthetics with steroids can be injected.

1.5.4 Effects

In a small retrospective study, nine patients with intractable trigeminal neuralgia underwent peripheral trigeminal nerve block such as supraorbital, infraorbital, and mental nerve blocks [19]. All patients experienced immediate pain relief above 50%, and seven patients experienced completely pain-free or mild paresthesia. Six patients experienced lasting pain relief (1–8 months). Further investigation of conventional RF thermocoagulation of the mental nerve is needed.

1.5.5 Complications

Pain at the injection site, edema, hematoma, dizziness, and infection can be possible side effects. To prevent edema or hematoma, compression of the injection site for over 5 min is mandatory.

1.6 Mental Nerve Neurolysis

1.6.1 Indications

Trigeminal neuralgia, cancer pain, cluster headache, or atypical facial pain [9].

1.6.2 Methods

Blind Technique

The patient is placed in the supine position. A mental nerve block can be administered by palpation of the mental foramen. The chin is disinfected below the second premolar where the procedure will be performed. The physician palpates the patient's chin below the second premolar and should detect the mental foramen. After identification of the mental foramen, the physician's second or third finger should be placed and maintained over the mental foramen. Then, a 25-gauge needle is inserted slowly into the mental foramen. After assessing no aspiration of blood, 0.5–1 mL of local anesthetics is injected.

After 15–20 min, block efficacy is confirmed, and 0.2–0.5 mL of a neurolytic agent (phenol, alcohol, or glycerol) is injected. To prevent hematoma or edema, physicians should instruct the patient to press on the injection site with gauze for at least 5 min.

Ultrasound Guidance Technique

Recently, ultrasound guidance blocks have been commonly used. Thus, this procedure can be performed more accurately and safely. A linear probe or a hockey stick probe was used. The physician places the probe on the patient's chin (the mental foramen is located below the second premolar.) and detects the mental foramen (Fig. 4). To determine the mental branch of the inferior alveolar artery, a physician can use color Doppler imaging [18]. After checking the artery position, a 25-gauge needle in-plane technique was inserted into the mental foramen. Sometimes, the mental nerve can be identified using ultrasound. After placing the needle near the nerve or mental foramen, inject 0.5–1 mL of local anesthetics. After 15–20 min, block efficacy is confirmed, and 0.2–0.5 mL of a neurolytic agent (phenol, alcohol, or glycerol) is injected. The needle insertion out-of-plane technique can also be used.

1.6.3 Effects

It is difficult to find the investigation of mental nerve neurolysis. In the investigation of alcohol neurolysis for inferior alveolar nerve, the mean effect was 19 months [20].

1.6.4 Complications

Pain at the injection site, anesthesia dolorosa, edema, hematoma, dizziness, and infection can be possible side effects. To prevent edema or hematoma, compression of the injection site for over 5 min is mandatory.

2 Sphenopalatine Ganglion Block [1]

2.1 Anatomy

The sphenopalatine ganglion (pterygopalatine ganglion) is located in the pterygopalatine fossa (Fig. 5A) and the largest peripheral parasympathetic ganglion. In the pterygopalatine fossa, the anterior part is the maxillary sinus, the posterior part is the medial pterygoid plate, the medial part is the palatine bone and pterygopalatine foramen, and the superior part is the sphenoid sinus. It supplies the paranasal sinus, lacrimal gland, nasal cavity, gingiva, pharynx, and hard palate. It is associated with the branches of the maxillary nerve, and the sensory root is derived from the sphenopalatine branches of the maxillary nerve. It also consists of sympathetic efferent fibers from the superior cervical ganglion.

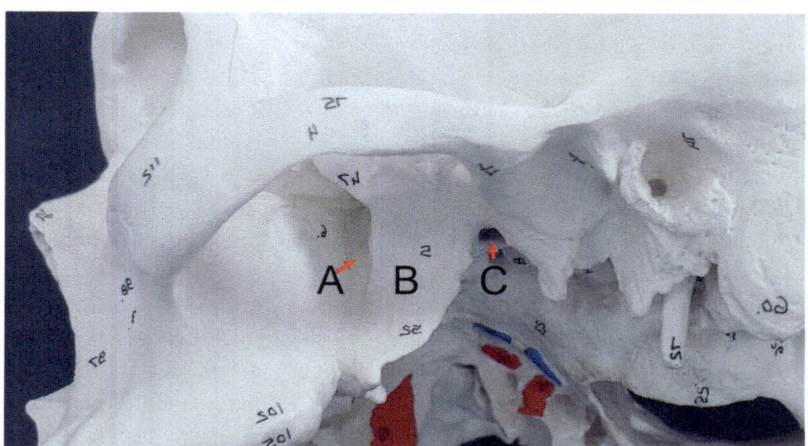

Fig. 5 Lateral side of skull. (A) pterygopalatine fossa, (B) pterygoid plate, (C) foramen ovale

2.2 Indications

Trigeminal neuralgia, migraine, cluster headache, atypical facial pain, postherpetic neuralgia, cancer pain, trigeminal nerve injury.

2.3 Methods [21]

There are transnasal, transoral, and transcutaneous approaches for sphenopalatine ganglion block.

2.3.1 Transnasal Approach

The patient is placed in the supine position with the neck extension.

Dip a 9 cm cotton swab was placed in a local anesthetic, such as 4% lidocaine, and inserted into the nasal cavity parallel to the zygomatic arch. The measurement of the distance from the opening of the nares to the mandibular notch directly below the zygoma can be used to estimate the depth of advancement needed. The tip of the cotton swab is laid on the nasopharyngeal mucosa, posterior to the middle nasal turbinate. A second cotton swab may be placed slightly posterior and superior to the initial applicator. However, a second cotton swab was not mandatory. A response is typically observed in 5–10 min. However, the cotton swab may be left in position for 30–45 min.

2.3.2 Transoral Approach

The transoral approach involves injection through the greater palatine foramen (GPF). The GPF was located just inside the gum line of the third molar. A curved dental needle passes through the GPF in the posterior portion of the hard palate. The needle moves 2.5 cm upward and backward. Then, 1–2 mL of local anesthetics with/without steroids were injected.

2.3.3 Infrazygomatic Approach

This approach can be used by C-arm fluoroscopy guidance.

The patient is placed in a supine position. Disinfect the lateral face near and below the zygomatic arch.

To make the bilateral pterygomaxillary fissure overlap in the lateral view, move the patient's head or C-arm fluoroscopy. The skin entry point can be the midpoint of the pterygomaxillary fissure. If the coronoid process of the mandible covers most of the pterygomaxillary fissure, the entry point can be above the sigmoid notch of the mandible. After skin infiltration with local anesthetics, a 10 cm 23 or 25 gauge needle was inserted into the target point (the midpoint of the pterygopalatine fossa) in the lateral view. Needles can generally be advanced toward the inside, upward, and front of the target point. The direction is determined in the lateral views, and the depth was checked on the PA views. If a physician feels resistance at any time, he should take the needle out slightly and change the direction. The terminal needle position in the AP view was immediately adjacent to the ipsilateral nasal wall (Fig. 6). If it was confirmed that the needle was located in the pterygopalatine fossa, 0.5–1 mL of contrast media is administered to ensure that there was no intravascular or nasal injection. If there is no problem, inject 1–2 mL of local anesthetics with/without steroids.

2.3.4 Pulsed RF Treatment

If the effect of the nerve block is short, pulsed RF treatment can be performed. Although the RF needle is larger than the block needle, the insertion technique is the same as above. The RF needle with a 0.2–0.5 cm active tip was positioned at the pterygopalatine fossa; the physician started 50 Hz and 1 V sensory stimulation and found stimulation of the roof of the nose. Then, move the needle little by little until the ganglion is found with a stimulation of 0.3–0.5 V. Stimulation below 0.5 V means that the needle is quite close to or in contact with the ganglion. Pulsed RF treatment was performed for 10 min.

Conventional RF Thermocoagulation

If the effect of the nerve block is short, conventional RF thermocoagulation can be performed. The insertion technique is the same as the pulsed RF treatment described above. An RF needle with a 0.5–1 cm active tip was positioned at the pterygopalatine fossa; the physician started

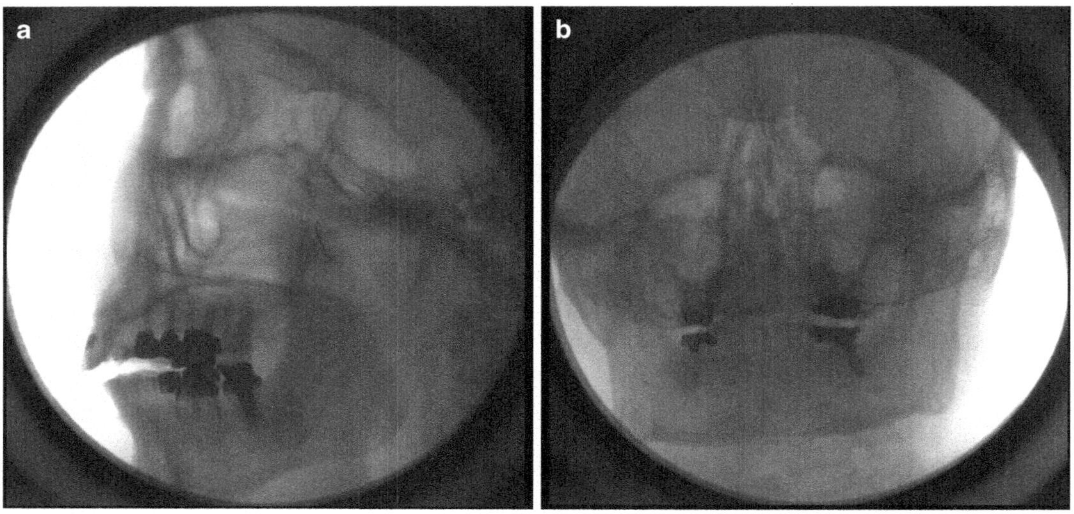

Fig. 6 Needle tip position of sphenopalatine ganglion block in lateral view (**a**) and PA view (**b**)

50 Hz and 1 V sensory stimulation and found stimulation of the roof of the nose. Then, move the needle little by little until the ganglion is found with a stimulation of 0.3–0.5 V. Stimulation below 0.5 V means that the needle is quite close to or in contact with the ganglion. After injection of local anesthetics, conventional RF thermocoagulation at 60–80 °C was performed for 2 min several times. In general, the procedure starts at a low temperature and gradually increases with temperature. Finally, 1–2 mL of local anesthetics with steroids can be injected.

2.4 Effects

Some studies have investigated the effect of sphenopalatine ganglion block on trigeminal neuralgia [22, 23]. However, further evaluation with a large number of patients and long-term studies are needed.

In patients with intractable facial and head pain, pain was completely relieved in 35% of patients, and mild to moderate pain relief was achieved in 42% of patients [24]. Further evaluation of the long-term effect of pulsed RF treatment of the sphenopalatine ganglion is needed. There are some case series about the effect of conventional thermocoagulation of the sphenopalatine ganglion [25]. Further evaluation of conventional RF thermocoagulation of the sphenopalatine ganglion is needed.

2.5 Complications

Pain at the injection site, edema, hematoma, dizziness, headache, infection, bradycardia, diplopia, and epistaxis (transnasal approach) can be possible side effects.

3 Major Branch Block of the Trigeminal Nerve, Pulsed RF Treatment, and Percutaneous Neurolysis for Major Branch of Trigeminal Nerve

3.1 Maxillary Nerve Block and Pulsed RF Treatment [1]

3.1.1 Anatomy

The maxillary nerve is one of the three major branches of the trigeminal nerve. It is a pure sensory nerve. It begins at the middle of the trigeminal ganglion and passes through the lateral wall of the cavernous sinus. Then, it exits from the skull though the foramen rotundum. The branch before the foramen rotundum was the middle meningeal nerve. The branches after the foramen rotundum are branches to the pterygopalatine ganglion, zygomaticofacial nerve, zygomaticotemporal nerve, pterygopalatine nerve, posterior superior alveolar nerve, greater and lesser palatine nerve, anterior superior alveolar nerve, middle superior alveolar nerve, and external nasal branch.

In pterygopalatine fossa, maxillary nerve is placed above the sphenopalatine ganglion.

3.1.2 Indications

Trigeminal neuralgia, atypical facial pain, postherpetic neuralgia, cancer pain, trigeminal nerve injury.

3.1.3 Methods

The methods of maxillary nerve block are similar to the infrazygomatic approach of the sphenopalatine ganglion. However, the endpoint of the needle tip was different. The target point of the sphenopalatine ganglion block is the midpoint of the pterygopalatine fossa, and that of the maxillary nerve block is the upper part of the pterygopalatine fossa. Therefore, the needle tip goes upward compared to the sphenopalatine ganglion block.

Infrazygomatic Approach

This approach can be used by C-arm fluoroscopy guidance.

The patient was placed in a supine position. Disinfect the lateral face near and below the zygomatic arch.

To make bilateral pterygomaxillary fissure overlap in lateral view, move the patient's head or C-arm fluoroscopy. The skin entry point can be the midpoint of the pterygomaxillary fissure. If the coronoid process of the mandible covers most of the pterygomaxillary fissure, the entry point can be above the sigmoid notch of the mandible. After skin infiltration with local anesthetics, a 10 cm 23 or 25 gauge needle was inserted into the target point (the upper part of the pterygopalatine fossa) in the lateral view. Needles can usually be advanced toward the inside, upward, and front of the target point. The direction was checked in the lateral views, and the depth was checked on the PA views. If a physician feels resistance at any time, he should take the needle out slightly and change the direction. The terminal needle position in the AP view was adjacent to the ipsilateral nasal wall (Fig. 7). If paresthesia appeared in the maxillary nerve distribution area during needle insertion, the needle was stopped and the position was checked by C-arm fluoroscopy. If it was confirmed that the needle was located in the upper

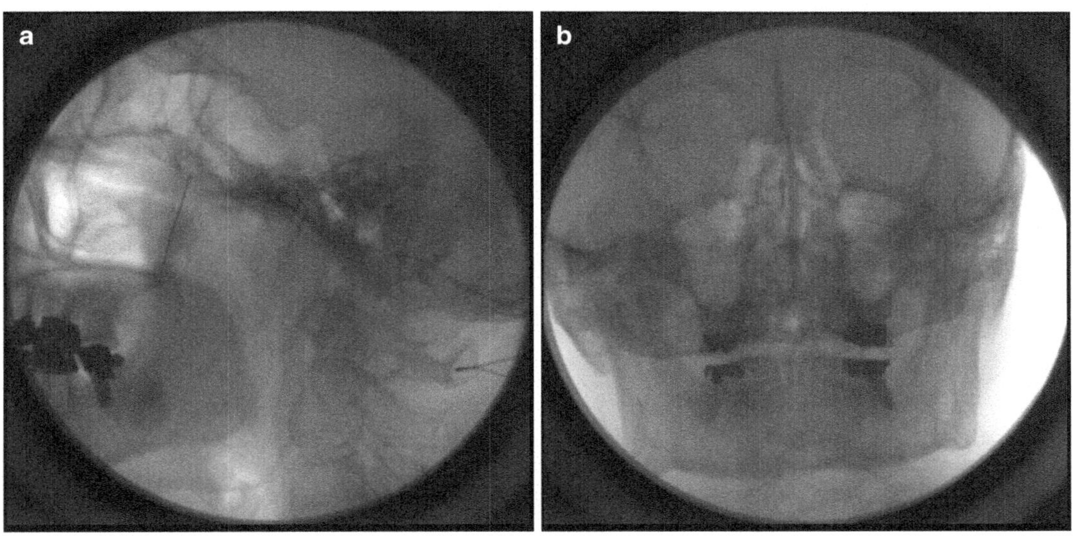

Fig. 7 Needle tip position of maxillary nerve block and neurolysis in lateral view (**a**) and PA view (**b**)

part of the pterygopalatine fossa, 0.5–1 mL of contrast media is administered to ensure that there was no intravascular injection. If there is no problem, inject 1–2 mL of local anesthetic with/without steroids.

Pulsed RF Treatment
If the effect of the nerve block is short, pulsed RF treatment can be performed. Although the RF needle is larger than the block needle, the insertion technique is the same as above. The RF needle with a 0.2–0.5 cm active tip was positioned at the upper part of the pterygopalatine fossa, and the physician started 50 Hz and 1 V sensory stimulation and found stimulation of the maxillary nerve. Then, move the needle little by little until the maxillary nerve is found with a stimulation of 0.3–0.5 V. Stimulation below 0.5 V means that the needle is quite close to or in contact with the nerve. Pulsed RF treatment was performed for 10 min.

Conventional RF Thermocoagulation
If the effect of the nerve block is short, conventional RF thermocoagulation can be performed. The insertion technique is the same as the pulsed RF treatment described above. An RF needle with 0.5–1 cm active tip is positioned near the maxillary nerve, the physician starts 50 Hz and 1 V sensory stimulation and stimulates the maxillary nerve. Then, move the needle little by little until the nerve is found with a stimulation of 0.3–0.5 V. Stimulation below 0.5 V means that the needle is quite close to or in contact with the nerve. After injection of local anesthetics, conventional RF thermocoagulation at 60–80 °C was performed for 2 min several times. In general, the procedure starts at a low temperature and gradually increases with temperature. Finally, 1–2 mL of local anesthetics with steroids can be injected.

3.1.4 Effects

Clinically, the maxillary nerve is an effective treatment for trigeminal neuralgia. However, there are few articles on maxillary nerve block and pulsed RF treatment for trigeminal neuralgia. Further evaluation of the maxillary nerve block and pulsed RF treatment is needed.

In 25 patients with trigeminal neuralgia of the maxillary branch, conventional RF thermocoagulation was effective [26]. During the follow-up period (mean, 14.74 months), nine (36%) patients recurred and the symptoms were well managed with repeat procedures. Complete pain relief was achieved in 85 (97.7%) of 87 patients with idiopathic trigeminal neuralgia of the maxillary nerve [27]. Fifteen (17.2%) patients experienced recurring pain during the mean follow-up period of 44.3 months. In a prospective comparison with conventional RF thermocoagulation through the foramen rotundum versus the foramen ovale, thermocoagulation of the maxillary nerve through the foramen rotundum had better efficacy and fewer complications than Gasserian ganglion ablation [28].

3.1.5 Complications

Pain at the injection site, edema, hematoma, dizziness, headache, infection, bradycardia, diplopia, and paralysis of the abducens nerve can be possible side effects. After conventional RF thermocoagulation, 23 out of 25 patients had facial numbness; however, this was tolerable [26]. There were no other complications. After conventional RF thermocoagulation, no severe complications occurred, except for hypoesthesia of V2 distribution in all patients (100%) and facial hematoma in 10 (11.5%) patients [27].

3.2 Percutaneous Neurolysis for Maxillary Nerve

3.2.1 Indications

Trigeminal neuralgia, cancer pain, cluster headache, or atypical facial pain [9].

3.2.2 Methods

The methods of maxillary nerve block are similar to the infrazygomatic approach of the sphenopalatine ganglion. However, the endpoint of the needle tip was different. The target point of the sphenopalatine ganglion block is the midpoint of the pterygopalatine fossa, and that of the maxillary nerve block is the upper part of the pterygopalatine fossa. Therefore, the needle tip goes upward compared to the sphenopalatine ganglion block.

Infrazygomatic Approach

This approach can be used by C-arm fluoroscopy guidance.

The patient was placed in a supine position. Disinfect the lateral face near and below the zygomatic arch.

To make bilateral pterygomaxillary fissure overlap in lateral view, move the patient's head or C-arm fluoroscopy. The skin entry point can be the midpoint of the pterygomaxillary fissure. If the coronoid process of the mandible covers most of the pterygomaxillary fissure, the entry point can be above the sigmoid notch of the mandible. After skin infiltration with local anesthetics, a 10 cm 23 or 25 gauge needle was inserted into the target point (the upper part of the pterygopalatine fossa) in the lateral view. Needles can usually be advanced toward the inside, upward, and front of the target point. The direction was checked in the lateral views, and the depth was checked on the PA views. If a physician feels resistance at any time, he should take the needle out slightly and change the direction. The terminal needle position in the AP view was adjacent to the ipsilateral nasal wall (Fig. 7). If paresthesia appeared in the maxillary nerve distribution area during needle insertion, the needle was stopped and the position was checked by C-arm fluoroscopy. If it was confirmed that the needle was located in the upper part of the pterygopalatine fossa, 0.5–1 mL of contrast media is administered to ensure that there was no intravascular injection. If there is no problem, inject 0.5–1.5 mL of local anesthetic. After 15–20 min, block efficacy is confirmed, and 0.2–0.5 mL of a neurolytic agent (phenol, alcohol, or glycerol) is injected.

3.2.3 Effects

With regard to alcohol neurolysis of the infraorbital nerve, Wakasugi [11], Wilkins [12], and Kim et al. [29] reported a mean effect duration of 17 months, 12 months, and 16.8 months, respectively.

3.2.4 Complications

Pain at the injection site, anesthesia dolorosa, edema, hematoma, dizziness, headache, infection, bradycardia, diplopia, and paralysis of the abducens nerve can be possible side effects.

3.3 Mandibular Nerve Block and Pulsed RF Treatment [1]

3.3.1 Anatomy

The mandibular nerve is the largest of the three major branches of the trigeminal nerve. It is a mixed nerve that includes the sensory and motor nerves. It begins at the lower lateral part of the trigeminal ganglion and exits from the skull through the foramen ovale. The branches are meningeal branch, and masseteric, nervus spinosus, anterior and posterior deep temporal, buccal, lateral pterygoid, lingual, auriculotemporal, and inferior alveolar nerves.

3.3.2 Indications

Trigeminal neuralgia, atypical facial pain, postherpetic neuralgia, cancer pain, trigeminal nerve injury.

3.3.3 Methods

Lateral Extraoral Route, Coronoid Approach (Blind Technique)

The coronoid approach of mandibular nerve block can be performed using a blind technique or C-arm fluoroscopy guidance.

The patient is placed in a supine position. The lateral face is disinfected near and below the zygomatic arch. The entry point is below the zygomatic arch on a vertical line passing through the center of the sigmoid notch of the mandible. The needle is inserted perpendicular to the skin. If the needle goes approximately 4–5 cm, it meets the lateral pterygoid plate (Fig. 5B). This position is 1 cm anterior to the foramen ovale (Fig. 5C). Afterward, the needle is pulled back slightly and moved posterior slowly to the outside of the pterygoid plate. If paresthesia appears in the mandibular nerve distribution area, the needle is stopped, and blood aspiration is assessed. If there is no problem, inject 1–2 mL of local anesthetic with/without steroids.

Lateral Extraoral Route, Coronoid Approach (C-Arm Fluoroscopy Guidance)

The patient is placed in a supine position. The lateral face is disinfected near and below the zygomatic arch. To make the bilateral posterior margin of the pterygoid plate overlap in the lateral view, the patient's head or C-arm fluoroscopy is moved. The entry point is the same as that of the blind technique. The needle is advanced to the upper posterior part of the pterygoid plate and contacted. The needle is then pulled back slightly and moved posterior slowly to the foramen ovale. If paresthesia appears in the mandibular nerve distribution area, the needle is stopped, and blood aspiration is assessed.

The needle depth can be assessed by C-arm fluoroscopy with a submentovertex view or anteroposterior oblique view. The physician can advance the needle near the foramen ovale by performing C-arm fluoroscopy. If there is no problem, inject 1–2 mL of local anesthetic with/without steroids.

Perioral Approach

This approach can be used by C-arm fluoroscopy guidance.

The patient is placed in the supine position and his head extended by approximately 45°. If the pillow is placed under the patient's shoulder, it is easier to lean his head extension (Fig. 8). The perioral face is disinfected laterally from the lip commissure. To make the bilateral temporomandibular joint or posterior margin of the pterygoid plate overlap in the lateral view, the patient's head is moved. This can be helpful for assessing needle depth in the lateral view. Then, the image intensifier or flat panel detector is moved at 15–25° laterally to the painful side and 15–30° of caudal inclination (Fig. 9). The skin entry point corresponds to the foramen ovale 2–3 cm lateral to the lip commissure. The target point is lower than the lateral margin of the foramen ovale. Needles can generally be advanced inside and upwards to the target point. The direction and depth are assessed in the anteroposterior oblique views and on the lateral views, respectively. The terminal needle position in the anteroposterior oblique view is immediately adjacent to the target point or foramen ovale (Fig. 10). If paresthesia appears in the mandibular nerve distribution area during needle insertion, the needle is stopped, and the position is determined using C-arm fluoroscopy. If it is confirmed that the needle is located in the target point or immediately adjacent to foramen ovale, 0.5–1 mL of contrast media is administered to ensure that there is no intravascular. If there is no problem, inject 1–2 mL of local anesthetic with/without steroids.

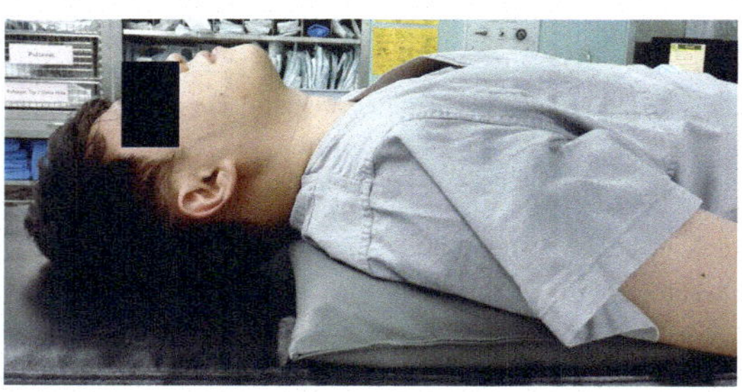

Fig. 8 Pillow is placed under the shoulder for assisting in extending the head approximately 45°

Pulsed RF Treatment

If the effect of the nerve block is short, pulsed RF treatment can be performed. Although the RF needle is larger than the block needle, the insertion technique is the same as above. The RF needle with a 0.2–0.5 cm active tip is positioned adjacent to the foramen ovale, and the physician initiates 50 Hz and 1 V sensory stimulation and detects stimulation of the mandibular nerve. Then, the needle is gradually moved until the mandibular nerve is detected with a stimulation of 0.3–0.5 V. Stimulation below 0.5 V indicates that the needle is in close proximity to or in contact with the nerve. Pulsed RF treatment can be performed for 10 min.

Conventional RF Thermocoagulation

If the effect of the nerve block is short, conventional RF thermocoagulation can be performed. The insertion technique is the same as the pulsed RF treatment described above. An RF needle

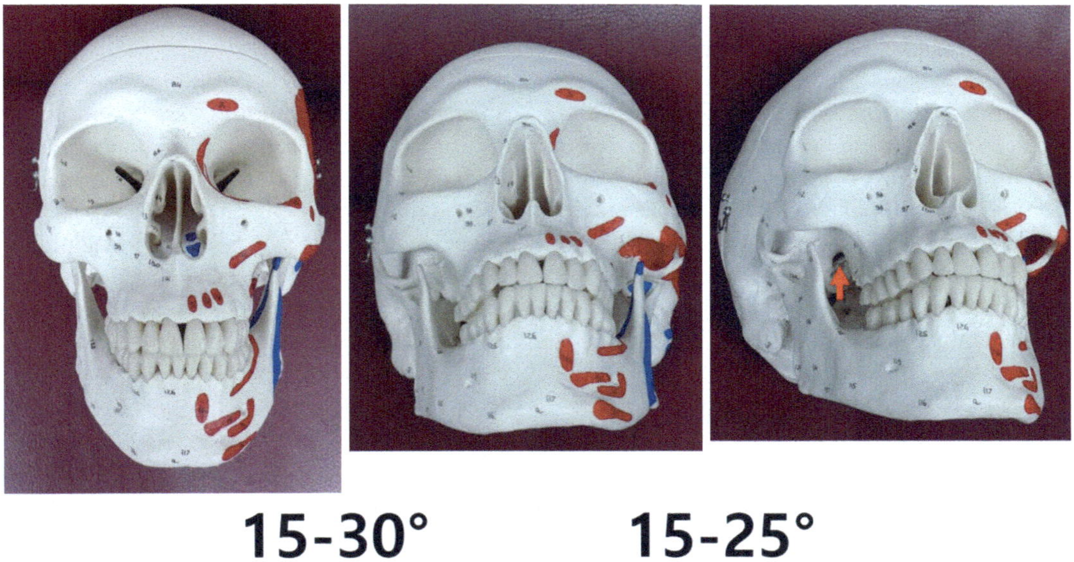

Fig. 9 The motion of image intensifier or flat panel detector to determine foramen ovale: move at 15–25° laterally to the painful side and 15–30° of caudal inclination, red arrow: foramen ovale

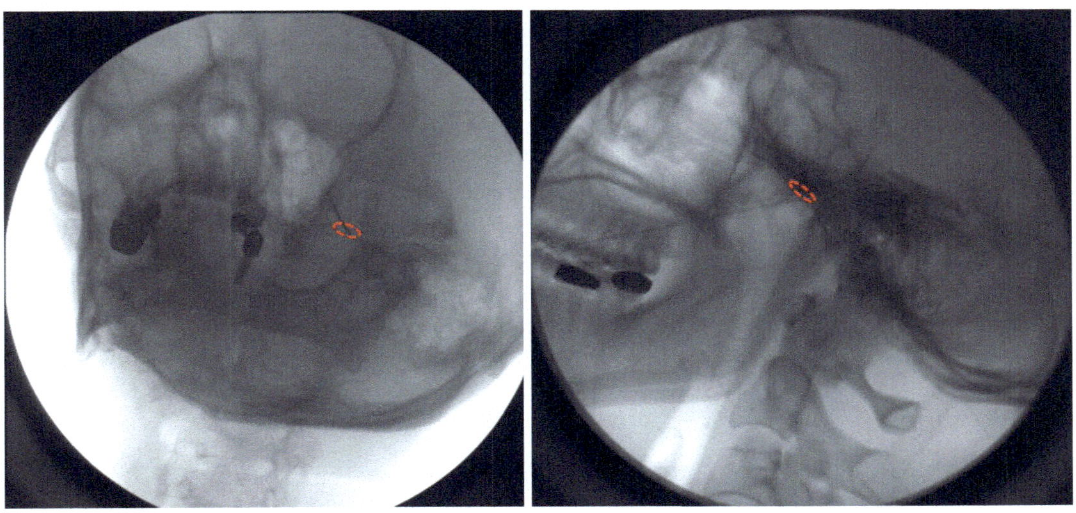

Fig. 10 The needle tip position of mandibular nerve block. Red dotted ovale: foramen ovale

with 0.5–1 cm active tip is positioned near the mandibular nerve, the physician initiates 50 Hz and 1 V sensory stimulation and stimulates the mandibular nerve. Then, the needle is gradually moved until the nerve is detected with a stimulation of 0.3–0.5 V. Stimulation below 0.5 V indicates that the needle is in close proximity or in contact with the nerve. After injection of local anesthetics, conventional RF thermocoagulation at 60–0 °C can be performed for 2 min several times. In general, the procedure initiates at a low temperature and gradually increases with temperature. Finally, 1–2 mL of local anesthetics with steroids can be injected.

3.3.4 Effects

Pulsed RF treatment of the mandibular nerve was effective in patients with refractory TN [30]. The therapeutic effects lasted for over 6 months and 1 year, and medications including carbamazepine could be discontinued or reduced. Further evaluation of the mandibular nerve block and pulsed RF treatment is needed.

Conventional RF thermocoagulation of the mandibular nerve was performed in 107 patients with trigeminal neuralgia of the mandibular nerve [31]. Of these, 104 patients experienced immediate complete pain relief, while two were cured after the second procedure.

The effects and complications of monopolar and bipolar disorders were compared in 26 patients with extracranial RF thermocoagulation of the mandibular branch [32]. During the immediate postoperative period, both groups achieved 100% complete pain relief. During up to 27 months follow-up, complete pain relief persisted in the bipolar group, and one patient recurred at 14 months.

3.3.5 Complications

Pain at the injection site, edema, hematoma, dizziness, headache, infection, epidural or subarachnoid injection, taste impairment, paralysis of the facial nerve, asymmetric face, and paralysis of the masseter muscle can be possible side effects.

No intracranial hemorrhage not infection complications occurred.

In 107 patients after extracranial RF thermocoagulation of the mandibular nerve, no intracranial hemorrhage or infection complications occurred, except for facial hematoma in 21 cases [31].

After conventional RF thermocoagulation, the complications of the bipolar and monopolar groups were not significantly different [32].

3.4 Percutaneous Neurolysis for Mandibular Nerve

3.4.1 Indications

Trigeminal neuralgia, cancer pain, cluster headache, or atypical facial pain [9].

3.4.2 Methods

Lateral Extraoral Route, Coronoid Approach (Blind Technique)

The coronoid approach of mandibular nerve block can be performed using a blind technique or C-arm fluoroscopy guidance.

The patient is placed in a supine position. The lateral face is disinfected near and below the zygomatic arch. The entry point is below the zygomatic arch on a vertical line passing through the center of the sigmoid notch of the mandible. The needle is inserted perpendicular to the skin. If the needle goes approximately 4–5 cm, it meets the lateral pterygoid plate (Fig. 5B). This position is 1 cm anterior to the foramen ovale (Fig. 5C). Afterward, the needle is pulled back slightly and moved posterior slowly to the outside of the pterygoid plate. If paresthesia appears in the mandibular nerve distribution area, the needle is stopped, and blood aspiration is assessed. If there is no problem, inject 0.5–1.5 mL of local anesthetic. After 15–20 min, block efficacy is confirmed, and 0.2–0.5 mL of a neurolytic agent (phenol, alcohol, or glycerol) is injected.

Lateral Extraoral Route, Coronoid Approach (C-Arm Fluoroscopy Guidance)

The patient is placed in a supine position. The lateral face is disinfected near and below the zygomatic arch. To make the bilateral posterior margin of the pterygoid plate overlap in the lateral view, the patient's head or C-arm fluoroscopy is moved. The entry point is the same as that of the blind technique. The needle is advanced to the upper posterior part of the pterygoid plate and contacted. The needle is then pulled back slightly, and moved posterior slowly to the foramen ovale. If paresthesia appears in the mandibular nerve distribution area, the needle is stopped, and blood aspiration is assessed.

The needle depth can be assessed by C-arm fluoroscopy with a submentovertex view or anteroposterior oblique view. The physician can advance the needle near the foramen ovale by performing C-arm fluoroscopy. If there is no problem, inject 0.5–1.5 mL of local anesthetic. After 15–20 min, block efficacy is confirmed, and 0.2–0.5 mL of a neurolytic agent (phenol, alcohol, or glycerol) is injected.

Perioral Approach

This approach can be used by C-arm fluoroscopy guidance.

The patient is placed in the supine position and his head extended by approximately 45°. If the pillow is placed under the patient's shoulder, it is easier to lean his head extension (Fig. 8). The perioral face is disinfected laterally from the lip commissure. To make the bilateral temporomandibular joint or posterior margin of the pterygoid plate overlap in the lateral view, the patient's head is moved. This can be helpful for assessing needle depth in the lateral view. Then, the image intensifier or flat panel detector is moved at 15–25° laterally to the painful side and 15–30° of caudal inclination (Fig. 9). The skin entry point corresponds to the foramen ovale 2–3 cm lateral to the lip commissure. The target point is lower than the lateral margin of the foramen ovale. Needles can generally be advanced inside and upwards to the target point. The direction and depth are assessed in the anteroposterior oblique views and on the lateral views, respectively. The terminal needle position in the anteroposterior oblique view is immediately adjacent to the target point or foramen ovale (Fig. 10). If paresthesia appears in the mandibular nerve distribution area during needle insertion, the needle is stopped, and the position is determined using C-arm fluoroscopy. If it is confirmed that the needle is located in the target point or immediately adjacent to foramen ovale, 0.5–1 mL of contrast media is administered to ensure that there is no intravascular. If there is no problem, inject 0.5–1.5 mL of local anesthetic. After 15–20 min, block efficacy is confirmed, and 0.2–0.5 mL of a neurolytic agent (phenol, alcohol, or glycerol) is injected.

3.4.3 Effects

With regard to alcohol neurolysis of the infraorbital nerve, Wakasugi [11], Wilkins [12], and Kim et al. [29] reported a mean effect duration of 21 months, 16 months, and 23.4 months, respectively. Han et al. reported that V3 and V2 + 3 neurolysis using alcohol produced longer pain relief than other neurolyses such as V2, supraorbital nerve, infraorbital nerve, and major branch with supraorbital or infraorbital nerve [33]. In an investigation of simultaneous peripheral and major branch neurolysis using alcohol, the prevalence of sensory discomfort, difficulty in mastication, tinnitus, ptosis, excessive salivation, and diplopia was 7.3%, 1.1%, 0.7%, 0.2%, 0.6%, and 0.4%, respectively [33]. Repeated alcohol neurolysis was effective in recurrent cases [29, 33, 34].

3.4.4 Complications

Pain at the injection site, anesthesia dolorosa, edema, hematoma, dizziness, headache, infection, epidural or subarachnoid injection, taste impairment, paralysis of the facial nerve, asymmetric face, and paralysis of the masseter muscle can be possible side effects.

4 RF Thermocoagulation of Trigeminal Ganglion or Rootlet [1, 35] and Percutaneous Neurolysis of Trigeminal Ganglion

4.1 RF Thermocoagulation of Trigeminal Ganglion or Rootlet

4.1.1 Anatomy [36]

The trigeminal nerve is the largest cranial nerve. The trigeminal ganglion is located in Meckel's cave, a cavern in the petrosal part of the temporal bone on the floor of the middle cranial fossa, formed by a pocket of the dura mater. Three large nerves arise from the trigeminal ganglion: the ophthalmic nerve (V1), maxillary nerve (V2), and mandibular nerve (V3). The trigeminal ganglion is a sensory ganglion, and a thin bundle of trigeminal motor fibers passing through the ganglion accompanies the trigeminal nerve medially and the mandibular nerve rostrally from the ganglion.

The fascicles of nerve fibers separate aggregations of neurons that belong to the three parti-

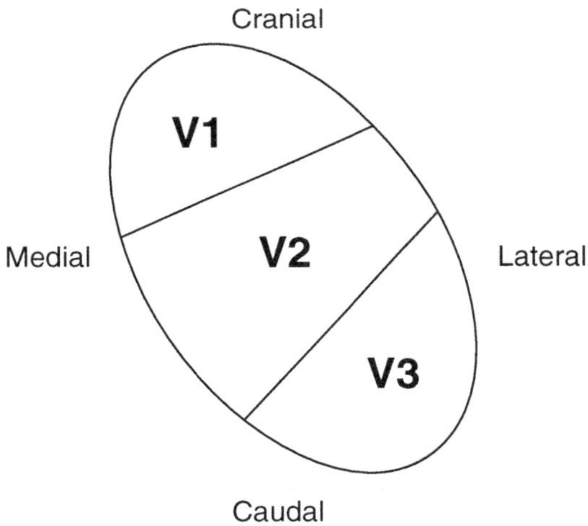

Fig. 11 The separated fascicles of nerve fibers within trigeminal ganglion

tions, V1–V3, which can be distinguished according to their location within the ganglion. In horizontal sections, the ophthalmic division is located cranio-medially, the maxillary division centrally, and the mandibular division caudal-laterally (Fig. 11). Therefore, during RF thermocoagulation of the trigeminal ganglion or rootlet, physicians should position each trigeminal nerve division and advance the RF needle toward the symptom-related area.

The proximal trigeminal ganglion is connected by rootlets, which exist in the form of floating in the CSF.

4.1.2 Indication

Trigeminal neuralgia.

Some physicians perform RF thermocoagulation of the trigeminal ganglion or rootlet in patients with atypical facial pain, postherpetic neuralgia, cancer pain, or trigeminal nerve injury. However, there is a possibility that the symptoms may worsen after the procedure, so these patients should carefully decide whether to perform the procedure.

4.1.3 Methods

The painful process is performed under sedation, and but stimulation is found while the patient is awake.

RF Thermocoagulation of the Trigeminal Ganglion

With the patient in a supine position on the operating table, a pillow beneath the shoulders, and the head hyperextended, electrocardiography, pulse oxygen saturation monitoring, and noninvasive blood pressure monitoring were initiated, and oxygen was supplied at 5 L/min through a facial mask. After ascertaining the foramen ovale on the lesion side using a C-arm fluoroscope, the area was anesthetized with 1% lidocaine, and a curved RF needle using a 0.2–1 cm active tip was inserted approximately 2–3 cm away from the mouth angle using a perioral approach. Using the C-arm fluoroscope to ascertain the needle position on oblique and lateral images, the needle was advanced to the front of the foramen ovale. After injecting propofol (1.0–1.5 mg/kg) and fentanyl (1 mg/kg) for sedation, the needle was introduced into the foramen ovale and positioned the trigeminal ganglion. When the patient regained consciousness, the physician checked stimulation at a frequency of 50 Hz at 0.3–0.5 V. If the stimulus occurs somewhere other than the pain area, the needle position is changed, and the stimulation is checked. The patient was then re-anesthetized with propofol 1.0 mg/kg, and RF thermocoagulation was performed 3–5 times for 60–120 s at 60–80 °C. Propofol was injected for the first RF thermocoagulation application; no further propofol injections were administered thereafter. After the procedure, the patients were observed for 1 day for side effects and complications.

RF Thermocoagulation of the Trigeminal Rootlet

The insertion technique is the same as RF thermocoagulation of the trigeminal ganglion. However, the active tip positions different. It should be advanced through the trigeminal ganglion and positioned at the rootlets in the CSF. The needle was introduced into the foramen ovale and passed through the trigeminal ganglion. The fluoroscope was used to ascertain that the needle was at the petroclival junction, and/or cerebrospinal fluid flow from the needle was con-

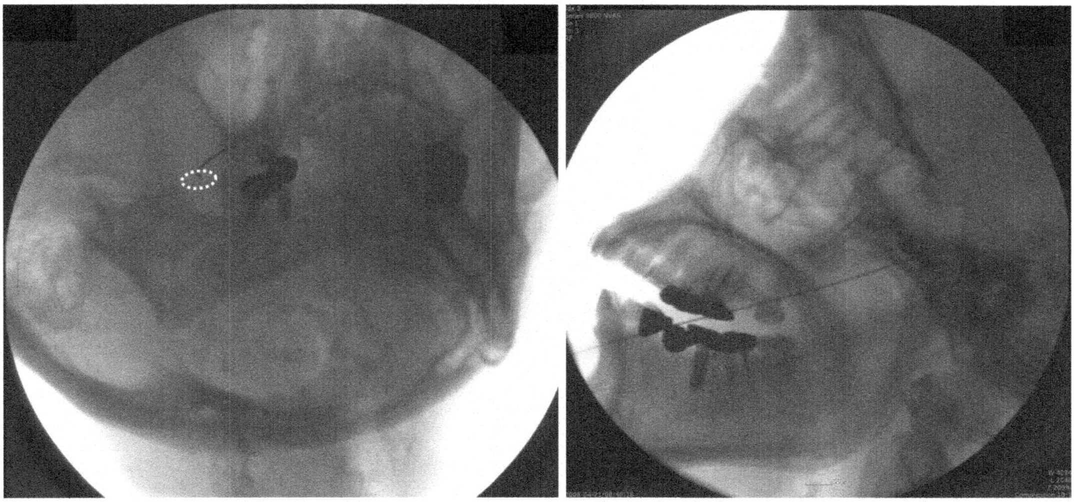

Fig. 12 Needle tip position of radiofrequency (RF) thermocoagulation of trigeminal rootlet and retrogasserian neurolysis, white dotted ovale: foramen ovale

firmed (Fig. 12). When the patient regained consciousness, physician located the needle tip at the source of pain by slowly rotating a curved radiofrequency needle stimulated at a frequency of 50 Hz at 0.3–0.5 V. To detect the stimulation of pain legion, the active tip can be advanced or pulled back slowly. To prevent brain injury, the active tip should not proceed more than 2 mm above the petroclival junction. The patient was then re-anesthetized using propofol 1.0 mg/kg, and RF thermocoagulation was performed 3–5 times for 60–120 s at 60–80 °C. Propofol was injected for the first RF thermocoagulation application; no further propofol injections were administered thereafter. After the procedure, the patients were observed for 1 day for side effects and complications.

4.1.4 Effects

In a multicenter retrospective study of 1481 patients with trigeminal neuralgia, the median RFS was 136 months [37]. The rate of RFS was 85.3% at 1 year, 74.6% at 3 years, 68.0% at 5 years, and 54.9% at 10 years.

In the 1600 patients with idiopathic trigeminal neuralgia (mean follow-up period: 68.1 months), acute pain relief was achieved in 97.6% of patients, and complete pain relief was achieved at 5 years in 57.7% of the patients [38]. At 5 years, pain relief was reported in 92% of patients who underwent a single or multiple procedures.

4.1.5 Complications

Pain at the injection site, edema, hematoma, dizziness, headache, infection, meningitis, taste impairment, numbness or decreased facial sensation, loss of corneal reflex, paralysis of the facial nerve, asymmetric face, and paralysis of the masseter muscle can be possible side effects.

Complications included diminished corneal reflex in 91 (5.7%) patients, masseter weakness, and paralysis in 66 (4.1%), dysesthesia in 16 (1%), anesthesia dolorosa in 12 (0.8%), keratitis in 10 (0.6%), and transient paralysis of cranial nerves III and VI in 12 (0.8%) patients. Permanent cranial nerve VI palsy was observed in two patients, cerebrospinal fluid leakage in two, carotid-cavernous fistula in one, and aseptic meningitis in one patient [38]. According to a review article [39], if V1 is involved, to decrease the risk of corneal reflex weakness or disappearance, a temperature of ≤65 °C is recommended. If V2 and/or V3 are involved, temperatures of 65–70 °C are more suitable to effectively control pain and decrease the probability of adverse reactions. Too high temperature (≥80 °C) should be avoided because it can critically damage the tissue and is associated with irreversible complications.

4.2 Percutaneous Neurolysis of Trigeminal Ganglion

4.2.1 Indication

Trigeminal neuralgia, cancer pain, cluster headache, or atypical facial pain [9].

4.2.2 Methods [40]

The painful process can be performed under sedation and checking effect or side effects is found while the patient is awake. According to a previous study [9], CSF aspiration is not necessary for trigeminal neurolysis. However, the trigeminal ganglion is located in the CSF, and no aspiration indicates that the needle tip has either not penetrated the dura or is located in the trigeminal ganglion. If the needle tip has not penetrate the dura, trigeminal ganglion neurolysis is unsuccessful. However, if the needle tip is located in the trigeminal ganglion, the injected neurolytic solution can spread in the CSF despite there being no aspiration of CSF. Therefore, I recommend retrogasserian neurolysis after confirming CSF aspiration for trigeminal ganglion neurolysis.

With the patient in a supine position on the operating table, a pillow beneath the shoulders, and the head hyperextended, electrocardiography, pulse oxygen saturation monitoring, and noninvasive blood pressure monitoring were initiated, and oxygen was supplied at 5 L/min through a facial mask. After ascertaining the foramen ovale on the lesion side using a C-arm fluoroscope, the area was anesthetized with 1% lidocaine, and a curved RF needle using a 0.2–1 cm active tip was inserted approximately 2–3 cm away from the mouth angle using a perioral approach. Using the C-arm fluoroscope to ascertain the needle position on oblique and lateral images, the needle was advanced to the front of the foramen ovale. After injecting propofol (1.0–1.5 mg/kg) and fentanyl (1 mg/kg) for sedation, the needle was introduced into the foramen ovale and positioned in the cistern of Meckel's cave (Fig. 12) and cerebrospinal fluid flow from the needle was confirmed. Nonionic, water-soluble contrast can be injected to confirm the needle position. Contrast media was gradually injected under fluoroscopy (cisternography) to fill the cistern, and the dose to the cistern was noted. Usually, the capacity of the cistern is 0.3–0.5 mL [40]. After confirming the volume of the cistern, the injected contrast media was aspirated and the same volume of chemical neurolytic was injected. Phenol (6%) and alcohol can be used, but glycerol appears to be the most commonly used agent for neurolysis of the trigeminal ganglion [9]. To check for side effects, neurolytic agents can be injected after the patient regains consciousness. After glycerol injection, the patient turned his head slightly to the injection side and bent his neck for 2 h while sitting. To prevent hematoma formation, the patient pressed the injection site for 10–30 min. Immediately after glycerol injection, the head was bent at 45–60° if the affected part was V1, and if it was V2 or V3, the head was facing forward. After the procedure, the patients were observed for 1 day for side effects and complications.

4.2.3 Effects

In a study of percutaneous retrogasserian glycerol neurolysis in 43 patients, the mean effect duration was 15.5 months [40]. In another study of percutaneous retrogasserian glycerol neurolysis in 80 cases (follow-up duration, 38–54 months), the median pain-free interval was 32 months [41]. In a study of percutaneous retrogasserian glycerol neurolysis in 4012 patients, the immediate success rate was 97.1%, and after 10 years, the total success rate was 81.18% [42]. In this study, the presence of CSF outflow during the procedure was correlated with immediate and long-term outcomes [42]. Repeated glycerol neurolysis was effective in recurrent cases [42].

4.2.4 Complications

Pain at the injection site, anesthesia dolorosa, edema, hematoma, dizziness, headache, infection, meningitis, taste impairment, numbness or decreased facial sensation, loss of corneal reflex, paralysis of the facial nerve, asymmetric face, and paralysis of the masseter muscle can be possible side effects.

Complications included definite hypesthesia of the face (63%), unpleasant dysesthesia (29%), and anesthesia dolorosa (2.5%) [41]. In an investigation of 4012 patients, 24.5% of patients experienced mild headache for 1–2 days after glycerol injection, and 1.2% of patients experienced nausea, vomiting, and severe headache [42]. Fever and blisters that healed spontaneously within a week without any treatment were reported in 47.6% of the patients. Other complications included slow corneal reflex (6.3%), retrobulbar hemorrhage (0.05%), aseptic meningitis (0.12%), and transient paresis (0.05%) [42].

References

1. Society TKP. Keystone of pain intervention. Seoul: Median Book; 2016.
2. Kim JH. Ultrasound guidance nerve block. DaeHan Medical Book; 2019.
3. Woo SW, Lee HJ, Nahm FS, Lee PB, Choi EJ. Anatomic characteristics of supraorbital foramina in Korean using three-dimensional model. Korean J Pain. 2013;26:130–4.
4. Dach F, Eckeli AL, Ferreira Kdos S, Speciali JG. Nerve block for the treatment of headaches and cranial neuralgias - a practical approach. Headache. 2015;55(Suppl 1):59–71.
5. Tsui BC. Ultrasound imaging to localize foramina for superficial trigeminal nerve block. Can J Anaesth. 2009;56:704–6.
6. Luo F, Lu J, Ji N. Treatment of refractory idiopathic supraorbital neuralgia using percutaneous pulsed radiofrequency. Pain Pract. 2018;18:871–8.
7. Ren H, Shen Y, Luo F. Treatment of supraorbital neuralgia using ultrasound-guided radiofrequency Thermocoagulation of the supraorbital nerve: a retrospective study. J Pain Res. 2020;13:251–9.
8. Xie K, Liu S, Huang B, Yao M. Effects of supraorbital foramen variations on the treatment efficacy of radiofrequency therapy for V1 trigeminal neuralgia: a retrospective study. Pain Res Manag. 2020;2020:8142489.
9. Day M. Neurolysis of the trigeminal and sphenopalatine ganglions. Pain Pract. 2001;1(2):171–82.
10. Choe H. Alcohol neurolysis for the treatment of trigeminal neuralgia. Korean J Pain. 1989;2:45–8.
11. Wakasugi B. Treatment of trigeminal neuralgia and facial spasm. Neurosurgeons. 1983;2:203–8.
12. Wilkins RH. Tic doulourex. Contemp Neurosurg. 1986;8:1–6.
13. Ben Aziz M, Cascella M. Peripheral neurolytic blocks. In: StatPearls. Treasure Island (FL), StatPearls Publishing; 2022.
14. Luo F, Lu J, Shen Y, Meng L, Wang T, Ji N. Effectiveness and safety of pulsed radiofrequency treatment guided by computed tomography for refractory neuralgia of infraorbital nerve: a pilot study. Pain Physician. 2015;18:E795–804.
15. Jia Y, Chen Z, Ren H, Luo F. The effectiveness and safety of 42°C pulsed radiofrequency combined with 60°C continuous radiofrequency for refractory infraorbital neuralgia: a prospective study. Pain Physician. 2019;22:E171–e9.
16. Luo F, Wang T, Shen Y, Meng L, Lu J, Ji N. High voltage pulsed radiofrequency for the treatment of refractory neuralgia of the infraorbital nerve: a prospective double-blinded randomized controlled study. Pain Physician. 2017;20:271–9.
17. Gregg JM, Banerjee T, Ghia JN, Campbell R. Radiofrequency thermoneurolysis of peripheral nerves for control of trigeminal neuralgia. Pain. 1978;5:231–43.
18. Allam AE, Khalil AAF, Eltawab BA, Wu WT, Chang KV. Ultrasound-guided intervention for treatment of trigeminal neuralgia: an updated review of anatomy and techniques. Pain Res Manag. 2018;2018:5480728.
19. Perloff MD, Chung JS. Urgent care peripheral nerve blocks for refractory trigeminal neuralgia. Am J Emerg Med. 2018;36:2058–60.
20. Fardy MJ, Zakrzewska JM, Patton DW. Peripheral surgical techniques for the management of trigeminal neuralgia--alcohol and glycerol injections. Acta Neurochir. 1994;129:181–4. discussion 5
21. Alexander CE, Dua A. Sphenopalatine ganglion block. In: StatPearls. Treasure Island (FL), StatPearls Publishing. 2021, .
22. Peterson JN, Schames J, Schames M, King E. Sphenopalatine ganglion block: a safe and easy method for the management of orofacial pain. Cranio. 1995;13:177–81.
23. Candido KD, Massey ST, Sauer R, Darabad RR, Knezevic NN. A novel revision to the classical transnasal topical sphenopalatine ganglion block for the treatment of headache and facial pain. Pain Physician. 2013;16:E769–78.
24. Akbas M, Gunduz E, Sanli S, Yegin A. Sphenopalatine ganglion pulsed radiofrequency treatment in patients suffering from chronic face and head pain. Braz J Anesthesiol. 2016;66:50–4.
25. Ho KWD, Przkora R, Kumar S. Sphenopalatine ganglion: block, radiofrequency ablation and neurostimulation - a systematic review. J Headache Pain. 2017;18:118.
26. Xue T, Yang W, Guo Y, Yuan W, Dai J, Zhao Z. 3D image-guided percutaneous radiofrequency thermocoagulation of the maxillary branch of the trigeminal nerve through foramen rotundum for the treatment of trigeminal neuralgia. Medicine (Baltimore). 2015;94:e1954.
27. Ran B, Wei J, Zhong Q, Fu M, Yang J, Chen X, et al. Long-term follow-up of patients treated with percutaneous radiofrequency Thermocoagulation via the foramen rotundum for isolated maxillary nerve idiopathic trigeminal neuralgia. Pain Med. 2019;20:1370–8.
28. Xue TQ, Zhang QX, Bian H, Zhou PC, Liu C, Niu SF, et al. Radiofrequency thermocoagulation through foramen rotundum versus foramen ovale for the treatment of V2 trigeminal neuralgia. Pain Physician. 2019;22:E609–e14.

29. Chan Kim HKL, Yang SK, Lee HJ, Lee YC, Kim SM. Alcohol block in the treatment of trigeminal neuralgia: a retrospective study to assess its efficacy. Korean J Pain. 1996;9:83–8.
30. Thapa D, Ahuja V, Dass C, Verma P. Management of refractory trigeminal neuralgia using extended duration pulsed radiofrequency application. Pain Physician. 2015;18:E433–5.
31. Lin H, Cao G, Jin G, Yang Z, Huang C, Shao J, et al. Extracranial non-gasserian ganglion application of radiofrequency thermocoagulation on the mandibular branch of the trigeminal through the foramen ovale for trigeminal neuralgia. Pain Physician. 2021;24:E425–e32.
32. Huang B, Xie K, Chen Y, Wu J, Yao M. Bipolar radiofrequency ablation of mandibular branch for refractory V3 trigeminal neuralgia. J Pain Res. 2019;12:1465–74.
33. Han KR, Chae YJ, Lee JD, Kim C. Trigeminal nerve block with alcohol for medically intractable classic trigeminal neuralgia: long-term clinical effectiveness on pain. Int J Med Sci. 2017;14:29–36.
34. Kyung Ream Han CK, Kim DW, Cho OG, Cho HW. Long-term outcome of trigeminal nerve block with alcohol for the treatment of trigeminal neuralgia. Korean. J Pain. 2006;19:45–50.
35. Kim JH, Yu HY, Park SY, Lee SC, Kim YC. Pulsed and conventional radiofrequency treatment: which is effective for dental procedure-related symptomatic trigeminal neuralgia? Pain Med. 2013;14:430–5.
36. Messlinger K, Russo AF. Current understanding of trigeminal ganglion structure and function in headache. Cephalalgia. 2019;39:1661–74.
37. Zheng S, Li X, Li R, Yang L, He L, Cao G, et al. Factors associated with long-term risk of recurrence after percutaneous radiofrequency thermocoagulation of the gasserian ganglion for patients with trigeminal neuralgia: a multicenter retrospective analysis. Clin J Pain. 2019;35:958–66.
38. Kanpolat Y, Savas A, Bekar A, Berk C. Percutaneous controlled radiofrequency trigeminal rhizotomy for the treatment of idiopathic trigeminal neuralgia: 25-year experience with 1,600 patients. Neurosurgery. 2001;48:524–32. discussion 32-4
39. Hong T, Ding Y, Yao P. Long-term efficacy and complications of radiofrequency thermocoagulation at different temperatures for the treatment of trigeminal neuralgia. Biochem Res Int. 2020;2020:3854284.
40. Kim JSKJ, Kim YI, Lee SK, Park W, Kim SY. Percutaneous retrogasserian glycerol rhizolysis in the management of trigeminal neuralgia. Korean J Pain. 1992;4:137–41.
41. Fujimaki T, Fukushima T, Miyazaki S. Percutaneous retrogasserian glycerol injection in the management of trigeminal neuralgia: long-term follow-up results. J Neurosurg. 1990;73:212–6.
42. Chen L, Xu M, Zou Y. Treatment of trigeminal neuralgia with percutaneous glycerol injection into Meckel's cavity: experience in 4012 patients. Cell Biochem Biophys. 2010;58:85–9.

Percutaneous Radiofrequency Thermal Rhizotomy for Trigeminal Neuralgia

Byung-chul Son

Denervation of the perceptual area of trigeminal neuralgia has been considered as an effective method for the treatment of trigeminal neuralgia [1]. Initially, to control trigeminal neuralgia, chemical drugs such as alcohol were injected into the trigeminal nerve branch or peripheral nerve resection was performed. The subtemporal trigeminal rhizotomy or ganglionectomy also provided relatively long-term pain relief [2]. The first electrocoagulation using a radiofrequency probe in the trigeminal ganglion was reported by Kirschner in 1932 [3]. White and Sweet introduced a stable radiofrequency lesion generator to make accurate RF lesions [4]. Trigeminal deafferentation using thermal lesion had many feared sensory complications, such as anaesthesia dorolosa and neuroparalytic keratitis [1]. As experience was accumulated, it was found that damage to the afferent nerve caused by RF thermal lesion can be controlled through graded lesioning that induces hypoalgesia while reducing pain [1].

Although microvascular decompression is the most effective treatment for trigeminal neuralgia, but in case of patients with old age, systemic problems, or refuse surgery under general anesthesia, percutaneous radiofrequency thermal rhizotomy is an effective method in alleviation of pain [1]. Radiofrequency thermal rhizotomy is a simple method to control pain if only the foramen puncture is performed safely and accurately, and has the advantage that it can be easily performed again in case of recurrence [1, 5].

Unlike other percutaneous procedures such as balloon compression or glycerol injection, it has the advantage of being able to control the degree of thermal coagulation during the procedure. As a disadvantage, neuralgia involving V2 and V3 division can be effectively treated, but V1 neuralgia can not be performed due to complications of corneal anesthesia and keratitis [5]. Also, like other percutaneous procedures, there is a recurrence rate of 20% at 10 years [6]. In addition, there is a risk of excessive thermal coagulation or trigeminal neuropathic pain such as dysesthesia or anesthesia dorolosa during repeated coagulation [1]. In this chapter, I would like to discuss the techniques and the problems associated with percutaneous radiofrequency thermal rhizotomy, and prevention of complications.

B.-c. Son (✉)
Seoul St. Mary's Hospital, College of Medicine, The Catholic University of Korea, Seoul, Republic of Korea

Catholic Neuroscience Institute, College of Medicine, Catholic University of Korea, Seoul, Republic of Korea
e-mail: sbc@catholic.ac.kr

K. Park, K. R. Cho (eds.), *Trigeminal Neuralgia*, https://doi.org/10.1007/978-981-19-9171-4_19

1 Technique of Percutaneous Thermal Rhizotomy Under Sedation

The patient is taken to the operating room and a nasopharyngeal airway of an appropriate size for the patient is prepared. Monitoring of the vital sign is routinely performed [1]. A slight neck extension position in the supine position is taken to make it easier to obtain an image of the foramen ovale (Fig. 1a). The position of the foramen ovale is addressed using a fluoroscopic view before surgery is performed (Fig. 1b). Routine sterile draping is performed around the entry point of the cannulation.

The line of insertion is the junction of two planes from the insertion site: to a point 3.0 cm anterior to the ipsilateral tragus, and to a point at the medial border of the ipsilateral pupil (Härtel technique) (Fig. 1c). The cannula is carefully advanced into the base of the skull, and once it has touched the bone, it is placed in the foramen fossa using fluoroscopy. The cannula is introduced into the foramen ovale, and its position is confirmed through a lateral fluoroscopic view. (Fig. 1d and e) When the cannula enters through the foramen ovale, a brief tingling pain and jaw jerk are induced. When viewing lateral fluoroscopy, the correct position of the cannula tip is confirmed only when the clival line is aligned with the true lateral view (Fig. 1d). For alignment of the true lateral view, it is necessary to look closely at the profile of the sellar and orbital roof. For V3 pain, a straight electrode is placed 5 mm below the clival line, and for V2 pain, the electrode is placed on the clival line (Fig. 1d). For V1 pain, a straight electrode can be positioned more posteriorly and upward from the clival line, or a curved electrode can be used, but it is not recommended to perform thermal rhizotomy for V1 pain. Deeper penetration is necessary to approach V2 and V2, and a more superior trajectory is more like to achieve access to V1.

After confirming that the radiofrequency electrode is in a satisfactory position, stimulation testing is performed. Electrical stimulation was increased in the order of 0.5, 1.0, and 1.5 mA at 50 Hz, 1 ms setting to determine whether paresthesia was induced in the target dermatome. If paresthesia is induced in the pain dermatome, test lesion is induced at 40 ° for 60 s to check whether there are any special side effects. Thermal lesioning was performed at 70, 75, and 80 ° for 60 s each. After thermal lesioning, sensory testing of the patient is performed using a pin prick and light touch sensation. In the past, it was recommended to induce dense hypoalgesia, but recently, to reduce dyesthesia caused by thermal lesioning, the goal is to reduce the loss of the patient's ability to differentiate sharp and dull sensation.

If the target sensory loss is not confirmed, the sensory loss should be induced by increasing the thermal lesion by 5 °. Thermal lesion can be achieved by local lidocaine infiltration, but sedation can be done using a short-acting analgesic bolus such as propofol to reduce the patient's pain from thermal lesion. During thermal lesioning, continuous monitoring of blood pressure and pulse should be performed. When the sensory decrease due to thermal lesioning is confirmed and it is confirmed that the patient's existing pain is not induced, the radiofrequency lesion electrode is carefully removed and manual compression over the puncture site is performed for about 3 min. When the procedure is over, the patient can drink water, eat a liquid diet in the evening, and if nothing special happens, the patient can be discharged the next day.

2 Radiofrequency Thermal Rhizotomy Under General Anesthesia

Although Härtel's technique is a well-known method [5], it is basically a blind procedure, so cannulation may be difficult depending on the skill of the operator. Cooperating with the procedure without extending and moving the neck may be difficult for some patients. The fear, pain, and discomfort experienced by patients during cannulation are also significant. Accordingly, the pulse and blood pressure rise should be carefully monitored. In addition, although thermal coagulation under local anesthesia takes a short time, the pain felt by the patient is so great that patients

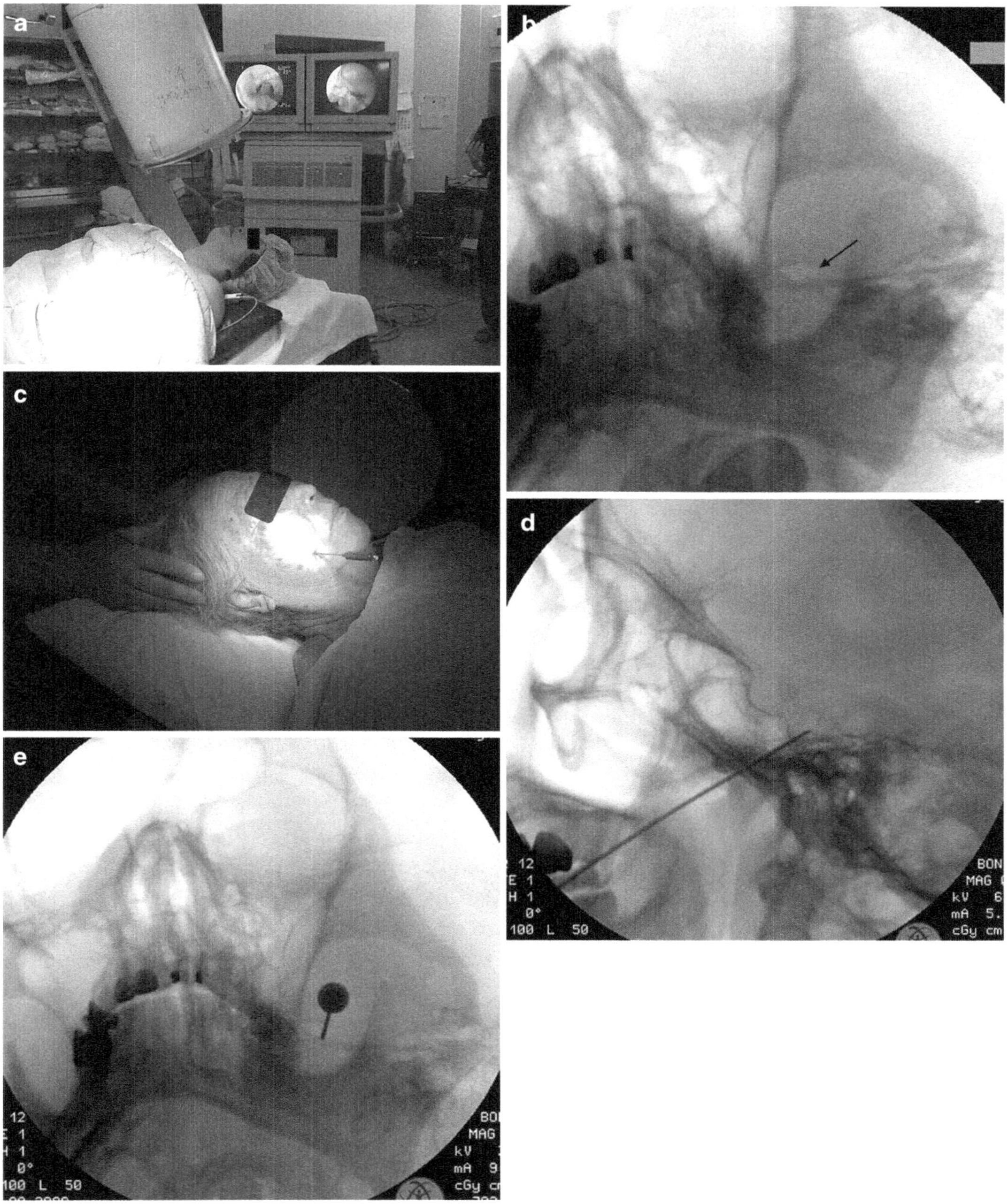

Fig. 1 Procedure of percutaneous radiofrequency thermal rhizotomy. (**a**) A photograph showing an operative scene for percutaneous radiofrequency thermocoagulation under fluoroscopic image-guidance. Note the caudocephalic tilting of x-ray tube. (**b**) A fluoroscopic image showing the foaramen ovale (black arrow). With 55° caudocephalic tilting of fluoroscopy and 20° head rotation to ipsilateral side, the foramen ovale is just lateral to a line through that lateral wall of the orbit. (**c**) An intraoperative photograph showing a cannula inserted through the cheek. (**d**) A fluoroscopic image showing a cannula located in the foramen ovale. (**e**) A fluoroscopic image of skull lateral view showing a cannula reaching a clival line. When an cannula reaches the clival line, stimulation-induced paresthesia is usually induced in the V2 segment. If V3 rather than V2 paresthesia is induced, a lesioning probe should be advanced further

who have undergone thermal coagulation once under local anesthesia do not want to undergo thermal coagulation again, even if it is a percutaneous procedure [5].

Therefore, in the case of the author, it is recommended that radiofrequency thermal coagulation be performed under general anesthesia [5]. This is because, since thermal coagulation is not performed on the first branch, the localization of the second and third branches can be easily confirmed by the position of the electrode on the fluoroscopic view. As a disadvantage, it is difficult to confirm damage to the motor branch. For this reason, it is recommended not to use muscle relaxants even under general anesthesia. The anesthesia time is as short as 30 min, so the patient does not feel pain and there is no burden. The procedure is simpler than repeated sedation and awakening using profopol and fentanyl.

Accurate cannulation of the foramen ovale and positioning of the lesioning electrode are of paramount importance, as the patient does not wake up to check. In order to accurately confirm the position of the foramen ovale on fluoroscopy, the oblique submentovertical view using Gaber's zygomatic point is basically used [5, 7]. The patient lies in supine position with neck slightly extended. The head is roated 20° away from the ipsilateral side, with the central x-ray beam directed at the foramen ovale at an angle 55° caudal to the orbitomeatal line. With this 55° caudocephalic tilting of fluoroscopy and 20° head rotation, the foramen ovale is just lateral to a line through that lateral wall of the orbit (Fig. 1a and b). It is important to keep the central beam angled at least 40°caudal to the orbitomeatal line. With less angulation, the foramen ovale may be superimposed on the petrous bones, thus obscuring the image (Fig. 1b). If the foramen ovale may be superimposed on the mandibular ramus, decreasing the angle of rotation of the head will place the foramen medial to the anterior ridge of the ramus (Fig. 1e).

As a general precaution, it is recommended that the needle be directed at the anterolateral aspect of the foramen ovale and "walked" into the foramen [7]. This decreases the possibility of going too far posteromedially in the proximity of the carotid artery. The image intensifier can then be rotated for a lateral image to permit judgement of the depth of penetration of needles. After local infilteration of 2% lidocaine along the trajectory of cannulation over the skin and subcutaneous tissue, the cannula was introduced under fluoroscopic guidance. After verification of depth of penetration of foramen ovale, test stimulation was given in 2 Hz to check the threshold of masseter contraction [5]. After confirming the high threshold of masseter contraction, radiofrequency heat lesion was made at 70 °C, 75 °C, and 80 °C for 60 s each. After finishing the thermal lesion, the electrode can be carefully removed and manual compression is given.

3 Outcome and Complications

Results of percutaneous thermal rhizotomy vary [1]. The various results appear to be due to the temperature of the thermal lesioning and complications. For the strength of thermal lesion, lesioning making sufficient to induce dense hypoalgesia was recommended initially. However, it is known that the greater the sensory loss, the less recurrence but an increase in the frequency of complications such as dysesthesia and anesthesia dorolosa [1]. Therefore, it is recommended to induce heat lesions enough to cause sensory loss of mild hypoalgesia.

In general, thermal rhizotomy provides immediate pain relief in 90% of cases immediately after the procedure. The long-term recurrence rate varies depending on the report, but it is generally known that the recurrence rate is 50% at 3 years. Since radiofrequency thermal lesion is a thermal neuroablative treatment for the trigeminal nerve, sensory loss and paresthesia are inevitable. Paresthesia or dysesthesia is the most common complication despite successful relief of evoked neuralgic pain. Paresthesia is known to occur after surgery with a frequency of about 20%, and dysesthesia is a rare but serious complication of thermal lesion. Among them, if dysesthesia accompanying hypoalgesia is severe, the most dangerous sensory complication called anesthesia dorolosa may occur [1]. Currently, when anesthesia dorolosa is not controlled with drugs, there is no clear treatment. Therefore, it is recommended that thermal lesion be performed with an intensity that does not induce dense hypoalgesia. Masseter weakness is also common after thermal rhizotomy. However, it is usually temporary and permanent weakness is rarely encountered.

Thermal lesion for V1 division pain is no longer recommended due to the risk of complications such as keratitis or herpes zoster. This is because there are alternative treatments such as balloon compression, radiosurgery and definitive treatments such as microvascular decompression. Accidental puncture of the foramen lacerum and the internal carotid artery due to mis-cannulation of the foramen ovale can be prevented with accurate fluoroscopic verification during cannulation.

4 Conclusion

Percutaneous radiofrequency thermal rhizotomy is a good treatment method that can safely and effectively control pain in trigeminal neuralgia if accurate cannulation is possible using C-arm fluoroscopy under local or general anesthesia. Sensory complications can be avoided if heat lesions that cause dense analgesia are avoided.

References

1. Burchiel KJ. Chapter 45. Percutaneous radiofrequency trigeminal gangliolysis for trigeminal neuralgia. In: Burchiel KJ, editor. Surgical management of pain. 2nd ed. New York: Thieme; 2015. p. 463–9.
2. Cushing HW. A method of total extirpation of the Gasserian ganglion for trigeminal neuralgia. By a route through the temporal fossa and beneath the middle meningeal artery. JAMA. 1900;34:1035–41.
3. Kirschner M. Elektrocoagulation des ganglion gasseri. Zentralbl Chir. 1932;47:28–41.
4. White JC, Sweet WH. Pain and the neurosurgeon. Springfield, IL: Charles C. Thomas; 1969. p. 322–30.
5. Son BC, Kim HS, Kim IS, Yang SH, Lee SW. Percutaneous radiofrequency thermocoagulation under fluoroscopic image-guidance for idiopathic trigeminal neuralgia. J Korean Neurosurg Soc. 2011;50:446–52.
6. Taha JM, JMJ T, CRT B. A prospective 15-year-follow up of 154 consecutive patients with trigeminal neuralgia treated by percutaneous stereotactic radiofrequency thermal rhizotomy. J Neurosurg. 1995;83:989–93.
7. Gerber AM. Improved visualization of the foramen ovale for percutaneous approaches to the gasserian ganglion. J Neurosurg. 1994;80:156–9.

Percutaneous Balloon Compression and Glycerol Rhizotomy

Myung Ki Lee

This chapter presents the historical background, action mechanism, techniques, indications, results, and complications of percutaneous balloon compression and glycerol rhizotomy for the treatment of trigeminal neuralgia. These techniques will also be compared with other surgical methods for trigeminal neuralgia. Furthermore, practical advice on techniques to minimize complications during surgery is discussed.

1 Balloon Compression

1.1 Historical Background

Percutaneous balloon compression is a technique derived from mechanical injury caused by balloon compression of the trigeminal ganglion and retrogasserian ganglion root. Shelden and Pudenz successfully relieved trigeminal neuralgia by opening Meckel's cave and compressing the posterior root fibers with a blunt dissector through temporal craniotomy in 1955 [1]. Mullan modified this to a percutaneous technique for controlled compression of the trigeminal ganglion through the foramen ovale with a Forgarty-type balloon catheter in 1978; its description was reported by Mullan and Lichor in 1983 [2]. This technique made the percutaneous trigeminal nerve-compression approach through the foramen ovale less risky.

M. K. Lee (✉)
Department of Neurosurgery, On General Hospital, Busan, South Korea

1.2 Action Mechanism

The histopathological changes that occurred after trigeminal balloon compression in New Zealand rabbits indicated that balloon compression selectively injures large myelinated fibers that mediate light touch involved in the sensory trigger [3]. Thus, compression reduces the sensory neural input from the face. However, compression selectively avoids injury to the small unmyelinated and unmyelinated nociceptive fibers that mediate the corneal reflex. Thus, compression is especially helpful in the treatment of first-division pain.

1.3 Indications

Balloon compression is relatively well tolerated by the elderly and patients without a history of cardiac arrhythmia who are considered candidates for brief general anesthesia. The patients should also be aware that the procedure will produce facial numbness. Young patients are also candidates if they are willing to accept it. The main indication is classic or typical trigeminal neuralgia. Secondary trigeminal neuralgia asso-

K. Park, K. R. Cho (eds.), *Trigeminal Neuralgia*, https://doi.org/10.1007/978-981-19-9171-4_20

ciated with multiple sclerosis or mass lesion is another indication. In general, the method is especially helpful for first-division and multidivisional pain and uncooperative patients. Postherpetic neuralgia patients with predominant paroxysmal pain and/or allodynia may benefit from balloon compression, except for herpetic patients with predominant burning or deafferentation pain. The procedure can be performed without greater technical difficulty on failed or recurrent cases in the treatment of microvascular decompression, gamma knife radiosurgery, and percutaneous procedures. Contralateral jaw weakness is a relative contraindication because compression often causes temporary masseter weakness.

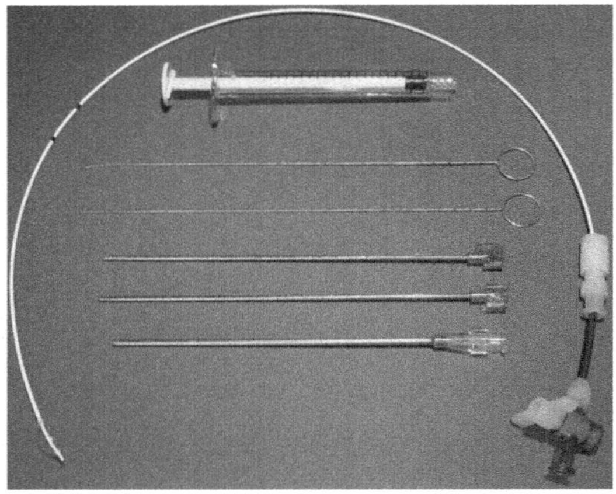

Fig. 1 Trigeminal balloon compression cannula kit

1.4 Techniques and Equipment

Balloon compression is performed by using either volume control or pressure monitor. The balloon can be inflated with radiopaque contrast dye either with a 1-mL tuberculin syringe or with a calibrated insufflator syringe with attached pressure transducer.

The volume-controlled technique, an original technique described by Mullan [2], is performed in the operation room using a C-arm fluoroscopy unit. The fluoroscopy unit is initially placed in the full submental position and then rotated into the lateral projection. In this method, a No. 14 needle for liver biopsy and a No. 4 Fogarty balloon catheter are used. The volume and compression time of the balloon catheter requires surgeon experience.

The pressure-controlled technique, developed by Brown [4], is performed in the angiography suite with biplane imaging. Three views of radiologic imaging are used to position the balloon accuracy: (1) modified submental view, (2) modified anterior–posterior (Caldwell) view, and (3) lateral view. Two disposable kits are used [5]. One has an introducing cannula, sharp and blunt obturators, curved and straight guiding stylets, and a No. 4 balloon catheter (Cook, INC., Bloomington, IN, USA) (Fig. 1). The second contains an insufflation syringe, an attachment transducer, and a digital pressure monitor (Merit Medical, Inc., Salt Lake City, UT, USA). Pressure measurement provides a guide to measure the appropriate degree of trigeminal nerve compression. The proper intraluminal balloon pressure is 1200–1400 mmHg.

1.5 Preoperative Evaluation

All patients undergo a routine diagnostic assessment via skull radiography including a submental vertex view, CT, and magnetic resonance imaging (MRI). The preoperative MRI of the posterior fossa with and without gadolinium-DTPA is helpful in confirming the diagnosis of primary or secondary trigeminal neuralgia. Preoperative facial CT, including three-dimensional CT, using the orbitomeatal plane is useful in determining a plane of percutaneous approaches to the foramen ovale (Fig. 2) [6, 7]. The morphological shape and location of the foramen ovale and its surrounding structures, including the condylar process of the mandible, external auditory meatus, and their anatomical configuration, are investigated. The procedure is performed under a brief general anesthesia. Because most of the patients are elderly or otherwise physically infirm, appropriate medical and cardiological consultation is obtained to assess the cardiovascular risks for intraoperative bradycardia, arrhythmia, and hypertension.

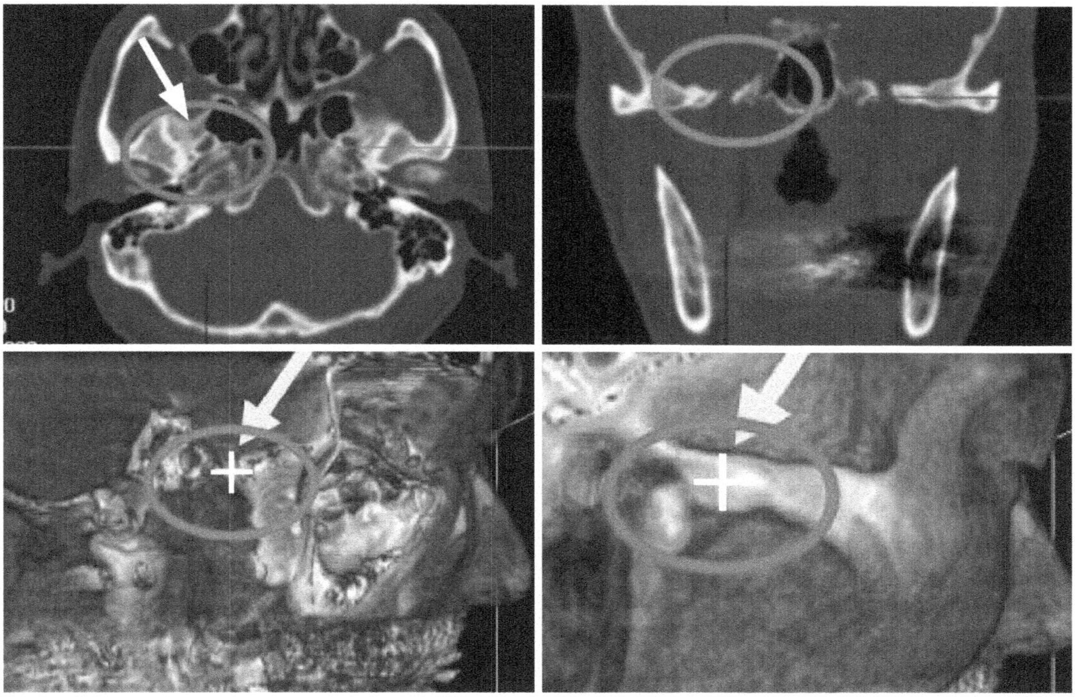

Fig. 2 Preoperative facial CT including three-dimensional CT demonstrating the intended target for percutaneous needle puncture to the foramen ovale

1.6 Preparation of Patient and Anesthesia

Oral antihypertensive medication is given to patients with hypertension. Premedication with an antibiotic and atropine (0.4 mg) is administered intravenously and intramuscularly, respectively, 30 min to 1 h before operation. General anesthesia is induced with propofol and maintained using either isoflurane or sevoflurane. Remifentanil or dexmedetomidine is used as an adjuvant for intraoperative and postoperative pain control. Pacing pads for external cardiac pacemaker are positioned on the chest in patients at risk of bradyarrhythmia. Continuous arterial blood pressure monitoring is done through the cannulation of the radial artery or dorsalis pedis artery. It is important to minimize the trigeminal cardiac reflex or trigeminal vagal response, such as bradycardia, and fluctuating blood pressure during the procedure [8, 9]. Atropine and antihypertensive agents should be prepared to manage it. Unwanted cardiovascular risk can also be controlled by a deeper level of anesthesia before foramen ovale insertion.

1.7 Operative Procedure

1.7.1 Position of Patient and C-Arm

After general anesthesia with intratracheal intubation, the patient is placed in the neutral supine position with neck extension to 40–50 ° (Fig. 5a). It is necessary to elevate the shoulders using a pillow or suitable pad to permit adequate extension of the neck and immobilize the head using a donut-shaped pillow with a strip of adhesive tape. A portable C-arm fluoroscopy unit is positioned for the true lateral view of the skull. The accuracy of the position can be checked based on the mandibular shadow in lateral projection radiography. An oblique submental imaging is then obtained, while the patient remains positioned in the neutral supine position. The foramen ovale can be visualized by 15–20 ° of ipsilateral angulation from the mid-sagittal plane, while the central ray is directed about 2.5–3 cm lateral to the angle of the mouth on the affected side (Fig. 3a). After the direct identification of the foramen, the C-arm fluoroscopy unit is changed to true lateral projection. Two sides of the mandible should be exactly superimposed. The patient's eyes are taped with instillation of eye ointment. The face is antiseptically prepared.

1.7.2 Foramen Ovale Puncture

Needle insertion was performed in accordance with the modified Hartel guidelines. The cheek point for entry (2.5–3.0 cm lateral from the angle of the mouth and 1 cm inferior to the occlusal plane), the orbital point (2.5 cm lateral from the nasion or the medial canthus), and the zygomatic point (the measured values from facial CT regarding the external auditory canal and anterior border of the condylar process of the mandible) are marked with a sterile pen. The air space of a No. 4 Fogarty catheter is filled with radiographic contrast using a 1-mL tuberculin syringe. The catheter is then inserted into the needle cannula to a point marked on the shaft of the catheter beyond the cannula tip.

The skin at the entry point is injected with lidocaine, and the skin is slightly punctured by a No. 14 needle. A 21-gauge nerve block needle with a 150-mm-long shaft is then introduced and advanced in a submucosal plane with a gloved index finger inside the oral cavity to avoid penetration into the oral cavity. The lateral projection of the C-arm fluoroscopy unit is checked to ensure the proper position and trajectory of the needle to the two targets of the foramen ovale and the trigeminal porus of Meckel's cave. The foramen ovale is targeted at the zygomatic point, about 0.5 cm anterior to the anterior border of the condylar process of the mandible. The trigeminal porus is targeted at just the superior clival line to the petroclival junction. The clival trajectory point in relation to trigeminal nerve selectivity is indicative of lateral radiographic landmarks for localizing each division (Fig. 4). The needle is advanced vertically to the orbital point on the face, while horizontally heading to the zygomatic point and the clival point in lateral projection of the C-arm fluoroscopy unit. As soon as the needle touches the base of the skull or punctures the foramen ovale, C-arm fluoroscopy is changed to oblique submental projection to visualize the foramen ovale. The needle is withdrawn slightly and redirected to the desired target of the fora-

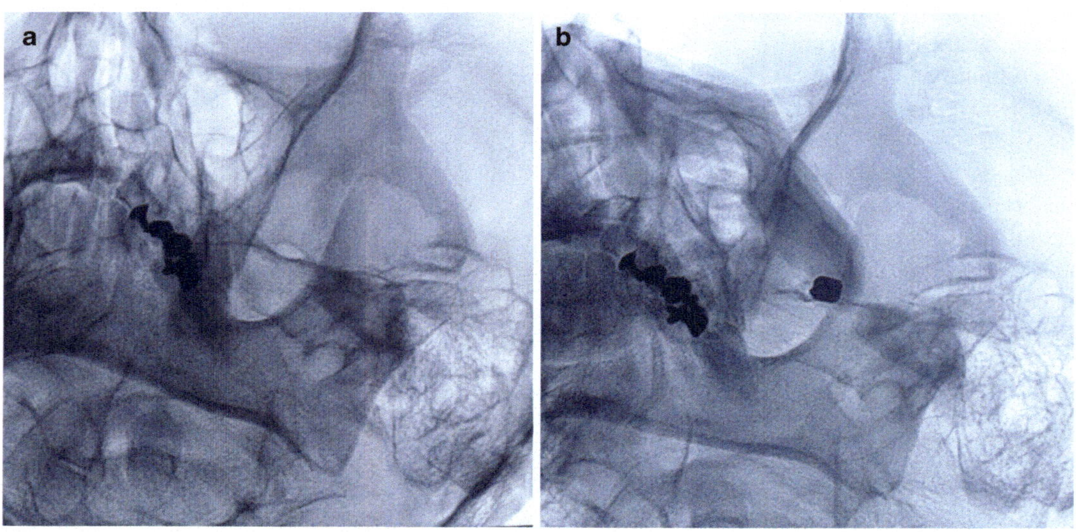

Fig. 3 (**a**) An oblique submental projection with 15 ° of ipsilateral angulation in the neutral supine position with the neck extension showing the foramen ovale. (**b**) Needle puncture of the foramen ovale

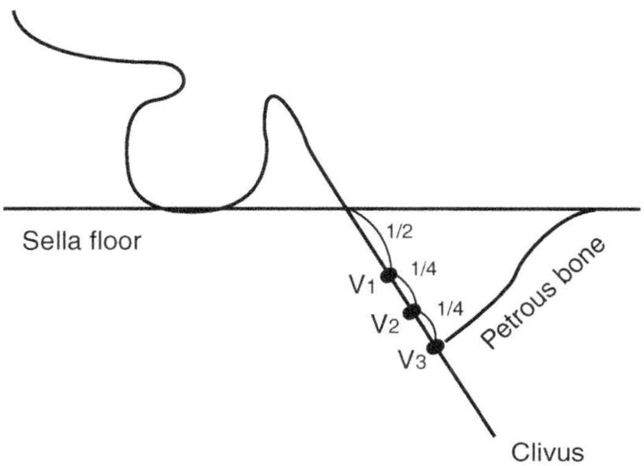

Fig. 4 Clival trajectory point in relation to trigeminal nerve selectivity. Two points half and quarter along the clival line from the intersection of the sella floor to the clival line to the juncture of the clivus and petrous ridge corresponding to the V1 and V2 targets, respectively. The juncture of the clivus and petrous ridge corresponding to the V3 target

men, just medial to the midpoint (Fig. 3b). The puncture of the foramen is felt by the surgeon. The C-arm fluoroscopy unit is then changed to true lateral projection. After the 21-gauge needle enters the foramen ovale to reach the clival point, the trigeminal cistern is identified by injecting 1 mL of mixed agents (0.5 mL lidocaine and 0.5 mL contrast medium) using a 1 mL syringe (Fig. 5b, c). The injection of the agents helps to identify the needle position and to minimize the trigeminal vagal response.

1.7.3 Meckel's Cave Cannulation and Trigeminal Porus Compression

After cutting the hub part of the 21-gauge needle with a cutter, a 14-gauge cannula is advanced to the external orifice of the foramen ovale through the shaft of the needle (Fig. 5d). Penetration

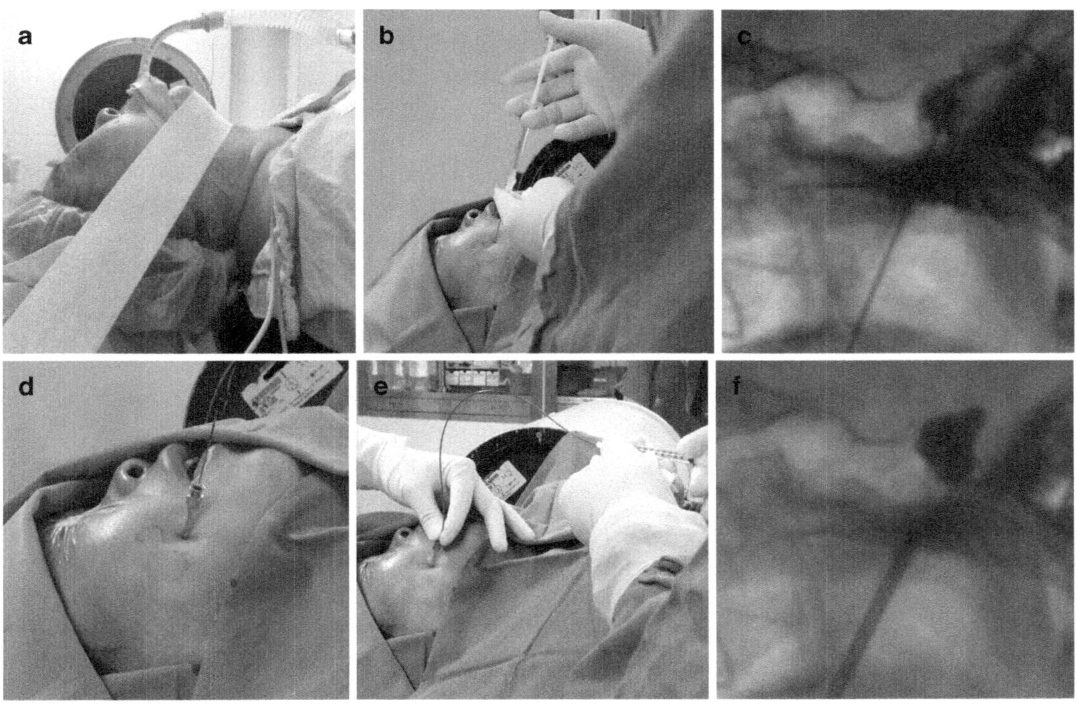

Fig. 5 The steps of balloon compression procedure. (**a**) Patient's neutral supine position with neck extension, (**b**) Injection of contrast medium and lidocaine after the foramen ovale puncture using a 21-gauge needle, (**c**) Trigeminal cisternography, (**d**) No. 14 needle cannulation through the shaft of the 21-gauge needle, (**e**) No. 4 French Fogarty balloon catheter inflation using a 1 mL syringe with contrast medium, (**f**) The pear shape of a distended balloon indicating trigeminal porus compression

beyond the foramen is avoided with the 14-gauge needle. The cannula is held in position by an assistant with one hand. The No. 4 French Fogarty balloon catheter is inserted through the 14-gauge cannula to the clival line. After the stylet is removed from the balloon catheter, the balloon catheter is then inflated by slowly injecting 0.3 mL of radiopaque contrast using a 1-mL syringe (Fig. 5e). At this step, the heart rate, blood pressure, and balloon location are checked. Atropine and antihypertensive agents may be used to treat bradycardia and hypertension, respectively. Bradycardia can be controlled rapidly by the deflation of the distended balloon. When the balloon is in proper position, it is inflated by slowly injecting the contrast dye until a small nipple protrudes into the posterior fossa through the porus trigeminus, the entrance of Meckel's cave, which communicates between the temporal fossa and the posterior fossa (Fig. 5f).

When a pear-shaped balloon is achieved with about 0.5–0.7 mL of contrast, nerve compression is maintained for 1 min. The shape and position of the balloon are checked in relation to the neighboring bone landmarks; if its shape and position are not correct, the balloon is immediately deflated and the needle is repositioned. The maximum liquid capacity volume of the catheter is 0.75 mL, but a risk of rupture is expected after reaching 1.0 mL. After compression, the balloon catheter and cannula are removed and the cheek is compressed for a few minutes.

1.8 Results

Initial or early pain relief is about 92%. Long-term pain relief appears to be approximately 76% at 3 years. Complications are noted mostly as mild or transient, but occasional serious vascular complications could occur because of the large size of the needle used. Early morbidity includes trigeminal motor weakness or masseter muscle weakness (66%), troublesome dysesthesia (10%), cranial nerve deficits (1.5%), meningitis (2.6%), and vascular complications (2%). Long-term complications include troublesome dysesthesia (6%), masseter muscle weakness (5%), corneal analgesia (0.6%), and cranial nerve palsy (0.6%). Repeated surgery after recurrence is generally safe and effective, but the results are not as good as in the first-time procedure. Denser numbness and masseter muscle weakness have become more frequent in repeated surgery. Chen (2011) reported the recurrence rates after balloon compression for trigeminal neuralgia in 130 patients: 14% (2 years), 18.9% (3 years), 29.5% (5 years), and 37.7% (10 years) [10].

Brown (2005) reported the results of 65 procedures over 4 years based on balloon compression pressure monitoring for the treatment of trigeminal neuralgia [5]. The mean intraluminal compression pressure was 1160 ± 62 mm Hg, and the mean duration of compression was 1.15 ± 0.27 min. The trigeminal depressor response (92%), initial pain relief (92%), and recurrence rate (16%) occurred. Mild numbness (83%) immediately after surgery, persistent non-troublesome numbness (17%), and minor dysesthesia (4%) were observed, whereas moderate or severe numbness did not occur. Mild masseter muscle weakness (24%) occurred and resolved within a maximum period of 1 year. No patient experienced anesthesia dolorosa, corneal keratitis, or other cranial nerve deficits. These morbidity rates are lower than those reported in the literature when pressure monitoring was not used.

1.9 Complication Avoidance

The surgical results and complications of balloon compression are related to needle placement, catheter location, balloon shape, and the compression time of the balloon [6]. Surgical complications, such as cardiovascular stress, masseter muscle weakness, severe dysesthesia, diplopia, carotid cavernous fistula, intratemporal hemorrhage, and infection, could also be related to avoidable technical errors [11–15]. Balloon mislocation outside Meckel to avoidable also be avoided, and its atypical shape must be recognized early.

The inflated balloon shows four shapes: pear, dumbbell, oval, and cylindrical (Fig. 6) [6]. When properly positioned at Meckel's cave entrance, the

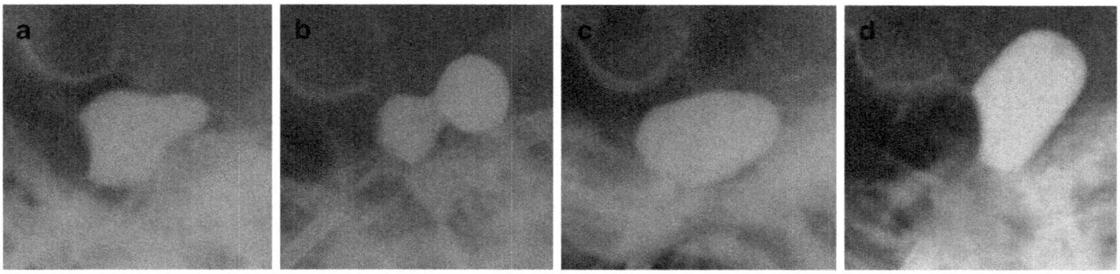

Fig. 6 The shape of ballooning. (**a**) Typical pear shape, (**b**) dumb-bell shape, (**c**) round or oval shape, (**d**) cylindrical shape

balloon compresses the retrogasserian trigeminal nerve against the petrous bone inferior and the cerebellar tentorium superior, resulting in a pear shape. It has been reported that the pear-shaped appearance is predictive of success. The catheter tip can enter the posterior fossa, and the balloon is inflated to a dumbbell shape, partly within the posterior fossa and partly within the cave. Even if this is done successfully, the migration of the catheter into the posterior fossa is always a concern since annoying dysesthesia may result from the maximal compression of the retrogasserian fibers. To achieve optimum results, the catheter is withdrawn slightly or compression time is decreased by less than 1 min. An oval shape may appear because of the large size of the cave, adhesion or merely balloon compression within the ganglion, and the wrong position of the catheter tip. The advance or repositioning of the catheter may help. A cylindrical shape appears from the subtemporal placement of the catheter, which is positioned laterally to Meckel's cave. The catheter needs to be repositioned medially instead of the prolonged compression of the balloon.

The optimal volume and compression time are not firmly established from 0.4 to 0.9 mL and from 1 to 6 min, respectively. For Mullan and Lichtor (1983), the volume was usually 0.7 mL for 1 min [2]. For Bergenheim (2103), a pear-shaped balloon was inflated with 0.5–0.7 mL for 1.5–3 min [16]. For Abdennebi and Guenane (2014), the balloon was inflated with 0.7 mL for 6 min [17]. In our case [6], symptomatic dysesthesia did not occur following compression for 1 min with the pear-shaped balloon. However, with the double balloon shape, compression for 1 min caused severe dysesthesia in 25% of the cases. A dumbbell-shaped balloon can be achieved with 0.4–0.5 mL for 40–50 seconds to obtain a good functional outcome. This may be related to the fact that compression time or balloon shape is critical to the development of adverse annoying dysesthesias. Compression with a duration longer than 1 min with the pear-shaped balloon increases numbness and reduces recurrence but increases the risk of dysesthesia. When treating trigeminal neuralgia with percutaneous surgery, it is advisable to avoid excessive sensory abnormalities to prevent recurrence. Favorable results have been achieved with a compression time of 1 min routinely, but a prolonged compression time of more than 1.5 min causes more dysesthesia [4, 6].

2 Percutaneous Glycerol Rhizotomy

2.1 Historical Background

Percutaneous glycerol rhizotomy is a technique derived from chemical injury caused by glycerol injection into the trigeminal cistern. The beneficial effects of glycerol have been discovered accidentally. Leksell and Hakanson injected a mixture of glycerin and tantalum powder into the trigeminal cistern to serve as a permanent marker to create a visible target for gamma knife radiosurgery in Stockholm. When the targeting solution is injected prior to performing the radiosurgery procedure, patients obtained often free from their trigeminal pain. Based on these observations,

Hakanson introduced the method of injecting glycerol into the trigeminal cistern for the treatment of trigeminal neuralgia in 1981 [18].

2.2 Action Mechanism

Glycerol is a weak alcohol that injures both the myelinated and unmyelinated axons of the nerve. The highly viscous anhydrous glycerol used in operation has potent neurolytic properties due to its hypertonicity, which may act mainly on the large myelinated or tactile fibers affecting the trigger mechanism for paroxysmal pain over time and thereby prevent aberrant impulses to the thin nociceptive fibers, and the rate of the alteration of osmolarity is critical for the effect on the nociceptive fibers [19, 20]. Eide and Stubhaug (1999) suggested that partial deafferentation, with the impairment of thin and large fiber-mediated sensations and abnormal temporal summation of pain, refers to the increased perception of pain with repetitive noxious stimuli, which is present in the trigger area of patients with trigeminal neuralgia [21]. Relief of pain after glycerol injection depends on the normalization of the abnormal temporal summation of pain, which is independent of the general impairment of sensory perception.

2.3 Indications

Glycerol rhizotomy is indicated as a choice in elderly or weak patients with symptoms of typical trigeminal neuralgia and those who have failed medical treatment. Because glycerol injection does not require general anesthesia, it can be a good option for someone with heart or lung problems and others who cannot tolerate general anesthesia. In this procedure, the patient can be more deeply anesthetized compared with radiofrequency rhizotomy. The main indication is classic or idiopathic trigeminal neuralgia. Secondary trigeminal neuralgia associated with multiple sclerosis or mass lesion is also an indication. Patients need to accept that glycerol injection causes facial numbness. Young patients are also candidates if they are willing to accept them. Patients with paroxysmal pain after a failed microvascular decompression or other percutaneous procedures or glycerol injection can also receive reinjections easily.

2.4 Techniques and Equipment

Glycerol rhizotomy is an inexpensive method that requires very little special equipment. A spinal needle (18-, 20-, or 22-gauge), a tuberculin syringe (1 mL), water-soluble contrast dye, anhydrous glycerol (99.9%), a portable C-arm, and/or tantalum powder is needed. The precise anatomic localization of the target is done using trigeminal cisternography. The permanent marking of the cistern is recommended by Hakanson and can be obtained using a mixture of 2 mL of glycerol and 0.5 g of sterile tantalum power. This makes it easier to identify the cistern and serves as a guide if reinjections are needed. The original technique of Hakanson has been modified by various neurosurgeons. Some surgeons do not inject contrast [22], relying on the fluoroscopic findings and cerebrospinal fluid (CSF) drainage, and others do not directly visualize the injection of glycerol into the trigeminal cistern with radiopaque tantalum powder [23, 24]. This surgical approach is essentially the same as that described for other percutaneous techniques to approach the foramen ovale with the Hartel technique.

2.5 Operative Procedure

A 20-gauge needle is advanced to the foramen ovale in the supine position with the neck extended as previously described. It is helpful to visualize the foramen ovale using an oblique submental projection of the portable C-arm. After the position of the needle tip is confirmed in the center of the medial half of the foramen, the depth of the needle tip is then checked in the lateral projection of the C-arm fluoroscopy unit. The free flow of CSF from the needle should be confirmed to ascertain the needle tip position in the trigeminal cistern. If CSF is not observed, the needle can be advanced incrementally to the clival line. If CSF drainage is observed, or the needle position is correct radiographically without it, trigeminal cisternography is performed under a sitting position with the neck slightly flexed. The sitting position helps keep a contrast agent within the cistern. The contrast dye is injected slowly with a 1-mL tuberculin syringe until it escapes to the posterior fossa. If the cistern outline is not visualized, the needle tip needs to be repositioned more medially. The average volume of the trigeminal cistern is 0.25 mL and rarely exceeds 0.4 mL [25]. When the intracisternal position of the needle is identified, the contrast agent is evacuated from the cistern by spontaneous drainage through the needle or in the supine position with the neck extended. Furthermore, the cistern may be flushed with about 2 mL of saline until the cistern is emptied radiographically.

Glycerol injection is also performed in the sitting position in the same manner as the injection of contrast dye. The volume of glycerol injected is based on the cisternal volume measured and the trigeminal pain distribution [18, 26]. Glycerol is floated above the retained contrast owing to the different densities of contrast and glycerol. For patients with V3 pain, approximately one-half of the cistern is filled with glycerol, and the optimal needle position is in the lowest part of the cistern. For V2 and V3 pains, approximately two-thirds of the cistern is filled with a small volume of glycerol (0.15–0.2 mL); for V1, V2, and V3 pains, the cistern is filled completely. In isolated V1 pain, contrast dye can be left at approximately two-thirds of the cistern to protect the lower division fibers. About 99.9% of anhydrous glycerol is injected slowly, with 0.05 mL increments or approximately a drop. An initial bolus of approximately 0.2 mL is injected. After observing the patient's reaction, facial pinprick sensation and corneal reflex are tested after 3–5 min, and 0.05 mL glycerol is injected until a mild sensory loss is obtained and/or a total of 0.3-mL glycerol is injected [22]. If the corneal reflex is decreased or the patient complains of paresthesia in the

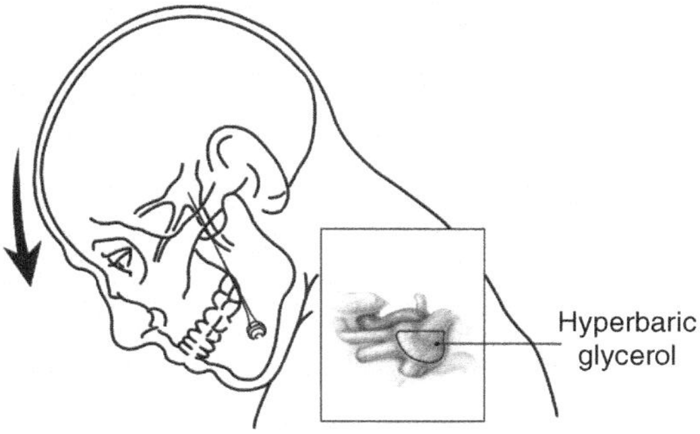

Fig. 7 Patient positioning for glycerol infusion in the trigeminal cistern

eye and the trigeminal neuralgia pain is not within the first division, no further glycerol is injected. If V1 sensory loss is observed, the evacuation of glycerol from the cistern within 10 min after the onset of V1 analgesia is recommended to avoid persistent corneal anesthesia [19]. After glycerol has been injected, the needle and syringe are removed together. The patient is kept in the upright position with the neck flexed for about 1 h after the procedure to maximize the exposure of the trigeminal ganglion and nerves to the glycerol (Fig. 7).

2.6 Results

Immediate or early complete pain relief is 90%. The average risk of early recurrence (<2 years) appears to be approximately 20%, and the rate of late recurrence (>2 years) within 5–10 years may reach 50% [19]. Long-term complications of corneal analgesia (5%), troublesome dysesthesia (4%), anesthesia dolorosa (2.3%), and masseter muscle weakness (1%) can be observed [27]. Glycerol injection can be repeated several times with no increase in morbidity [24, 28].

Pollock (2005) reported 98 patients who underwent glycerol rhizotomy [29]. Fifty patients (51%) had previously undergone surgery. In six patients (6%), the trigeminal cistern could not be defined and the procedure was aborted. The 1- and 3-year chances of an excellent facial pain outcome without medications were 61% and 50%, respectively. Mild paresthesia or numbness was noted in 53% of the patients. Forty-six patients (53%) experienced either mild numbness/paresthesia in 39 patients (52.3%) or dysesthesia in seven patients (0.7%). Herpes simplex perioralis developed in 12% of the patients. Harries (2011) reported 179 patients who underwent repeat glycerol rhizotomy [28]. An overall success rate of 92.1% in the improvement of facial pain was recorded. Nine patients had reduced facial sensation postoperatively. No cases of anesthesia dolorosa were observed. The mean time to repeat injection was 22.9 months. Of those requiring repeat glycerol injections within 6 months, 23% had multiple sclerosis. No significant increase in the complications with repeat procedures was observed in patients having up to six procedures. Although the initial success rate of repeat injections is similar to that of the initial injection, the duration of effectiveness subsides.

2.7 Complication Avoidance

The key to the avoidance of complication is correct needle placement and the incremental injection of glycerol with intermittent facial sensory monitoring. What is the optimal amount of glycerol injected? Hakanson's usual dose of glycerol is approximately 0.22–0.28 mL, with a maximum dose of 0.25 mL [18, 26]. A dose of more than 0.3 mL usually results in more pronounced sensory deficits [4, 26]. In the case of previous destructive procedures, the injected amount of glycerol should be reduced. It is important to know the exact amount of glycerol injected. Calculating the needle dead volume first is required. A 20-gauge spinal needle generally contains a dead volume of about 0.1 mL of fluid. Where is the appropriate anatomical targeting point of the foramen ovale punctured for the branch selectivity of trigeminal neuralgia? The anatomical targeting of V1 is more efficiently achieved by inserting the needle in the medial third of the foramen; for V2 targeting, in the middle of the foramen; and for V3 targeting, in the lateral third of the foramen [30]. What additional measures should be taken if the CSF is not visible when a spinal needle perforates the foramen ovale? These additional measures include the following: (a) The needle is advanced incrementally to the clival line to confirm the spontaneous drainage of CSF. (b) The needle tip probably lies subtemporarily and needs to be repositioned more medially. If one needle already has penetrated the foramen, the other new needle can readily be inserted in the medial part of the foramen ovale. (c) Trigeminal cisternography is performed to confirm the intracisternal tip location. What are positive prognostic indicators during glycerol rhizotomy? Factors that predict good outcomes include easy penetration of the foramen ovale, free flow of CSF, normal appearance of the trigeminal cistern, ipsilateral V1 pain during the injection of glycerol, and mild hypesthesia on the pain site [29]. When is reinjection necessary if the patient's pain relief is insufficient after glycerol injection? Incomplete pain relief seems in most cases to be the result of technical problems during the procedure. Approximately half of the patients are relieved of their paroxysmal pain within the first day of the procedure, whereas the others may take up to 2 days or 3 weeks for the full effect to occur [25, 19]. Reinjections should not be performed up to 3 weeks after the initial procedure.

2.8 Comparison of Percutaneous Ablative Procedures

Radiofrequency rhizotomy has a very high initial success rate and lower recurrence rate and has compatible results with microvascular decompression [27]. However, it has a highly likely risk of sensory disturbance, such as severe numbness and dysesthesia. Radiofrequency lesioning provides the most selective and graded lesion among the percutaneous techniques. Target localization does well in lower divisions, especially V3 lesion, and carries the highest risk of corneal anesthesia in V1 pain. Balloon compression is especially useful in patients with V1 pain and multiple divisions, and carries the highest risk of trigeminal motor dysfunction. It does not result in corneal anesthesia [23, 5, 6]. It is relatively easy to perform under general anesthesia for a brief period and does not require patient cooperation. However, the radiofrequency method, as well as glycerol rhizotomy, does require cooperation. Glycerol rhizotomy remains a useful tool for paroxysmal facial pain, particularly in elderly patients, weak patients, or those with multiple sclerosis [25, 19]. Glycerol injection provides a lower risk of sensory disturbance, severe numbness, and dysesthesia, although it usually presents with a higher recurrence rate compared with either radiofrequency lesion or balloon compression. It carries little risk for severe side effects, even with repeat procedures.

3 Conclusion

Three well-established percutaneous ablative techniques, namely, radiofrequency rhizotomy, glycerol rhizotomy, and balloon compression, are aimed at the trigeminal ganglion or trigeminal nerve roots in treating trigeminal neuralgia, but no consensus has been reached as to which is best. The choice of percutaneous procedures is related to the factors of patient age, health, the location of pain, any prior operations, advantages and disadvantages of each method, and preferences of the patient and physician. The neurosurgeon has to select the right weapon for the right patient.

These procedures share the same results as those treatments with a risk of complications related to needle placement and lesion-making method. Even if trigeminal neuralgia recurs, the percutaneous procedures can be easily performed, along with other surgical methods, so it is desirable to have fewer side effects as much as possible when performing the percutaneous surgery. The percutaneous procedures resulted in an efficacy rate above 90% in treating trigeminal neuralgia among patients with acceptable morbidity. In general, they are relatively simple, safe, and cost-effective compared with microvascular decompression, making percutaneous surgery a viable option.

References

1. Shelden CH, Pudenz RH, Freshwater DB, Crue BL. Compression rather than decompression for trigeminal neuralgia. J Neurosurg. 1955;12:123–6.
2. Mullan S, Lichtor T. Percutaneous microcompression of the trigeminal ganglion for trigeminal neuralgia. J Neurosurg. 1983;59:1007–12.
3. Brown JA, Hoeflinger B, Long PB, Gunning WT, Rhoades R, Bennett-Clarke CA, et al. Axon and ganglion cell injury in rabbits after percutaneous trigeminal balloon compression. Neurosurgery. 1996;38:993–1004.
4. Brown JA. Percutaneous technique. In: Youmans JR, editor. Neurological surgery, vol. 3. 5th ed. New York: Saunders; 2004. p. 2996–3004.
5. Brown JA, Pilitsis JG. Percutaneous balloon compression for the treatment of trigeminal neuralgia: results in 56 patients based on balloon compression pressure monitoring. Neurosurg Focus. 2005;18:E10.
6. Park SS, Lee MK, Kim JW, Jung JY, Kim IK, Ghang CG. Percutaneous balloon compression of trigeminal ganglion for the treatment of idiopathic trigeminal neuralgia: experience in 50 patients. J Korean Neurosurg Soc. 2008;43:186–9.
7. Thatikunta M, Eaton J, Mohammed N, Nauta HJ. Intraoperative CT for neuronavigation guidance and confirmation of foramen ovale cannulation for glycerol trigeminal rhizotomy: a technical report and case Series. Cureus. 2020;12:e8100.
8. Brown JA, Preul MC. Trigeminal depressor response during percutaneous microcompression of the trigeminal ganglion for trigeminal neuralgia. Neurosurgery. 1988;23:745–8.
9. Meuwly C, Golanov E, Chowdhury T, Erne P, Schaller B. Trigeminal cardiac reflex: new thinking model about the definition based on a literature review. Medicine. 2015;94:e484.
10. Chen JF, Tu PH, Lee ST. Long-term follow-up of patients treated with percutaneous balloon compression for trigeminal neuralgia in Taiwan. World Neurosurg. 2011;76:586–91.
11. Arrese I, Lobato RD, Alen JF, Lagares A, Miranda P. Acute subdural and intratemporal hematoma as a complication of percutaneous compression of the gasseiran ganglion for trigeminal neuralgia. Neurocirugia. 2005;16:177–82.
12. Córdoba JLD, Bach MG, Isach N, Piles S. Percutaneous balloon compression for trigeminal neuralgia: imaging and technical aspects. Reg Anesth Pain Med. 2015;40:616–22.
13. Lee SW, Lee MK, Kim WJ, Lee GS, Kim YS. Abducens nerve palsy following percutaneous balloon compression for idiopathic trigeminal neuralgia: case report and technical considerations. J Kor Soc Ster Func Neurosurg. 2014;10:110–2.
14. Lopez BC, Hamlyn PJ, Zakrzewska JM. Systemic review of ablative neurosurgical techniques for the

treatment of trigeminal neuralgia. Neurosurgery. 2004;54:973–82.
15. Urculo E, Alfaro R, Arrazola M, Astudillo E, Rejas G. Trochlear nerve palsy after repeated percutaneous balloon compression for recurrent trigeminal neuralgia: case report and pathologenic considerations. Neurosurgery. 2004;54:505–8.
16. Bergenheim AT, Asplund P, Linderoth B. Percutaneous retrogasserian balloon compression for trigeminal neuralgia: Review of critical technical details and outcomes. World Neurosurg. 2013;79:359–68.
17. Abdennebi B, Guenane L. Technical considerations and outcome assessment in retrogasserian balloon compression for treatment of trigeminal neuralgia. series of 901 patients. Surg Neurol Int. 2014;5:118.
18. Håkanson S. Trigeminal neuralgia treated by the injection of glycerol into the trigeminal cistern. Neurosurgery. 1981;9:638–46.
19. Linderoth B, Håkanson S. Retrogasserian glycerol rhizolysis in trigeminal neuralgia. In: Schmideck HH, Sweet HH editors. Operative neurosurgical techniques: Indications, methods, and results, vol. 2. 4th ed. New York: Saunders; 2000. p. 1552–59.
20. Pal HK, Dinda AK, Roy S, Banerji AK. Acute effect of glycerol on peripheral nerve: an experimental study. Br J Neurosurg. 1989;3:463–9.
21. Eide PK, Stubhaug A. Relief of trigeminal neuralgia after percutaneous retrogasserian glycerol rhizolysis is dependent on normalization of abnormal temporal summation of pain, without general impairment of sensory perception. Neurosurgery. 1998;43:462–72.
22. Young RF. Glycerol rhizolysis for treatment of trigeminal neuralgia. J Neurosurg. 1988;69:39–45.
23. Asplund P, Blomstedt P, Bergenheim AT. Percutaneous balloon compression vs percutaneous retrogasserian glycerol rhizotomy for the primary treatment of trigeminal neuralgia. Neurosurgery. 2016;78:421–8.
24. Bender M, Pradilla G, Batra S, See A, Bhutiani N, James C, et al. Effectiveness of repeat glycerol rhizotomy in treating recurrent trigeminal neuralgia. Neurosurgery. 2012;70:1125–34.
25. Kondziolka D, Lunsford LD. Percutaneous retrogasserian glycerol rhizotomy for trigeminal neuralgia: technique and expectations. Neurosurg Focus. 2005;18:E7.
26. Patel A, Lunsford DL. Percutaneous retrogasserian glycerol rhizotomy. In: Burchiel KJ, editor. Surgical management of pain. Thieme; 2002. p. 865–73.
27. Taha JM, Tew JM. Percutaneous rhizotomy in the treatment of intractable facial pain. In: Schmideck HH, Sweet HH, editors. Operative neurosurgical techniques: indications, methods, and results, vol. 2. 4th ed. W.B. Saunders; 2000. p. 1537–51.
28. Harris AM, Mitchell RD. Percutaneous glycerol rhizotomy for trigeminal neuralgia: safety and efficacy of repeat procedures. Br J Neurosurg. 2011;25:268–72.
29. Pollock BE. Percutaneous retrogasserian glycerol rhizotomy for patients with idiopathic trigeminal neuralgia: a prospective analysis of factors related to pain relief. J Neurosurg. 2005;102:223–8.
30. Peris-Celda M, Graziano F, Russo V, Mericle RA, Ulm AJ. Foramen ovale puncture, lesioning accuracy, and avoiding complications: microsurgical anatomy study with clinical implications. J Neurosurg. 2013;119:1176–93.

Stereotactic Radiosurgery for Trigeminal Neuralgia

Kyung Rae Cho

1 Introduction

The cause of trigeminal neuralgia is hypothesized as demyelination of trigeminal nerve sensory fibers within the proximal nerve root [1], either by vessels or other mass-like lesions. When definite offending vessel is identified from imaging, the treatment of choice could be microvascular decompression surgery. However, there are numerous exceptions who cannot or does not want to have surgery. Exceptions can be one with excessive comorbid conditions, no definite offending vessel found from imaging, recurred TN after MVD, and secondary TN from tumorous condition nearby trigeminal nerve. Treatment options for TN other than MVD are percutaneous procedures (balloon micro compression, glycerol injection, radiofrequency thermocoagulation), and external beam stereotactic radiosurgery (SRS) [2]. In means of less invasiveness, SRS is frequently used to treat TN. Gamma knife (GK) is most frequently used in the neurosurgical field; however, Cyberknife (CKR) and linear accelerator (LINAC) based SRS are also frequently used. As dosage and coverage of each modality differs, clinical outcomes also are different. In this chapter, we will discuss about the use of SRS for TN mostly focused on the result of GKS but will also include differences between CKR and LINAC.

K. R. Cho (✉)
Department of Neurosurgery, Konkuk University Medical Center, Konkuk University School of Medicine, Seoul, Republic of Korea

2 Mechanism of Pain Relief and History of SRS in TN

The mechanism of SRS is often referred as a rhizotomy being conceptually comparable to other methods for lesioning nerves that involve either thermal or mechanical energy. However, in a more microscopic viewpoint, SRS has an effect on nervous amyelinic, low caliver cells associated to nociceptive sensibility, and to the destruction of the ionic channels and relative blockade of electrical conduction [3]. Furthermore, by using tractography radial diffusivities changed markedly after SRS suggesting that SRS primarily affects myelin [4]. Those changes in the trigeminal nerve after radiation may alter the conduction of nerve fibers and result in terrible painful symptoms.

In 1951 the concept of RS was introduced by the Swedish neurosurgeon Lars Leksell. He treated TN patient with a prototype guiding device linked to a dental X-ray machine and "stereotactic gangliotomy" was performed similar to the percutaneous technique [5]. Twenty years later he published the result using stereotactically focused radiation targeted to the trigeminal ganglion in order to treat a small number of patients with TN [6]. As external beam technology and

K. Park, K. R. Cho (eds.), *Trigeminal Neuralgia*, https://doi.org/10.1007/978-981-19-9171-4_21

neuroimaging evolved, technologies such as the Gamma Knife, linear accelerator (LINAC), and CyberKnife RS (CKR) developed and reported their outcomes [2].

3 Clinical Outcome of SRS for TN

Most of the studies reported outcomes using Barrow Neurological Institute Pain Intensity (BNI) scale or a variation. BNI I, complete pain relief without medication; II, occasional pain not requiring medication; III, some pain but adequately controlled with medications; IV, some pain inadequately controlled with medication; V, continued severe pain or no pain relief [7].

3.1 Freedom from Pain

Tuleasca et al. [2] reviewed literature on 45 GKS, 9 CKR, and 11 LINAC-based treatment. The freedom from pain (FFP) with or without medication was achieved in 84.8% (66.6~100%), 87.3% (70~100%), and 79.3% (50~100%) in GKS, LINAC, and CKR each respectively. FFP without medication was achieved in 53.1% (28.6~100%), 49.3%(17.3~76%), and 56.3(40~72%) in GKS, LINAC, and CKR, respectively. The difference in the FFP response between each device was not significant. Differing from MVD and other percutaneous procedures, SRS delayed response after radiation. The mean time to pain relief ranged from 15 to 78 days in GKS and 28 to 81 days for LINAC but there were no specific report for CKR-treated patients. The maximum interval for pain relief is reported upto 480 days however generally considered 180 days after radiosurgery [2].

3.2 Long-Term Result

Unlike GKS, long-term efficacy of pain relief is rarely found in CKR and LINAC treatment group. GKS showed 22~59.7% pain relief in 7 years[8–10] follow-up and 30~67.7% in 10 years without new use of medication or other surgical procedures [10–12]. Good prognostic factors for long-term outcome were advanced age, previous MVD, higher prescription dose, no previous surgical treatments, and classical trigeminal pain features [10, 12]. Mousavi et al. [11] retrospectively reviewed 121 patients with TN treated with GKS primarily and concluded earlier GKS within 3 years of symptom onset led to a shorter time to pain relief, a longer interval of pain relief off medication, and longer adequate pain control.

3.3 Complications

Trigeminal nerve dysfunction is major possible toxicity in radiation to the trigeminal nerve. The most common complication is hypesthesia which onset among the studies was 21.7%, 27.6%, and 29.1% for GKS, LINAC, and CKR, respectively. Bothersome or very bothersome hypesthesia (BNI III or IV) was reported in 3.1% (0~17.3%) in GKS, one study reported 13.6% in LINAC and 9.3%(5.9~12%) in CKR. The difference between GKS and other SRS (CKR and LINAC) showed a significant difference ($p = 0.05$). The difference in the onset of hypesthesia between devices was not significant however studies of CKR and LINAC are limited in time and may be underestimated. The mean time to hypesthesia onset in the GKS group ranged from 6 to 36 months, there are insufficient data on other modalities [2]. While hypesthesia is a most common complication and other complications are rarely reported from GKS-treated patients, other treatment-related complications were observed in CKR and LINAC-treated patients, such as anesthesia dolorosa, dysgeusia, dry eye syndrome, neurotrophic keratopathy, decreased corneal reflex, trismus, dysesthesias, hearing impairment, and masticator weakness are reported rarely in the literatures [3, 13–16].

Factors that may affect the toxicity are the target selection, the length of the irradiated nerve, and the prescribed dose. Most fearful complications in SRS for TN could be related to the radiation to the ventral brainstem. Thus an intracisternal target is preferred rather than REZ target in the means of complication [17, 18]. A longer portion of the irradiated nerve may lead to a higher complication rate [16, 19]. And dose higher than 90 Gy seems to have increased complication rate than a dose lower than 90 Gy [20].

Radiation delivered to the brainstem was associated with a higher complication rate. Matsuda et al. [21] reported maximal dose to the brainstem(cutoff > 25 Gy), as well as the position of the isocenter(cutoff < 4.5 mm) was significantly related to the complications. Furthermore, a brainstem volume of more than 28 mm^3 receiving more than 12 Gy of radiation was related to complications. Many other reports support that higher doses related to a higher complication rate [13, 22].

3.4 Recurrence

Mean recurrence rates were 24.6% (0~52.2%), 32.3% (19~63%), and 25.8% (15.8–33%) in GKS, LINAC, and CKR group. For BNI III and IV, the recurrence rate of GKS was significantly low than that of LINAC but not significant from the result of CKR. Time to recurrence ranged from 6 to 48 months for GKS and 7.5–20.4 months for LINAC and 9 months in the CKR group [2]. Length of the trigeminal nerve, Ponto-trigeminal angle, trigeminal volume, target location, shot-emergence distance, and ratio between nerve length and targeting length were evaluated as anatomical factors related to the recurrence [17, 18, 22–24]. Factors related to the radiosurgical planning were prescription dose, the number of isocenters and beam channel blocking (plug use) were considered; more recently integral dose (depending on the volume of trigeminal nerve being examined), trigeminal volume receiving ≥80% of the maximal dose, calibration dose rate, and biologically effective dose were also considered as factors related to the recurrence [2, 23, 25–29]. Barzaghi et al. [23] reported long-lasting pain relief was achieved in 56.2% and 47.7% in 5 and 10 years, respectively while 89.3% had good pain control at 6 months after GKS. They found factors related to long-lasting pain relief were BNI I–II (74.9%) over BNI IIIa–IIIB (42%) and the pain relief period was longer in slow responders (69.1%) than fast responders (42%). They also found a dose lower than 80 Gy, a calibration dose rate < 2.5 Gy/min, and an isocenter-emergence distance >8 mm adopting retrogasserian target were related to the poor outcome. Repeated GKS was also useful in recurred cases, durability of pain relief was not inferior to previous GKS but patients who had a good outcome from previous GKS also had better pain relief at repeated treatment. Treatment-related complications such as hypesthesia of the affected face were also increased [30, 31].

4 Target Selection in SRS for TN

The goal for SRS in TN is to place radiation on the trigeminal nerve at the prepontine cistern. It is not difficult to target the nerve because the trigeminal nerve can be well visualized by modern MRI techniques. However, there are a few different targets considered, gasserian ganglion (GG) target, retrogasserian target, and REZ target. And consideration for targeting includes radiation dosage affected to brainstem. The gasserian target was firstly selected by Leksell but moved to the REZ [3]. Linquist reported the outcome of 46 patients for which radiation target was set on GG and 18% of whom had maintained pain relief at 2 years [2]. The anterior cisternal target, also called cisternal target, has been frequently used and reported by many authors [10, 26, 32–37]. Otherwise, the REZ has been the most consistent target also referred to as the "dorsal REZ" where the trigeminal nerve exits from the brain stem. Some authors make the choice of an anterior versus a posterior target based on the idea that the nerve is more radiosensitive at the REZ than at the anterior part. Matsuda et al. [38] compared anterior versus posterior target, receiving 80 Gy at the proximal trigeminal nerve (REZ) and anterior target receiving between 80 and 90 Gy at the retrogasserian portion of the trigeminal nerve. Median 30 months were followed up (range 3–88 months) and there was no difference in two

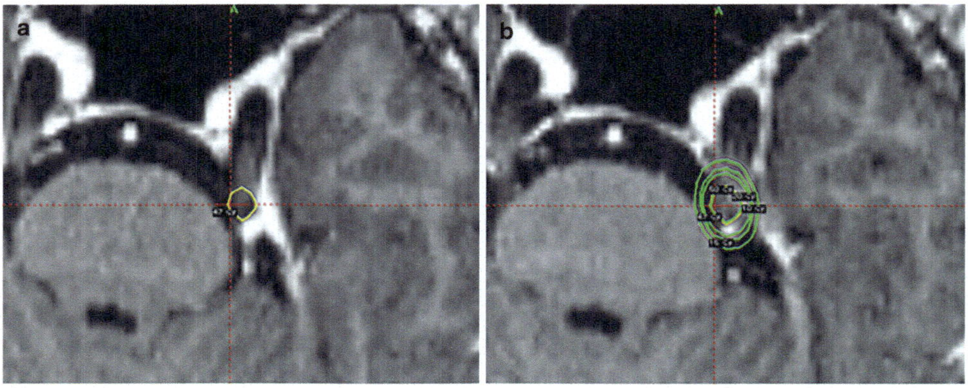

Fig. 1 Radiosurgery target and dosimetry of Gamma Knife Surgery for Trigeminal Neuralgia. (**a**, **b**) 4 mm collimator shot was placed on cisternal segment of trigeminal nerve. 47 Gy were prescribed at 55% isodose line, maximal dose was 85.5 Gy. 10 Gy isodose line slightly touched the brainstem. She had no immediate pain relief, but symptoms reduced by 50% in 3 months without any noticeable complications. (**c**, **d**) 4 mm collimator shot was placed on root entry zone (REZ). 64 Gy was prescribed at 75% isodose line in which maximal dose was 85.3 Gy. With blockage of radiation beam, massive radiation to the brainstem was avoided. However, still more than 15 Gy of radiation was delivered to the brain stem. Her symptom reduced gradually by 6 months without complications but recurred after a year. (**e**, **f**) Two 4 mm collimator shot was placed along the trigeminal nerve. 43 Gy of radiation was prescribed at 51% isodose line, 85 Gy maximum. Radiation was delivered through the whole segment of the nerve without massive radiation delivered to the brainstem. Her symptom disappeared after a year with medication without complications

groups (Initial and last follow-up score in anterior target, 81.6% and 67.4%, and posterior target, 92.2% and 68.6%) also there were no difference in complication (44.9% vs. 37.3%). Park et al. [17] also compared retrogasserian versus dorsal REZ target, with 39 cases followed up for 26.1 months (range 12–53 months). Anterior target received a median dose of 85 Gy (range 83~90) compared to 80 Gy in the posterior target (range 80–90 Gy). Initial FFP was comparable between the two groups, and the time to response was shorter in anterior group. Although anterior group received higher radiation, there was no bothersome complication at the anterior target while in the posterior group 13.1% of bothersome hypesthesia and 8.7% of dry eye syndrome [18]. Tuleasca et al. [2] concluded that anterior and posterior targets showed a similar result initially and maintain pain relief however increased risk of developing complication in REZ target.

Another consideration is the length of radiated portion of the nerve which are represented as the number of isocenters. Flickinger [25] reported similar pain relief but increased complications in two isocenter groups. Pollock et al. [39] reported the length of nerve irradiated did neither differ in efficacy nor in complication. However, other reports showed that patients treated with two isocenter were more likely to receive a higher radiation dose and result in better outcomes without increased complication [40]. Beam-blocking technique to the brainstem was analyzed by several authors, they concluded blocking results in an increase in the treated length of the nerve thus increasing the efficacy of treatment but also increasing the risk of complication which is opposite result to be expected [16, 27, 41]. Various target and their dosimetry are displayed in Fig. 1.

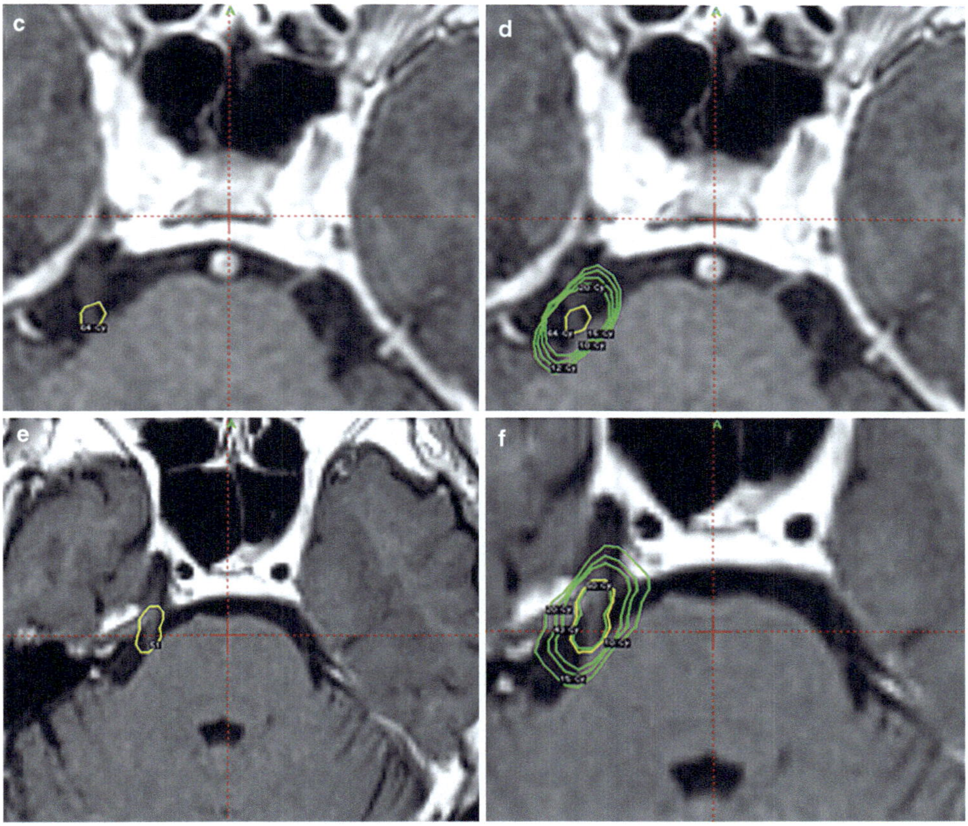

Fig. 1 (continued)

5 Optimal Dose of SRS for TN

Prescribed dose seems to be an absolute predictive factor for pain relief. Though dose prescription in GKS is usually done as one point with a single collimator CKR and LINAC prescribes a certain volume, the result may vary in the same prescribed dose. The mean maximal doses ranged from 71.1 to 90.1 Gy (prescribed at the 100% isodose line) for the GKS studies, from 70 to 90 Gy for LINAC studies, and from 64.3 to 80.5 Gy for CKR studies (the latter two prescribed at the 80% or 90% isodose lines, respectively). The ranges of maximal doses were as follows: 60–97 Gy (large majority 60–90 Gy, more being rather exceptional) for GKS, 50–90 Gy for LINAC, and 66–90 Gy for CKR [2]. Most studies report better outcome at higher prescribed dose [42–44]. However, maximal dose >90 Gy is related to the higher incidence of complication and is considered the upper margin of dose prescription [10, 12, 36, 39].

6 Conclusion

Recently, radiosurgery has been proposed for drug-resistant TN especially in case of the absence of other primary indications as well as surgically unsuitable patients [3]. To summarize the results of previous studies, as much radiation enters into the brainstem REZ, better pain relief can be achieved but bothersome complications can occur when it exceeds the limit. Yet there are no definite consensus to take SRS for the treatment of TN, patients are carefully determined which treatment should be the best option considering their age and the risk of surgery.

References

1. Love S, Coakham HB. Trigeminal neuralgia: pathology and pathogenesis. Brain. 2001;124(Pt 12):2347–60.
2. Tuleasca C, et al. Stereotactic radiosurgery for trigeminal neuralgia: a systematic review. J Neurosurg. 2018;130(3):733–57.
3. Marchetti M, et al. Radiosurgery for trigeminal neuralgia: the state of art. Neurol Sci. 2019;40(Suppl 1):153–7.
4. Hodaie M, et al. Tractography delineates microstructural changes in the trigeminal nerve after focal radiosurgery for trigeminal neuralgia. PLoS One. 2012;7(3):e32745.
5. Leksell L. The stereotaxic method and radiosurgery of the brain. Acta Chir Scand. 1951;102(4):316–9.
6. Leksell L. Sterotaxic radiosurgery in trigeminal neuralgia. Acta Chir Scand. 1971;137(4):311–4.
7. Rogers CL, et al. Gamma knife radiosurgery for trigeminal neuralgia: the initial experience of the Barrow neurological institute. Int J Radiat Oncol Biol Phys. 2000;47(4):1013–9.
8. Little AS, et al. Long-term pain response and quality of life in patients with typical trigeminal neuralgia treated with gamma knife stereotactic radiosurgery. Neurosurgery. 2008;63(5):915–23. discussion 923–4
9. Dhople AA, et al. Long-term outcomes of gamma knife radiosurgery for classic trigeminal neuralgia: implications of treatment and critical review of the literature. J Neurosurg. 2009;111(2):351–8.
10. Regis J, et al. Long-term safety and efficacy of gamma knife surgery in classical trigeminal neuralgia: a 497-patient historical cohort study. J Neurosurg. 2016;124(4):1079–87.
11. Mousavi SH, et al. Early radiosurgery provides superior pain relief for trigeminal neuralgia patients. Neurology. 2015;85(24):2159–65.
12. Kondziolka D, et al. Gamma knife stereotactic radiosurgery for idiopathic trigeminal neuralgia. J Neurosurg. 2010;112(4):758–65.
13. Smith ZA, et al. Dedicated linear accelerator radiosurgery for the treatment of trigeminal neuralgia. J Neurosurg. 2003;99(3):511–6.
14. Richards GM, et al. Linear accelerator radiosurgery for trigeminal neuralgia. Neurosurgery. 2005;57(6):1193–200. discussion 1193–200
15. Lim M, et al. CyberKnife radiosurgery for idiopathic trigeminal neuralgia. Neurosurg Focus. 2005;18(5):E9.
16. Villavicencio AT, et al. Cyberknife radiosurgery for trigeminal neuralgia treatment: a preliminary multicenter experience. Neurosurgery. 2008;62(3):647–55. discussion 647–55
17. Park SH, et al. The retrogasserian zone versus dorsal root entry zone: comparison of two targeting techniques of gamma knife radiosurgery for trigeminal neuralgia. Acta Neurochir. 2010;152(7):1165–70.
18. Xu Z, et al. Impact of target location on the response of trigeminal neuralgia to stereotactic radiosurgery. J Neurosurg. 2014;120(3):716–24.
19. Lim M, et al. Stereotactic radiosurgery using CT cisternography and non-isocentric planning for the treatment of trigeminal neuralgia. Comput Aided Surg. 2006;11(1):11–20.
20. Longhi M, et al. Gamma knife radiosurgery for trigeminal neuralgia: results and potentially predictive parameters--part I: Idiopathic trigeminal neuralgia. Neurosurgery. 2007;61(6):1254–60. discussion 1260–1
21. Matsuda S, et al. Gamma knife radiosurgery for trigeminal neuralgia: the dry-eye complication. J Neurosurg. 2002;97(5 Suppl):525–8.
22. Marshall K, et al. Predictive variables for the successful treatment of trigeminal neuralgia with gamma knife radiosurgery. Neurosurgery. 2012;70(3):566–72. discussion 572–3
23. Barzaghi LR, et al. Gamma knife radiosurgery for trigeminal neuralgia: role of trigeminal length and pontotrigeminal angle on target definition and on clinical effects. World Neurosurg. 2020;142:e140–50.
24. Hung YC, et al. Radiosurgery target location and individual anatomical variation in trigeminal nerves. J Neurosurg. 2014;121(Suppl):203–9.
25. Flickinger JC, et al. Does increased nerve length within the treatment volume improve trigeminal neuralgia radiosurgery? A prospective double-blind, randomized study. Int J Radiat Oncol Biol Phys. 2001;51(2):449–54.
26. Massager N, et al. Gamma knife surgery for idiopathic trigeminal neuralgia performed using a far-anterior cisternal target and a high dose of radiation. J Neurosurg. 2004;100(4):597–605.
27. Massager N, et al. Influence of nerve radiation dose in the incidence of trigeminal dysfunction after trigeminal neuralgia radiosurgery. Neurosurgery. 2007;60(4):681–7. discussion 687–8
28. Mousavi SH, et al. A proposed plan for personalized radiosurgery in patients with trigeminal neuralgia. J Neurosurg. 2018;128(2):452–9.
29. Wolf A, et al. The relationship of dose to nerve volume in predicting pain recurrence after stereotactic radiosurgery in trigeminal neuralgia. J Neurosurg. 2018;128(3):891–6.

30. Omar NB, et al. Repeat gamma knife stereotactic radiosurgery in the treatment of trigeminal neuralgia: a single-center experience and focused review of the literature. J Clin Neurosci. 2019;70:102–7.
31. Helis CA, et al. Results of a third gamma knife radiosurgery for trigeminal neuralgia. J Neurosurg. 2020;134(3):1237–43.
32. Dellaretti M, et al. Clinical outcomes after gamma knife surgery for idiopathic trigeminal neuralgia: review of 76 consecutive cases. J Neurosurg. 2008;109(Suppl):173–8.
33. Lucas JT Jr, et al. Predictive nomogram for the durability of pain relief from gamma knife radiation surgery in the treatment of trigeminal neuralgia. Int J Radiat Oncol Biol Phys. 2014;89(1):120–6.
34. Rand RW, et al. Leksell gamma knife treatment of tic douloureux. Stereotact Funct Neurosurg. 1993;61(Suppl 1):93–102.
35. Regis J, et al. Prospective controlled trial of gamma knife surgery for essential trigeminal neuralgia. J Neurosurg. 2006;104(6):913–24.
36. Regis J, et al. The very long-term outcome of radiosurgery for classical trigeminal neuralgia. Stereotact Funct Neurosurg. 2016;94(1):24–32.
37. Tuleasca C, et al. Patterns of pain-free response in 497 cases of classic trigeminal neuralgia treated with gamma knife surgery and followed up for least 1 year. J Neurosurg. 2012;117(Suppl):181–8.
38. Matsuda S, et al. Comparison of the results of 2 targeting methods in gamma knife surgery for trigeminal neuralgia. J Neurosurg. 2008;109(Suppl):185–9.
39. Pollock BE, et al. Stereotactic radiosurgery for idiopathic trigeminal neuralgia. J Neurosurg. 2002;97(2):347–53.
40. Alpert TE, et al. Gamma knife surgery for trigeminal neuralgia: improved initial response with two isocenters and increasing dose. J Neurosurg. 2005;102(Suppl):185–8.
41. Massager N, et al. Effect of beam channel plugging on the outcome of gamma knife radiosurgery for trigeminal neuralgia. Int J Radiat Oncol Biol Phys. 2006;65(4):1200–5.
42. Kondziolka D, et al. Trigeminal neuralgia radiosurgery: the University of Pittsburgh experience. Stereotact Funct Neurosurg. 1996;66(Suppl 1):343–8.
43. Shaya M, et al. Gamma knife radiosurgery for trigeminal neuralgia: a study of predictors of success, efficacy, safety, and outcome at LSUHSC. Surg Neurol. 2004;61(6):529–34. discussion 534–5
44. Kim YH, et al. Is it effective to raise the irradiation dose from 80 to 85 Gy in gamma knife radiosurgery for trigeminal neuralgia? Stereotact Funct Neurosurg. 2010;88(3):169–76.

Surgical Treatment of Trigeminal Neuralgia: Partial Sensory Rhizotomy

Ha-Young Choi and Eun-Jeong Koh

1 Introduction

The pain with the slightest movement during daily life in patients with trigeminal neruralgia (TN) is starting innocuous stimulation such as mastication, washing, and sudden contact with cold air in the face [1]. The pain nature, types according to the etiology, and treatment methods were mentioned in previous chapters [2]. In patients with medical intractability, common surgical techniques including radiofrequency ablation (RFA), stereotactic radiosurgery (SRS), percutaneous balloon compression (PBC), microvascular decompression (MVD), and partial sensory rhizotomy may be done according to its etiology. MVD is the most effective surgical method for treating patients with typical TN (caused by vascular compression of the trigeminal nerve root), with a recurrence rate between 6% and 47% [3–8]. For patients with idiopathic TN (no clear cause) and secondary TN (secondary to other neurological diseases, such as multiple sclerosis) [9, 10], PSR of a quite destructive operation has rarely been done in spite of its complications which is unable to control. The existing literature reported a recurrence rate between 30% and 50% after the first simple PSR [11–15]. Nevertheless, for patients that simple MVD is not applicable, PSR is often required in clinical practice [1].

2 Surgical Indications of the Partial Sensory Rhizotomy

1. Cases without offenders for doing MVD.
2. Recurrence after MVD.
3. Unavailable cases of microdissection.
4. Cases associated with multiple sclerosis.

As long as there are no appropriate surgical methods for patients with recurrence or existence of pain after MVD, PSR which is a somewhat destructive surgery may be done as an alternative procedure. In case of no significant compression against the trigeminal sensory root (absence of neurovascular compression), or in a case with no allowance of intraoperative safety and no guarantee of effective decompression, PSR also may be performed [13, 15–17].

H.-Y. Choi (✉) · E.-J. Koh
Department of Neurosurgery, Jeonbuk National University Medical School,
Jeonju, Jeonbuk, Republic of Korea
e-mail: hayoungc@chonbuk.ac.kr;
kohejns@jbnu.ac.kr

K. Park, K. R. Cho (eds.), *Trigeminal Neuralgia*, https://doi.org/10.1007/978-981-19-9171-4_22

3 Operative Technique

Operative techniques for skin incision, craniotomy, dural opening, and procedures of slack-down of the brain in the posterior fossa for MVD were mentioned in the earlier chapter.

Meticulous approach is necessary in the way to the trigeminal nerve in following the petrotentorial junction. It is important to manage the petrosal vein carefully being encountered, and not to tear down the vein in the junction with the dural entrance to the sinus, whether it is coagulated or preserved. The arachnoid overlying the fifth nerve was exposed and opened [18].

PSR (the "PSR group") of cutting the posterolateral (or inferolateral) two-thirds of the pars major of CNV in the juxtapontine area as close as possible to the brain stem was done in patients without vascular contact against the full length of the trigeminal nerve. Usual MVD and PSR (the "MVD + PSR group") were also performed in patients with vascular contact but no visualization of deformity of the nerve root [11, 18].

During sectioning of the trigeminal nerve, careful and sharp cut-off must be required to avoid mechanical damage to blood vessels and nerves (Fig. 1).

Intraoperative monitoring is helpful in defining the cutting area in the posterolateral or inferolateral portion of the trigeminal nerve [19]. Young and Wilkins reported the usefulness of the intraoperative monitoring (IOM) of brainstem auditory evoked responses and somatosensory evoked potentials [13]. Based on the IOM, Young and Wilkins underwent PSR with the section of one-third to one-half of the sensory root [13] in 74 (89%) of 83 patients and with the section of two-thirds of the nerve root in its caudolateral aspect about 2–5 mm from the pons in the remaining 9 patients (11%) [13]. Howng and Chang [17] reported that cutting the nerve section ranged from 20% to 70%. Bederson and Wilson [18] sectioned one-half to two-thirds of the portio major. Van Loveren et al. [20] reported a percutaneous stereotaxic rhizotomy.

4 Anatomy of TN; Schematic Drawing of the Anatomy of TN, MRI, and Operative Field

TN consists of three divisions. In the brain stem, the three divisions are located in order; anterior (ophthalmic), middle or intermediate (maxillary), and posterior (mandibular). When it comes out from the brain stem TN rotates laterally and it becomes different distribution from the spinal trigeminal nucleus; superomedial (ophthalmic), middle or intermediate (maxillary), and inferolateral (mandibular). Rotation of three divisions results in an inverted laminar arrangement in the brain stem and exterior to the brain stem (cisternal segment extending to Meckel's cave) (Figs. 2 and 3). This peculiar anatomical distribution of the TN shows the reason that PSR is done in the posterolateral (or inferolateral) two-thirds of the pars major of CNV as close as possible to the brain stem.

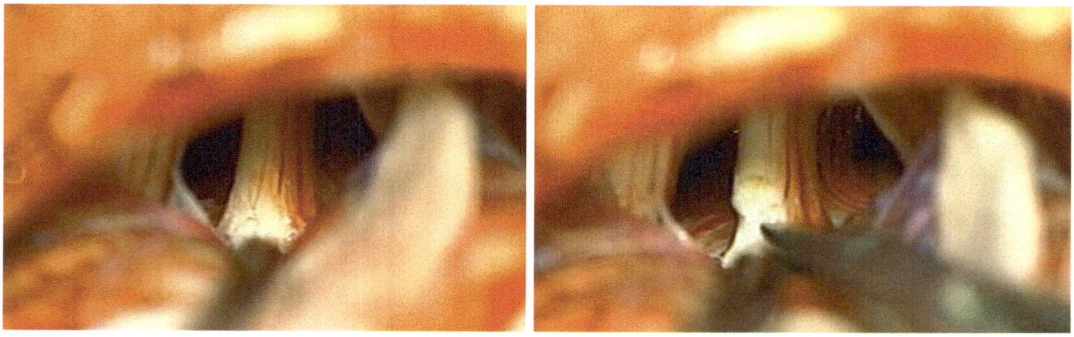

Fig. 1 (Lt. image showing trigeminal nerve before cutting, Rt. image showing lateral 2/3 sectioned trigeminal nerve)

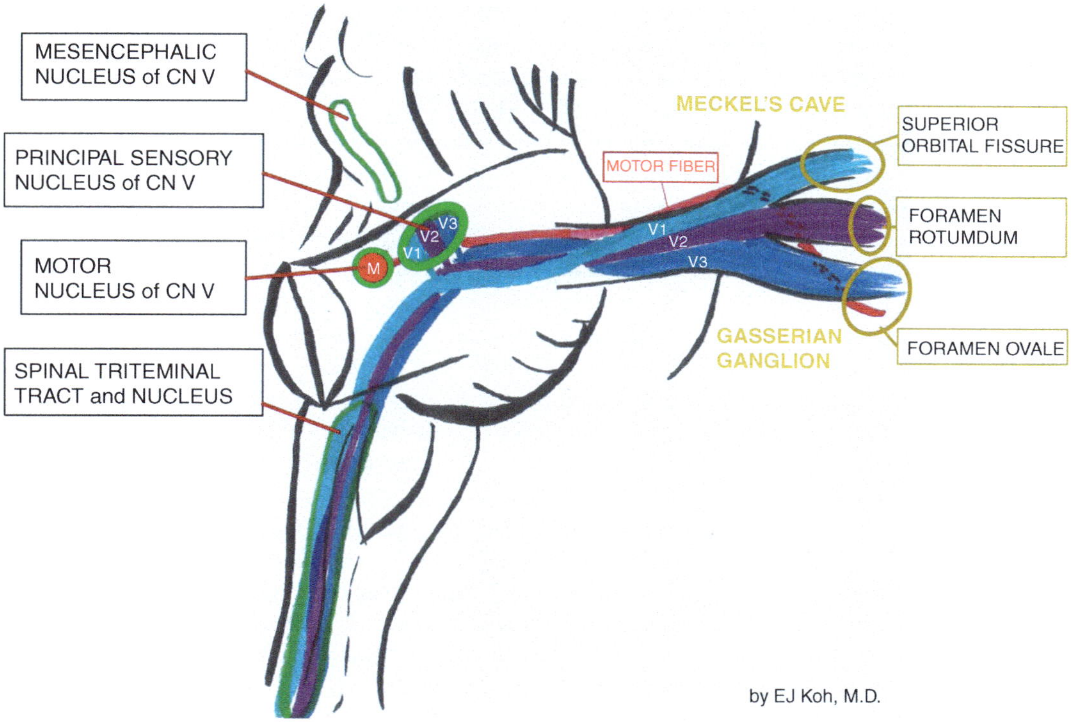

Fig. 2 Schematic drawing shows three divisions with medial rotation when it enters the brain stem (lateral rotation when it comes out from the brain stem)

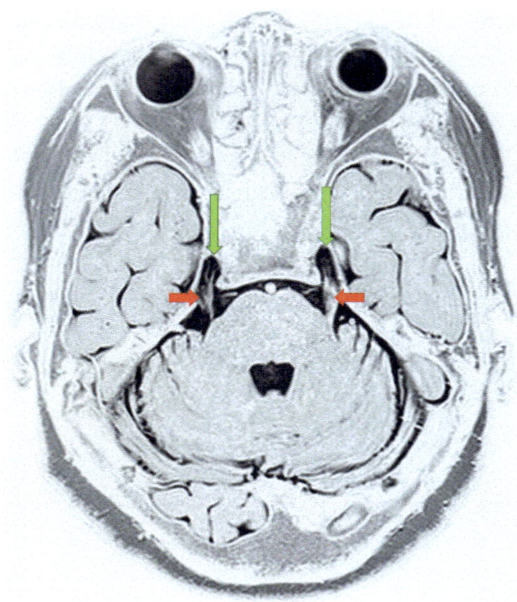

Fig. 3 MRI-axial inversion image at the level of Meckel's cave (yellow-green arrow: Meckel's cave, red arrow: Trigeminal nerve)

Arising from the motor nucleus of the trigeminal nerve within the mid portion of the pons anterolateral to the major sensory nucleus, axons exit the brain stem medial to the remaining portion of the nerve going to the cisternal space and extend to Meckel's cave. During extending to and locating within the gasserian ganglion they do not synapse and travel inferior to the ganglion. The motor branch joins the V3 division and exits the skull base through the foramen ovale to innervate the facial muscles [9] (Fig. 2).

Concerning the sensory changes in the face relating to the extent and area of the section of the trigeminal nerve in PSR, many authors reported different studies [11].

Dandy reported rare changes in the anterior segment of the ipsilateral eye with PSR at the caudal end (i.e., near the pons), contrary to PSR at the rostral portion by Frazier with frequent changes of anterior segment abnormalities [21–24]. Ley and Guitart [25] reported that preservation of tactility is more when total section of the trigeminal dorsal root is performed near the pons. These differences may arise from anatomic works [26–28] of dispersed trigeminal nerve root fibers according to a topographic somatotopy in their retrogasserian portion. Gudmundsson et al. [28] stated the reason for the variability of sensory loss after PSR at the pontine level, caused by the location of the first division fibers dorsomedial and the third division fibers caudolateral with variations of almost directly lateral to directly caudal to the first division fibers within the main sensory root.

Gudmundsson et al. insisted that preservation of tactility after PSR depends only on the individual differences in the degree of rotation of fibers into this portion of CNV and not on the existence of "accessory sensitive fibers" outside the main sensory roots and the functional somatotopy of the intracranial CNV. Nonetheless, some anatomic works [26, 27] reported grouping together the CNV root fibers according to their functional modality in the juxtapontine portion [22, 28, 29].

Intraoperatively, recognition of the pars major versus pars intermediaris is feasible to each other only at the juxtapontine level. Furthermore, the functional arrangement of the pars major and pars intermediaris and the existence of the pars major composed of nociceptive fibers explains analgesia without tactile anesthesia after PSR of the pars major with preservation of the pars intermediaris at the juxtapontine portion. On the other hand, because pars major fibers are organized according to a topographic somatotopy (i.e., considering the pars major with lateral rotation when it comes out of the brain stem at the juxtapontine level), physiopathologic preservation of corneal sensitivity can be explained [11]. Gudmundsson et al. [28] reported that intraoperative topographic mapping of the trigeminal nerve root using electrophysiological methods might be used as a guide for performing PSR.

5 Clinical Outcome and Postoperative Complications

The first goal of PSR is complete relief of the pain without minimal neurologic complications including sensory change of the face and loss of corneal reflex. A surgeon must consider which surgical technique gives the longest pain-free period with the fewest complication and good quality of life [11].

Estimation of surgical outcome based on the extent of PSR is hard to make out due to various definitions on the Extent of Rhizotomy. Analysis consisted of the great heterogeneity considering the section of the pars major or the entire nerve root, the level of rhizotomy (i.e., the distance between rhizotomy and pons), or the extent of rhizotomy (Fig. 4) in the literature. The para-

Reference	Number of Cases	Cases with Previous Procedure, N (%)	Median Follow-up (months)	Extent of Rhizotomy	Location of Rhizotomy	Pain Relief After Suregery (%)	Corneal Reflex Impairment/Hypesthesia (%)	Sensory Deficit (%)	Location of Sensory Deficit	Recurrence Rate
Young et al. [24] (*J Neurosurg* 1993)	83	35 (42)	72	1/3 to 1/2 ventrolateral of nerve root (89%) 2/3 of nerve root (11%)	2–5 mm from the pons	48	NA	67	96% V2 and V3	17% at 1 year and 2.6% each year thereafter
Bederson [25] (*J Neurosurg* 1989)	30	42% of the whole series of 246 patients (MVD and PSR)	61.2	Inferior 1/2 to 2/3 of pars major	NA	70	1.5	NA	NA	NA
Klun et al. [26] (*Neurosurg* 1992)	42	NA	62.4	1/3 or less of the pars major	As close as possible to the pons	86	0	100	NA	Total recurrence rate 50%
Zakrzewka et al. [27] (*Neurosurg* 2005)	53	21 (39.6)	68.4	NA	NA	NA	22 " eye problems"	48	NA	28% at 5 years
Ko et al. [28] (*J Neurosurg* 2015)	27	10 (37)	43.4	Longitudinal division along pars major and pars minor fibers	Internal neurolysis	85	NA	96	NA	42% at 1 year 53% at 5 years
Adams et al. [29] (*J Neurol Neurosurg Psychiatry* 1982)	55	84.2% of the whole series of 57 patients (MVD and PSR)	54	30%–100% of trigeminal nerve	Craniomedial portion or caudolateral portion	87.3	12.7	NA	NA	11.8% at 5 years
Terrier et al. (2017)	22	3 (13.6)	67.3	2/3 ventrolateral of pars major	As close as possible to the pons	86.4	0	22.7	60% one hemitongue, 20% V2 and V3, 20% V3	14.6% at 1 year 31.5% at 5 years

NA, not available; MVD, microvascular decompression; PSR, partial sensory rhizotomy.

Fig 4. Table from Terrier LM et al. world neurosurg. 2018 sep mount concern after PSR is sensory deficit and change of corneal reflex according to the extent of the section of CNV. Adams et al. [30] reported that loss of corneal reflex was observed in all patients with a total section of CNV even in patients with intact pars intermedia but intact corneal reflex was observed in all patients with a partial section. Young et al. [13] achieved the restoration of pain in only 48% with sections approximately from one-third to one-half of the nerve root in 89% of patients, and two-thirds in only 11% of patients. This study suggested low pain relief with less extensive section. Young et al. reported sensory deficit in 67% of patients. The higher rate of facial sensory change seemed to be related to the location of the sectioning. This study made a sense of being better sensory preservation as close to the pons as possible. Recently, Ko et al. [12] introduced internal neurolysis treating TN without neurovascular compression. A longitudinal division of the trigeminal nerve along its fibers including both the pars minor and the pars major was made. Tubbs et al. did a neurolysis of neural interconnections between the pars minor and pars major at the Meckel cave. This series restored pain-free survival at 1 and 5 years in 58% and 47%, respectively. Numbness or hypoesthesia of the face was in 96% of patients after this procedure.

The surgical outcome of restoration of pain and preservation of facial sense are varied by the presence of additional sensory roots and the existence of anastomosis between the motor and sensory root in most nerves but also the existence of anatomic connections between the trigeminal system on one side and the facial, glossopharyngeal, and vagal cranial nerves on the other side, both centrally and in the periphery [11, 25, 28]. Additionally, Gudmundsson et al. [28] insisted that variability in the degree of rotation of the sensory root entering the pons may also be related to the differences in the quantity of sensory loss after PSR.

In TN patients without vascular contact against the full length of the trigeminal nerve, PSR is an effective treatment modality, but it has rarely been carried out recently due to the higher incidence of dysesthesia in the face and recurrence of pain [31]. Facial hypoesthesia or numbness was a major issue of postoperative complication, which occurred in most or all reported patients [14, 15]. However, recent studies on PSR showed relatively good results in terms of pain control [18, 19, 32, 33]. Toda [19] has achieved excellent results of pain-free without medication, ranging from 48% to 86%. In Terrier et al.'s series [11], the cure rate was 54.5% and the efficacy rate was 72.7%. Pain recurred in one case. The results of their series were similar to those of previous studies [11].

In reviewing the recurrence of pain, Young and Wilkins reported as follows: In defining the failure as major persistence or recurrence of pain, the failure rate 1 year after surgery was 17% and yearly failure rates thereafter averaged 2.6%. Using the more stringent criterion of failure as any persistence or recurrence of pain, the failure rate at 1 year was 42%. Yearly failure rates after 1 year for this end point averaged 2.0% [13, 15, 17, 18, 34].

Besides major complications produced by PSR, other complications related to surgery onto the posterior fossa including CSF leakage, surgical site infection, meningitis (aseptic or bacterial), brain infarction, cerebellar edema, hematom, and CN VII and VIII deficit have been reported. Earlier chapters have mentioned how to avoid these complications.

6 Conclusion

One of the worst neuropathic pains leading to the slightest movement during daily life and even social disability in patients with trigeminal neuralgia (TN) is starting from innocuous stimulation [11]. TN is rarely a deadly disease and all surgical works must be functional surgery.

Great emphasis should be placed on improving the safety of operation and reduction of complications. Surgeons should be equipped with comprehensive knowledge and experience in retrosigmoid cranial nerve surgery.

Surgeons dealing with PSR must have an insight into the somatotopy of the trigeminal nerve in its juxtapontine portion, based on extensive literature reviewing electrophysiologic, anatomic, and historic surgical outcomes. In conclusion, PSR with the section of the ventrolateral two-thirds of the pars major of the trigeminal nerve at the pons provides excellent outcomes considering immediate pain relief, postoperative hypoesthesia, preservation of corneal reflex, and recurrence rate, compared with other ablative procedures for TN without vascular compression. This procedure is a standardized one and an interesting alternative to other ablative procedures for medically refractory TN patients without vascular compression.

References

1. Liu Y, Yu Y, Wang Z, Deng Z, Liu R, Luo N, Zhang L. Value of partial sensory Rhizotomy in the microsurgical treatment of trigeminal neuralgia through Retrosigmoid approach. J Pain Res. 2020;1(13):3207–15.
2. Arnold M. Headache classification committee of the international headache society (IHS) the international classification of headache disorders, 3rd edition. Cephalalgia. 2018;38(1):1–211.
3. Barker FG, Jannetta PJ, Bissonette DJ, Larkins MV, Jho HD. The long-term outcome of microvascular decompression for trigeminal neuralgia. N Engl J Med. 1996;334(17):1077–83. https://doi.org/10.1056/NEJM199604253341701.
4. Sindou M, Leston J, Howeidy T, Decullier E, Chapuis F. Micro-vascular decompression for primary trigeminal neuralgia (typical or atypical). Long-term effectiveness on pain; prospective study with survival analysis in a consecutive series of 362 patients [J]. Acta Neurochir. 2006;148(12):1235–45. https://doi.org/10.1007/s00701-006-0809-2.
5. Sarsam Z, Garcia-Fiñana M, Nurmikko TJ, Varma TR, Eldridge P. The long-term outcome of microvascular decompression for trigeminal neuralgia [J]. Br J Neurosurg. 2010;24(1):18–25. https://doi.org/10.3109/02688690903370289.
6. Oesman C, Mooij JJ. Long-term follow-up of microvascular decompression for trigeminal neuralgia [J]. Skull Base. 2011;21(5):313–22. https://doi.org/10.1055/s-0031-1284213.
7. Zhang H, Lei D, You C, Mao BY, Wu B, Fang Y. The long-term outcome predictors of pure microvascular decompression for primary trigeminal neuralgia [J]. World Neurosurg. 2013;79(5–6):756–62.
8. Burchiel KJ, Clarke H, Haglund M, Loeser JD. Long-term follow-up of microvascular decompression in trigeminal neuralgia. J Neurosurg. 1988;69:35–8.
9. Go JK, Kim PE, Zee CH. The trigeminal nerve. Semin Ultrasound CT MRI. 2001;22(6):502–20.
10. Kamel HA, Toland J. Trigeminal nerve anatomy: illustrated using examples of abnormalities. Am J Roentgenol. 2001;176(1):247–51.
11. Terrier L-M, Amelot A, François P, Destrieux C, Zemmoura I, Velut S. Therapeutic failure in trigeminal neuralgia: from a clarification of trigeminal nerve somatotopy to a targeted partial sensory rhizotomy[J]. World Neurosurg. 2018;117:138–45.
12. Ko AL, Ozpinar A, Lee A, Raslan AM, McCartney S, Burchiel KJ. Long-term efficacy and safety of internal neurolysis for trigeminal neuralgia without neurovascular compression[J]. J Neurosurg. 2015;122(5):1048–57. https://doi.org/10.3171/2014.12.JNS14469.
13. Young JN, Wilkins RH. Partial sensory trigeminal rhizotomy at the pons for trigeminal neuralgia. J Neurosurg. 1993;79(5):680–7. https://doi.org/10.3171/jns.1993.79.5.0680.
14. Zakrzewska JM, Lopez BC, S E K, Coakham HB. Patient reports of satisfaction after microvascular decompression and partial sensory rhizotomy for trigeminal neuralgia[J]. Neurol Surg. 2005;56(6):1304–11. https://doi.org/10.1227/01.neu.0000159883.35957.e0.
15. Klun B. Microvascular decompression and partial sensory rhizotomy in the treatment of trigeminal neuralgia: personal experience with 220 patients. Neurosurgery. 1992;30:49–52.
16. Delitala A, Brunori A, Chiappetta F. Microsurgical posterior fossa exploration for trigeminal neuralgia: a study on 48 cases. Minim Invasive Neurosurg. 2001;44:152–6.
17. Howng SL, Chang DS. Partial sensory rhizotomy as an alternative treatment of trigeminal neuralgia. Kaohsiung J Med Sci. 1998;14:492–7.
18. Bederson JB, Wilson CB. Evaluation of microvascular decompression and partial sensory rhizotomy in 252 cases of trigeminal neuralgia. J Neurosurg. 1989;71:359–67.
19. Toda K. Operative treatment of trigeminal neuralgia: review of current techniques. Oral Surg Oral Med Oral Pathol Oral Radiol Endod. 2008;106(6):788–805. 805.e1–6
20. van Loveren H, Tew JM Jr, Keller JT, Nurre MA. A 10-year experience in the treatment of trigeminal neuralgia. Comparison of percutaneous stereotaxic rhizotomy and posterior fossa exploration. J Neurosurg. 1982;57:757–64.
21. Dandy WE. An operation for the cure of tic douloureux. Partial section of the sensory root at the pons. Arch Surg. 1929;18:687–734.
22. Dandy WE. The treatment of trigeminal neuralgia by the cerebellar route. Ann Surg. 1932;96:787–95.
23. Alper MG. The anesthetic eye: an investigation of changes in the anterior ocular segment of the monkey caused by interrupting the trigeminal nerve at various levels along its course. Trans Am Ophthalmol Soc. 1975;73:323–65.

24. Frazier CH. Operation for the radical cure of trigeminal neuralgia: analysis of five hundred cases. Ann Surg. 1928;88:534–47.
25. Ley A, Guitart JM. Clinical observations on sensory effects of trigeminal dorsal root section. J Neurol Neurosurg Psychiatry. 1971;34:260–4.
26. Emmons WF, Rhoton AL. Functional subdivision of the trigeminal sensory root. Surg Forum. 1968;19:440–1.
27. Emmons WF, Rhoton AL. Subdivision of the trigeminal sensory root. J Neurosurg. 1971;35:585–91.
28. Gudmundsson K, Rhoton AL, Rushton JG. Detailed anatomy of the intracranial portion of the trigeminal nerve. J Neurosurg. 1971;35:592–600.
29. Jannetta PJ. Gross (mesoscopic) description of the human trigeminal nerve and ganglion. J Neurosurg. 1967;26:109–11.
30. Adams CB, Kaye AH, Teddy PJ. The treatment of trigeminal neuralgia by posterior fossa microsurgery. J Neurol Neurosurg Psychiatry. 1982;45:1020–6.
31. Zhang L, Zhang Y, Li C, Zhu S. Surgical treatment of primary trigeminal neuralgia: comparison of the effectiveness between MVD and MVD+PSR in a series of 210 patients. Turk Neurosurg. 2012;22(1):32–8.
32. Abhinav K, Love S, Kalantzis G, Coakham HB, Patel NK. Clinicopathological review of patients with and without multiple sclerosis treated by partial sensory rhizotomy for medically refractory trigeminal neuralgia: a 12-year retrospective study. Clin Neurol Neurosurg. 2012;114:361–5.
33. Koopman JS, de Vries LM, Dieleman JP, Huygen FJ, Stricker BH, Sturkenboom MC. A nationwide study of three invasive treatments for trigeminal neuralgia. Pain. 2011;152:507–13.
34. Swanson SE, Farhat SM. Neurovascular decompression with selective partial rhizotomy of the trigeminal nerve for tic douloureux. Surg Neurol. 1982;18:3–6.

Neuromodulation for Trigeminal Neuralgia

Jin-gyu Choi

1 Introduction

Trigeminal neuralgia (TN), used to be called Tic douloureux previously, is a chronic neuropathic pain disorder distributed in trigeminal nerve territory in the face. Prevalence ranges from 0.03 to 0.3% with female predominance [1]. According to the International Classification of Headache Disorders, 3rd edition (ICHD-3), it can be diagnosed by recurrent paroxysms of facial pain in the distribution(s) of one or more divisions of the trigeminal nerve, with no radiation beyond [2]. Pain lasts from a fraction of a second to 2 min and can be described as electrical shock-like, shooting, stabbing, or sharp in quality. However, in many cases, it is not easy to distinguish from other facial pain disorders such as painful trigeminal neuropathy (PTN) or persistent idiopathic facial pain (PIFP). In addition, nerve damage caused during the lesioning procedures for TN blurs the diagnostic boundaries. Because of these multiple causes and diagnostic ambiguity, the treatment of TN is not always easy.

The nomenclature describing trigeminal and facial pain has changed over time, and it is sometimes confusing when reviewing literature from multiple eras. ICHD-3 subdivides TN as classical, secondary, and idiopathic with different underlying causes. Unlike TN, PTN refers to a condition in which the main symptom is persistent burning or squeezing pain, indicating nerve damage. Painful trigeminal nerve dysfunction occurring after neuroablative lesioning for the treatment of TN, previously called anesthesia dolorosa, belongs to post-traumatic PTN. The diagnostic entity, previously referred to as atypical facial pain, corresponds to the PIFP in ICHD-3 [2].

Carbamazepine and other antiepileptic drugs are effective starting therapeutic agent for TN. In medically refractory cases, however, microvascular decompression (MVD) is considered as a curable surgical treatment for classical TN caused by a neurovascular conflict at the root entry zone of the trigeminal nerve. Percutaneous lesioning procedures or stereotactic radiosurgery (SRS) also can be applied according to age, individual medical condition, cost, and patient preference. Although it is rare, excision of space-occupying neoplasm is necessary for secondary TN caused by tumor. PTN patients are also treated pharmacologically, and in some cases, lesioning treatments can be tried, but the outcomes are not always good. Patients with refractory trigeminal pain who do not respond to the above treatment experience serious deterioration in the quality of life, and therefore sometimes it is referred to as "suicidal disease" [3].

Neuromodulation, defined as the alteration of nerve activity through targeted delivery of a

J.-g. Choi (✉)
Department of Neurosurgery, Yeouido St. Mary's Hospital, The Catholic University of Korea, Seoul, Republic of Korea

K. Park, K. R. Cho (eds.), *Trigeminal Neuralgia*, https://doi.org/10.1007/978-981-19-9171-4_23

stimulus, such as electrical stimulation or chemical agents to specific neurological sites in the body, can be considered as an alternative treatment for those patients with refractory TN or PTN, though it has limited clinical evidence. Just as neuromodulation used in the treatment of other refractory neuropathic pain is not to solve the cause of the disease but to control symptoms, neuromodulation for refractory trigeminal pain is performed only for the purpose of pain control. Therefore, neuromodulation for trigeminal or facial pain is often performed without a clear distinction of indication, and there are few reports of neuromodulation being used for the treatment of true TN. In this chapter, the types and indications of neuromodulation that have been used for trigeminal pain disorders and evidence from the literature will be reviewed.

2 Standard Treatment for Trigeminal Neuralgia

The current standard of care for TN can be found in published guidelines [4–7]. In all patients with TN, the first treatment should be pharmacological. Carbamazepine or oxcarbazepine is recommended first-line agent, while gabapentin, pregabalin, baclofen, and lamotrigine may be considered as alternative, adjuvant medications. Although there is no conclusion on how many drugs should be tried before invasive treatment is considered, it is essential to provide early information about the possibility of requiring surgical treatment if the patient is not satisfied or tolerated the pharmacological treatment.

Among invasive treatments including percutaneous lesioning procedures and SRS, MVD can be expected to provide the most effective and long-lasting pain relief. However, the cause of the pain must be a neurovascular conflict, and the patient must be willing and able to tolerate posterior fossa surgery.

Percutaneous neuroablative procedures include radiofrequency thermocoagulation, glycerol rhizolysis, and balloon compression targeted at the Gasserian ganglion of trigeminal nerve. The superiority of any of the three treatment modalities is unknown. Although it is less invasive than MVD, complications such as corneal hypoesthesia, numbness, and anesthesia dolorosa may occur after the procedure.

SRS is a minimally invasive lesioning treatment for TN with comparable efficacy to MVD and percutaneous procedures. It does not require generalized anesthesia or hospitalization and can be safely performed on patients with underlying diseases.

2.1 Refractory Trigeminal Neuralgia and Painful Trigeminal Neuropathy

Despite the recommended treatments described above, there exist refractory patients, and in these cases, the patient may experience a serious deterioration in the quality of life or may suffer from nerve damage caused by the treatment itself. In addition, it is known that the outcome of secondary treatment after a primary invasive procedure is poor with a high complication rate. Therefore, if the patient does not improve after the first operation or recurs after a temporary improvement, it is not easy to establish the next treatment plan.

According to a recently published systematic review that analyzed a total of 3897 patients from 46 studies, the rate of patients with persistent pain after primary MVD in drug-resistant TN was 24.2% [8]. Moreover, the outcome of revision MVD is known to be less effective with a higher complication rate compared to primary surgery [9, 10]. The frequency of pain remaining after SRS varied by study, and there were reports that pain remained at up to 71% without medication and up to 50% if the medication was taken after SRS [11]. In patients with percutaneous neuroablative treatment, the pain persisted in a median of 42% after radiofrequency thermocoagulation, 32% after balloon compression, and 72% after glycerol rhizolysis according to a recent systematic review [4].

Persisting neuralgic pain after any primary procedure is a problem, but post-traumatic PTN or anesthesia dolorosa being caused by nerve damage as a complication of neuroablative treatment is a catastrophe. There is no known effective treatment for anesthesia dolorosa, and most of the patients suffer from severe lifelong pain.

3 Neuromodulation

Neuromodulation controls the symptoms of a disease with changes that occur by giving electrical or chemical stimulation to target anatomical structures of the nervous system. Like the mechanism of neuromodulatory treatment in other intractable chronic pain disorders, the action mechanism of neuromodulation for refractory TN or PTN is unclear. As noted above, neuromodulation is not recommended as a standard treatment for TN. However, various types of neuromodulations have been developed and applied to patients, and since each has a different indication, technique, and invasiveness, an appropriately selected neuromodulatory modality can be helpful to intractable patients.

Transcranial magnetic stimulation (TMS) and transcranial direct current stimulation (tDCS) are minimally invasive neuromodulations for the treatment of trigeminal or facial pain. TMS uses magnetic energy on deep brain structure changing their neuronal activity. It can be performed in a single or repetitive session. tDCS delivers a weak electric current to the scalp. Both techniques have been applied to various pain disorders such as headache, trigeminal pain, and atypical facial pain. However, the evidence is limited, and the outcomes are variable. Nevertheless, it is a great advantage that it can be considered as a rescue or adjuvant treatment for intractable cases, regardless of the patient's age or medical condition because of the safety and less invasiveness of both treatments. On the other hand, to perform invasive neuromodulation, more caution is required in patient selection. The general recommendations for using neuromodulation for the treatment of TN or PTN are as follows

- When patient's quality of life is severely impaired due to chronic neuropathic pain.
- For classical TN patients, standard invasive treatment should be considered prior to neuromodulation.
- Patient's individual medical condition and age must be able to tolerate invasive neuromodulation.
- Patients should not have a psychiatric disorder that adversely affects the treatment outcome.
- Patients should understand and cooperate with the entire course of treatment, including trial stimulation.
- Successful trial stimulation is required before permanent implantation.

4 Motor Cortex Stimulation

Motor cortex stimulation (MCS) is an invasive treatment that has been reported to have a relatively favorable effect among neuromodulation procedures for the treatment of intractable facial pain. An electrical lead is placed in the epidural space just above the patient's motor cortex through either a small craniotomy or a burr hole. The motor cortex can be identified by observing the N20-P20 phase reversal of somatosensory evoked potential intraoperatively, and the final electrode position is confirmed by motor response using the implanted epidural lead. Transient intraoperative seizures, epidural hematoma, and stroke have been reported as major complications of MCS [12]. Although it is difficult to find any well-controlled prospective study on facial pain, multiple retrospective studies with a small number of cases have been reported to have favorable outcomes.

Myerson et al. reported a 60–90% pain improvement after MCS in all 5 patients with trigeminal neuropathic pain, although intraoperative generalized seizures were frequent [13]. According to Ebel et al., 6 out of 7 patients showed 50% or more pain relief after test stimulation, indicated for trigeminal neuropathic pain, so permanent implantation was performed, and 3 of them reported excellent or good long-term results [14]. Nguyen et al. emphasized the usefulness of the neuronavigation system in finding the motor cortex in their case series published in 2000 and reported good responses in 9 (75%) of 12 neuropathic facial pain patients [15]. Brown et al. published a prospective study in which MCS was performed on 10 patients with central and trigeminal neuropathic facial pain [16]. The causes of trigeminal neuropathic pain were postherpetic neuralgia and surgical nerve injury. Pain relief was achieved by 75% during a mean follow-up period of 10 months. Rache et al. reported 10 years of MCS experience, including 10 patients with trigeminal neuropathic pain [17]. Four patients had trigeminal neuropathic pain after lesioning procedure for TN, 3 patients after dental procedure, and 3 patients after tumor surgery, and among them, 5 patients (50%) responded with pain relief of 50% or more after MCS. In 2014, the case series published by Kolodziej et al. included 9 PTN patients, all showing at least 60% pain improvement [18].

The first randomized controlled trial was published in 2009 by Lefaucheur et al. [19]. This study was conducted for patients with refractory peripheral neuropathic pain in a randomized crossover design, and 13 out of a total of 16 participants completed 1 year follow-up. Of the 6 trigeminal pain patients who completed the study, 3 (50%) had good or satisfactory pain relief.

The case series presented by Raslan et al. included 8 patients with trigeminal neuropathic pain and 3 patients with trigeminal deafferentation pain (TDP) [20]. Of the three patients with TDP, two failed trial stimulation and one had unsatisfactory pain relief after permanent implantation. The authors described TDP as resistant to MCS.

Recently, there was a successful pilot study in which a burst waveform was applied to MCS [21], and a systematic review was published that a younger age contributes to a good prognosis of MCS [12].

5 Deep Brain Stimulation

Deep brain stimulation (DBS) is an invasive neuromodulatory treatment that controls symptoms of movement disorder, psychiatric disorder, epilepsy, or intractable pain with the effect obtained by electrically stimulating a specific target in the deep brain structure related to the pathophysiology. DBS for intractable pain was first performed in the 1950s. Although several DBS targets have been applied to patients with chronic pain, primary targets are the ventral posterior lateral nucleus/ventral posterior medial nucleus (VPL/VPM) of the thalamus and periaqueductal gray/periventricular gray (PAG/PVG).

Although there have been various advances in surgical technique, it is still standard to perform DBS using a stereotactic frame. The patient can receive MRI while wearing a stereotactic frame, or the target coordinates can be calculated by fusion of frame-applied CT with previously taken MRI using a stereotactic navigation workstation. The goal of surgery is to insert the intracranial electrode into the target structure through a small burr hole using a surgical stereotactic system. If the sensory thalamus is targeted, awaken surgery is required to check the sensory response of intraoperative macrostimulation. If it is confirmed that the stimulation-induced paresthesia is felt in the patient's pain area, the intracranial electrode is fixed. The distal lead is then externalized for trial stimulation or connected to a subclavian pulse generator. DBS outcomes for PTN and intractable facial pain are reported to be variable.

In 1973, Hosobuchi et al. inspired by the pain relief of intraoperative macrostimulation during previous VPM thalamotomies, performed VPM DBS in 5 patients with facial anesthesia dolorosa and reported satisfactory pain relief in 4 patients [22]. Green et al. reported a case in which pain was substantially relieved by simultaneous stimulation of VPL and PVG in a patient with postherpetic V1 trigeminal neuropathic pain [23]. Sims-Williams et al. compared PAG and centromedian-parafascicular (CmPf) nucleus stimulation in three anesthesia dolorosa patients [24]. In 3 patients, the mean pain relief was 56% after PAG stimulation and 67% after CmPf stimulation. Ben-Haim et al. reported a case series in which VPM and PAG stimulation were performed in 7 patients with intractable facial neuropathic pain [25]. The indications were deafferentation pain, PIFP, and poststroke pain, and all patients showed an average of 70% pain relief at 12 months after surgery. Six patients showed 50% or more pain relief.

Recently, Kashanian et al. reported the results of simultaneous VPM and PVG DBS in 9 patients with intractable facial pain [26]. Patients with 3 post-traumatic PTN, 3 poststroke pain, 2 postherpetic trigeminal pain, and 1 PIFP were included. One PIFP patient had the device removed due to extension line-related discomfort. All 8 patients who underwent permanent implantation showed improvement in pain compared to baseline, and 4 of them answered positively to the question of repeating DBS in the future.

Although it is difficult to find a large series of DBS for facial pain, general complications of DBS include intracerebral hemorrhage, infection, seizure, and hardware-related problems such as device damage or malfunction.

6 Peripheral Nerve Stimulation

Peripheral nerve stimulation (PNS) relieves pain by placing electrodes near a peripheral nerve at the site of pain and applying electrical stimulation to the nerve. PNS was first performed in 1962 for TN patients by Shelden et al. and their case series was published in 1967 [27]. Although there has been no significant change in the treatment mechanism, advances in technology have enabled minimal invasive and ultrasonography-guided electrode implantation, leading to the current PNS implantation [28, 29]. Several types of PNS target nerves have been used for facial pain, including the supraorbital nerve, infraorbital nerve, trigeminal branch, and gasserian ganglion. Although no randomized controlled trial has been reported to date, many clinical experiences have been published compared to other invasive neuromodulations for TN or PTN.

Meyerson and Håkanson (1986) performed gasserian ganglion stimulation in 14 patients with PTN after lesioning procedure [30]. Among them, 11 patients showed significant pain improvement during an average follow-up period of 4 years. Waldhauser and Steude reported that 54% of patients underwent permanent PNS implantation after successful pain relief in a large case series of gasserian ganglion stimulation in 149 patients with atypical TN, emphasizing the importance of trial stimulation [31]. Young published a case series in which trigeminal nerve root stimulation was applied to 23 patients with post-traumatic PTN [32]. During the mean follow-up period of 24 months, 12 of 23 patients (52%) showed more than 50% pain relief and 6 showed nearly complete pain relief. In another case series published by Kustermans et al., gasserian ganglion stimulation showed successful trial stimulation in 77.3% of 22 refractory PTN patients and long-term pain relief in 44% of patients at 24 months of follow-up.

Machado et al. reported the unfavorable outcomes of 10 patients treated with gasserian ganglion stimulation in post-traumatic PTN patients [33]. Eight patients underwent permanent implantation. However, only 3 patients maintained to have pain relief of more than 50% at 12 months after surgery.

Johnson and Burchiel published a pilot study in 2004 in which supraorbital nerve or infraorbital nerve stimulation was performed in patients with post-traumatic or postherpetic PTN [34]. Pain relief of more than 50% was shown in 70% of patients, and all patients in the post-traumatic group and half of the postherpetic group showed more than 50% pain relief. Stidd et al. reported that supraorbital or infraorbital nerve stimulation was performed in 3 trigeminal neuropathic pain patients, and good pain relief was maintained for up to 2 years in all patients [35].

Ellis et al. reported trigeminal branch stimulation in 35 patients with intractable facial pain in 2015 [29]. Indications included PTN, TN, headache, deafferentation pain, and supraorbital neuralgia. Electrodes were inserted at supraorbital, infraorbital, temporal, and mandibular locations. Seventeen out of 35 patients showed significant pain relief with trial stimulation and received permanent implantation. At an average follow-up of 15 months, pain relief was maintained in 73% of patients.

In 2019, McMahon et al. published a case series including only PIFP patients [36]. Twenty-three PIFP patients were treated with supraorbital stimulation for V1, infraorbital stimulation for V2, and trigeminal root stimulation for V3 pain [36]. Of these, 20 patients underwent permanent implantation, and 13 patients completed the follow-up. The mean VAS score was 5.69 ± 2.09 before surgery and 0.15 ± 0.55 after surgery respectively.

One of the advantages of PNS is that it is safe and has no life-threatening side effects. Electrode malfunction, extension wire malfunction, discomfort at the generator implanted site, inadequate pain relief, wound breakdown or skin erosion with hardware exposure, and infection are reported as complications of PNS for facial pain treatment [37].

Recently, reports of newly developed techniques such as burst stimulation [38], high-frequency stimulation [28], wireless stimulation [39], and peripheral nerve field stimulation [40, 41] have been introduced.

7 Spinal Cord Stimulation

Spinal cord stimulation (SCS) is one of the most widely performed neuromodulatory treatment for chronic intractable pain. Cylindrical or paddle-type electrode is inserted into the patient's epidural space and electrical stimulation is delivered to the dorsal column of the spinal cord. Although the mechanism of action of SCS has not been clearly elucidated, it is thought to be related to the gate-control theory of Melzack and Wall published in 1965 [42]. However, despite the favorable pain relief of SCS in various chronic pain disorders has been proved, the experience of SCS on trigeminal, and facial pain is limited. Several retrospective studies and case reports can be found.

In 1988, Barolat et al. reported that a 42-year-old male PTN patient with multiple sclerosis obtained complete pain relief by applying electrical stimulation through an electrode inserted into the C1-2 level epidural space [43]. Neuman et al. reported a case in which atypical facial pain improved coincidentally in a 45-year-old male patient who underwent thoracic SCS for angina pain in 2011 [44].

Tomycz et al. published a case series in which cervicomedullary paddle SCS was performed on 25 patients with head and facial pain [45]. Sixteen patients (64%) underwent permanent implantation with significant pain relief after trial stimulation. While trial stimulation was successful in 7 of patients with trigeminal deafferentation pain (70%), 4 of trigeminal neuropathic patients (80%), 2 patients with postherpetic pain (100%), and 1 patient with poststroke pain (100%), only 2 patients (28.6%) of occipital neuralgia underwent permanent implantation. Twelve out of 16 patients (75%) maintained SCS because it helped improve the quality of life for a long time, and 4 patients removed the system due to side effects or decreased efficacy.

A large case series of 121 patients published by Chivukula et al. in 2014 included 10 patients with TDP, 4 patients with trigeminal neuropathic pain, and 4 patients with postherpetic neuralgia, and they showed pain relief of 55.1%, 59.1%, and 61.1%, respectively [46]. Velasquez et al. also reported the results of upper cervical SCS in 12 trigeminal neuropathic pain patients [47]. During the mean follow-up period of 4.4 years, pain relief was 57.1% and the long-term failure rate was 24%.

Recently, new technologies and paradigms have been published. A case of successful treatment with high-frequency stimulation in a TNP patient refractory to conventional stimulation has been reported [48]. In another study, it has been reported that lateral stimulation is more effective than midline dorsal column stimulation, which is different from the conventional action mechanism of dorsal column stimulation. In the future, various studies on the indication, technology, and action mechanism of SCS for trigeminal pain are expected.

8 Conclusion

Although the evidence is limited, neuromodulation is a considerable treatment for refractory TN and PTN. Considering the rareness of the condition, the invasiveness and high cost of neuromodulatory treatment, it is not easy to conduct large-scale, well-controlled clinical trials. Nevertheless, as many experiences are published and new technologies are developed, the role of neuromodulation in the treatment of intractable trigeminal pain is expected to increase in the future.

References

1. De Toledo IP, Conti Reus J, Fernandes M, Porporatti AL, Peres MA, Takaschima A, et al. Prevalence of trigeminal neuralgia: a systematic review. J Am Dent Assoc. 2016;147(7):570–6 e2.
2. Headache Classification Committee of the International Headache Society (IHS) The international classification of headache disorders, 3rd ed. Cephalalgia. 2018;38(1):1–211.
3. Zakrzewska JM, Wu J, Mon-Williams M, Phillips N, Pavitt SH. Evaluating the impact of trigeminal neuralgia. Pain. 2017;158(6):1166–74.
4. Bendtsen L, Zakrzewska JM, Abbott J, Braschinsky M, Di Stefano G, Donnet A, et al. European academy of neurology guideline on trigeminal neuralgia. Eur J Neurol. 2019;26(6):831–49.
5. Gronseth G, Cruccu G, Alksne J, Argoff C, Brainin M, Burchiel K, et al. Practice parameter: the diagnostic evaluation and treatment of trigeminal neuralgia (an evidence-based review): report of the Quality Standards Subcommittee of the American Academy of Neurology and the European Federation of Neurological Societies. Neurology. 2008;71(15):1183–90.
6. Heinskou T, Maarbjerg S, Rochat P, Wolfram F, Jensen RH, Bendtsen L. Trigeminal neuralgia--a coherent cross-specialty management program. J Headache Pain. 2015;16:66.
7. O'Callaghan L, Floden L, Vinikoor-Imler L, Symonds T, Giblin K, Hartford C, et al. Burden of illness of trigeminal neuralgia among patients managed in a specialist center in England. J Headache Pain. 2020;21(1):130.
8. Holste K, Chan AY, Rolston JD, Englot DJ. Pain outcomes following microvascular decompression for drug-resistant trigeminal neuralgia: a systematic review and meta-analysis. Neurosurgery. 2020;86(2):182–90.
9. Bakker NA, Van Dijk JM, Immenga S, Wagemakers M, Metzemaekers JD. Repeat microvascular decompression for recurrent idiopathic trigeminal neuralgia. J Neurosurg. 2014;121(4):936–9.
10. Ravina K, Strickland BA, Rennert RC, Bakhsheshian J, Russin JJ, Giannotta SL. Revision microvascular decompression for trigeminal neuralgia and Hemifacial spasm: factors associated with surgical failure. J Neurol Surg B Skull Base. 2019;80(1):31–9.
11. Tuleasca C, Regis J, Sahgal A, De Salles A, Hayashi M, Ma L, et al. Stereotactic radiosurgery for trigeminal neuralgia: a systematic review. J Neurosurg. 2018;130(3):733–57.
12. Rapisarda A, Ioannoni E, Izzo A, Montano N. What are the results and the prognostic factors of motor cortex stimulation in patients with facial pain? A systematic review of the literature. Eur Neurol. 2021;84(3):151–6.
13. Meyerson BA, Lindblom U, Linderoth B, Lind G, Herregodts P. Motor cortex stimulation as treatment of trigeminal neuropathic pain. Acta Neurochir Suppl (Wien). 1993;58:150–3.
14. Ebel H, Rust D, Tronnier V, Böker D, Kunze S. Chronic precentral stimulation in trigeminal neuropathic pain. Acta Neurochir. 1996;138(11):1300–6.
15. Nguyen JP, Lefaucheur JP, Le Guerinel C, Fontaine D, Nakano N, Sakka L, et al. Treatment of central and neuropathic facial pain by chronic stimulation of the motor cortex: value of neuronavigation guidance systems for the localization of the motor cortex. Neurochirurgie. 2000;46(5):483–91.
16. Brown JA, Pilitsis JG. Motor cortex stimulation for central and neuropathic facial pain: a prospective study of 10 patients and observations of enhanced sensory and motor function during stimulation. Neurosurgery. 2005;56(2):290–7. discussion—7
17. Rasche D, Ruppolt M, Stippich C, Unterberg A, Tronnier VM. Motor cortex stimulation for long-term relief of chronic neuropathic pain: a 10 year experience. Pain. 2006;121(1–2):43–52.
18. Kolodziej MA, Hellwig D, Nimsky C, Benes L. Treatment of central deafferentation and trigeminal neuropathic pain by motor cortex stimulation: report of a series of 20 patients. J Neurol Surg A Cent Eur Neurosurg. 2016;77(1):52–8.
19. Lefaucheur JP, Drouot X, Cunin P, Bruckert R, Lepetit H, Creange A, et al. Motor cortex stimulation for the treatment of refractory peripheral neuropathic pain. Brain. 2009;132(Pt 6):1463–71.
20. Raslan AM, Nasseri M, Bahgat D, Abdu E, Burchiel KJ. Motor cortex stimulation for trigeminal neuropathic or deafferentation pain: an institutional case series experience. Stereotact Funct Neurosurg. 2011;89(2):83–8.
21. Sokal P, Harat M, Malukiewicz A, Kiec M, Switonska M, Jablonska R. Effectiveness of tonic and burst motor cortex stimulation in chronic neuropathic pain. J Pain Res. 2019;12:1863–9.
22. Hosobuchi Y, Adams JE, Rutkin B. Chronic thalamic stimulation for the control of facial anesthesia dolorosa. Arch Neurol. 1973;29(3):158–61.
23. Green AL, Nandi D, Armstrong G, Carter H, Aziz T. Post-herpetic trigeminal neuralgia treated with deep brain stimulation. J Clin Neurosci. 2003;10(4):512–4.
24. Sims-Williams HP, Javed S, Pickering AE, Patel NK. Characterising the analgesic effect of different targets for deep brain stimulation in trigeminal anaesthesia dolorosa. Stereotact Funct Neurosurg. 2016;94(3):174–81.
25. Ben-Haim S, Mirzadeh Z, Rosenberg WS. Deep brain stimulation for intractable neuropathic facial pain. Neurosurg Focus. 2018;45(2):E15.

26. Kashanian A, DiCesare JAT, Rohatgi P, Albano L, Krahl SE, Bari A, et al. Case series: deep brain stimulation for facial pain. Oper Neurosurg (Hagerstown). 2020;19(5):510–7.
27. Shelden CH, Pudenz RH, Doyle J. Electrical control of facial pain. Am J Surg. 1967;114(2):209–12.
28. Lerman IR, Chen JL, Hiller D, Souzdalnitski D, Sheean G, Wallace M, et al. Novel high-frequency peripheral nerve stimulator treatment of refractory postherpetic neuralgia: a brief technical note. Neuromodulation. 2015;18(6):487–93. discussion 93
29. Ellis JA, Mejia Munne JC, Winfree CJ. Trigeminal branch stimulation for the treatment of intractable craniofacial pain. J Neurosurg. 2015;123(1):283–8.
30. Meyerson BA, Håkanson S. Suppression of pain in trigeminal neuropathy by electric stimulation of the gasserian ganglion. Neurosurgery. 1986;18(1):59–66.
31. Waidhauser E, Steude U. Evaluation of patients with atypical trigeminal neuralgia for permanent electrode implant by test stimulation of the ganglion gasseri. Stereotact Funct Neurosurg. 1994;62(1–4):304–8.
32. Young RF. Electrical stimulation of the trigeminal nerve root for the treatment of chronic facial pain. J Neurosurg. 1995;83(1):72–8.
33. Machado A, Ogrin M, Rosenow JM, Henderson JM. A 12-month prospective study of gasserian ganglion stimulation for trigeminal neuropathic pain. Stereotact Funct Neurosurg. 2007;85(5):216–24.
34. Johnson MD, Burchiel KJ. Peripheral stimulation for treatment of trigeminal postherpetic neuralgia and trigeminal posttraumatic neuropathic pain: a pilot study. Neurosurgery. 2004;55(1):135–41. discussion 41–2
35. Stidd DA, Wuollet AL, Bowden K, Price T, Patwardhan A, Barker S, et al. Peripheral nerve stimulation for trigeminal neuropathic pain. Pain Physician. 2012;15(1):27–33.
36. McMahon JT, Tora MS, Bentley JN, Texakalidis P, Campbell MA, Keifer OP Jr, et al. Percutaneous trigeminal nerve stimulation for persistent idiopathic facial pain: a case series. World Neurosurg. 2019;126:e1379–e86.
37. Slavin K, Yin D, Rasskazoff S. Peripheral nerve stimulation for facial pain. In: Elliot Krames P, Peckham H, Rezai A, editors. Neuromodulation. 2nd ed. Saunders; 2018. p. 741–6.
38. Manning A, Ortega RG, Moir L, Edwards T, Aziz TZ, Bojanic S, et al. Burst or conventional peripheral nerve field stimulation for treatment of neuropathic facial pain. Neuromodulation. 2019;22(5):645–52.
39. Stokey BG, Weiner RL, Slavin KV, Hayek SM. Peripheral nerve stimulation for facial pain using wireless devices. Prog Neurol Surg. 2020;35:75–84.
40. Klein J, Siepmann T, Schackert G, Ziemssen T, Juratli TA. Peripheral nerve field stimulation in medically refractory trigeminal neuralgia attributed to multiple sclerosis. J Neurosurg. 2020;134(3):1244–50.
41. Jakobs M, Unterberg A, Treede RD, Schuh-Hofer S, Ahmadi R. Subcutaneous trigeminal nerve field stimulation for refractory trigeminal pain: a cohort analysis. Acta Neurochir. 2016;158(9):1767–74.
42. Melzack R, Wall PD. Pain mechanisms: a new theory. Science. 1965;150(3699):971–9.
43. Barolat G, Knobler RL, Lublin FD. Trigeminal neuralgia in a patient with multiple sclerosis treated with high cervical spinal cord stimulation. Case report Appl Neurophysiol. 1988;51(6):333–7.
44. Neuman SA, Eldrige JS, Hoelzer BC. Atypical facial pain treated with upper thoracic dorsal column stimulation. Clin J Pain. 2011;27(6):556–8.
45. Tomycz ND, Deibert CP, Moossy JJ. Cervicomedullary junction spinal cord stimulation for head and facial pain. Headache. 2011;51(3):418–25.
46. Chivukula S, Tempel ZJ, Weiner GM, Gande AV, Chen CJ, Ding D, et al. Cervical and cervicomedullary spinal cord stimulation for chronic pain: efficacy and outcomes. Clin Neurol Neurosurg. 2014;127:33–41.
47. Velásquez C, Tambirajoo K, Franceschini P, Eldridge PR, Farah JO. Upper cervical spinal cord stimulation as an alternative treatment in trigeminal neuropathy. World Neurosurg. 2018;114:e641–e6.
48. Floridia D, Cerra F, Corallo F, Di Cara M, Spartà S, Nania G, et al. Effectiveness of high-frequency cervical spinal cord stimulation in the treatment of refractory trigeminal neuropathy: a case report. Medicine (Baltimore). 2020;99(40):e22304.

Secondary Trigeminal Neuralgia

Min Ho Lee

1 Introduction

There are several causes of trigeminal neuralgia. Among them, the neurosurgeon described compression by the vessels around the trigeminal nerve as a neurovascular conflict syndrome. And this is being solved by microvascular decompression.

However, while treating patients, we often confront that trigeminal neuralgia occurs due to other causes than neurovascular conflict. Secondary TN occurs in up to 15% [1–3]. In this chapter, I would demonstrate secondary trigeminal neuralgia.

2 Tumor-Induced Trigeminal Neuralgia

The most easily encountered is compression by other tumors. According to the existing literature, trigeminal neuralgia caused by meningioma, trigeminal schwannoma, or dermoid cyst located in Meckel's cave or CPA region is reported. Secondary TN due to CPA tumors is less common than classic TN. The symptoms of tumor-induced TN appear earlier and surgery is performed at a younger age compared with classic TN. Secondary TN is caused more by direct compression than chemical irritation [4]. Although unrelated to tumor growth, it may be explained by the arachnoid adhesion around the trigeminal nerve [5].

Current treatment options for tumor-induced TN include rhizotomy, radiofrequency ablation, balloon compression, radiosurgery, and microsurgery when medication is not sufficient [6–12]. Direct removal of the causative tumor by microsurgery may be the most logical and effective method to control the pain [8, 11–13]. Microsurgical resection has the advantage of a decrease in both the tumor volume and the mass effect on the nerve. However, the tumors that cause these symptoms are all skull-based tumors, and the risk of surgery is quite high. In this case, other treatment modalities may be considered, especially stereotactic radiosurgery. I would describe each of these.

2.1 Meningioma and Schwannoma

Among the tumors that can develop around the trigeminal nerve, the most common are meningioma and schwannoma. Especially, petrous meningioma has been considered difficult to treat surgically because of its proximity to cranial nerves, the basilar artery, and the brainstem [14–

M. H. Lee (✉)
Department of Neurosurgery, Uijeongbu St. Mary's Hospital, The Catholic University of Korea, Seoul, South Korea
e-mail: minho919.lee@catholic.ac.kr

K. Park, K. R. Cho (eds.), *Trigeminal Neuralgia*, https://doi.org/10.1007/978-981-19-9171-4_24

16]. Trigeminal neuralgia is present in 5% of these petroclival meningioma patients [17, 18]. If the tumor is large, it can cause other symptoms besides trigeminal neuralgia, so surgical treatment should be given priority. However, if the tumor is small, it can be controversial. However, Park et al. [19] reported that microsurgical resection in small petroclival meningioma also showed providing prompt and medication-free pain relief compared to radiosurgery. Among them, an upper clival type tumor only has a single arachnoid plane of protection between the tumor and the brain stem. So, radiosurgery could be an option. On the other hand, since tentorium and petrous apex type tumors have a multilayer of arachnoid protection, the risk of surgical resection is relatively low, so microsurgical resection was recommended. Park et al. [20] compared and analyzed 35 microsurgery cases and 35 radiosurgery cases for petroclival meningioma. In the case where the mass was removed by microsurgery, 91% of patients no longer needed medication, and the recurrence rate of pain was also reported as 0%. On the other hand, in the group that underwent gamma knife radiosurgery, only 37% of the patients were able to discontinue the medication, and 23% of patients reported that the pain was recurred. Other previous studies also provide clear support that direct removal of mass effect by microsurgery has a higher rate of pain relief without medications [18]. However, as mentioned earlier, there are many important structures around, so the risk of surgery is very high. And, surgeons can consider radiosurgery as an alternative.

Patients with TS often suffer from numbness and hypoesthesia due to dysfunction of the trigeminal nerve in the distribution of the trigeminal branches. A tumor compressing the trigeminal root can also cause facial pain in some patients [21–23]. If the nerve fibers are injured during tumor resection, the facial numbness may not relieve, or even worsen, after the operation. The arachnoid plane should be recognized and protected during the operation so that nerve function can be preserved [24]. Li et.al reported the results of 43 cases of trigeminal schwannoma. Of the 29 patients with numbness, only 5 (17.2%) improved, whereas all 4 patients with TN improved (100%) [23]. Cho et al. [25] compared and analyzed the results of gamma knife radiosurgery for the treatment of trigeminal neuralgia caused by meningioma and schwannoma. There was no difference in the response rate between meningioma and schwannoma, but the recurrence rate was higher in the meningioma group.

Peciu-Fluorianu et al. [26] reviewed 13 previously published articles through meta-analysis research. As they concluded, stereotactic radiosurgery for TN secondary to benign brain tumors is associated with a favorable clinical course but less favorable than in idiopathic TN. Targeting both the nerve and the tumor seemed to achieve better long-term results. However, the complication rate was higher.

2.2 Case Illustration

Trigeminal schwannoma (Fig. 1).

Petrous meningioma (Fig. 2).

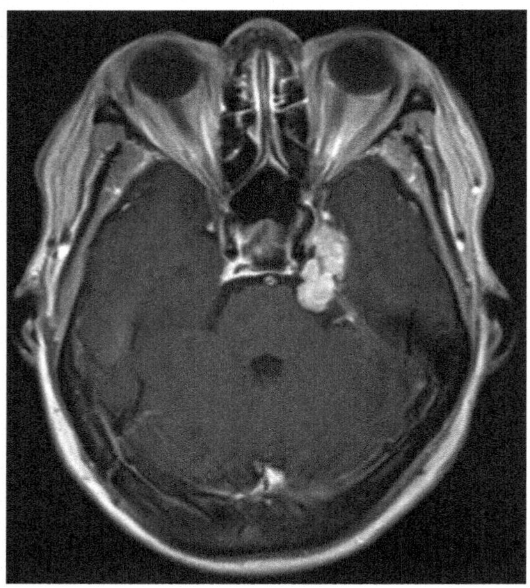

Fig. 1 A 63-year-old female patient, with trigeminal neuralgia, V2, Lt. The patient underwent surgery via transorbital approach. A facial pain was relieved but, numbness remained

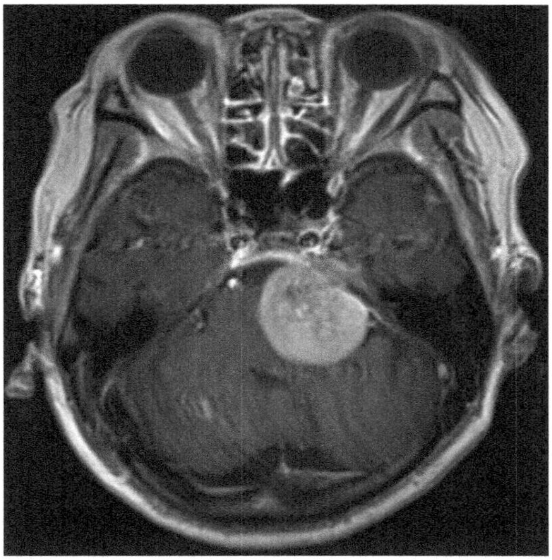

Fig. 2 A 78-year-old female patient, with trigeminal neuralgia, V2 and 3, Lt. The patient received surgery via retro-sigmoid approach. A facial pain was partially relieved

2.3 Dermoid Cyst

Dermoid cysts are benign slow growing masses accounting for 0.04–0.7% of all primary intracranial lesions [27] They are usually asymptomatic and appear incidentally on brain images. However, it can show various symptoms depending on the location, and in particular, when it becomes a rupture, it can cause abrupt symptoms [28–31]. Trigeminal neuralgia caused by dermoid cysts has been reported at the level of case reports [32–34]. Since dermoid cysts have not been proven effective with radiosurgery, surgical treatment should be prioritized if treatment is needed. And, in this situation, if the remnant remains, the possibility of recurring is very high, so vigorous removal is required.

3 Trigeminal Neuralgia Due to Multiple Sclerosis

Multiple sclerosis (MS) is a chronic inflammatory disease, causing demyelination and axonal degeneration in the central nervous system. Neuropathic pain is a common symptom in patients with MS. Trigeminal neuralgia is likely the most widely recognized neuropathic pain syndrome in MS. Prevalence ranges from 1.9% to 6.3% [35–37] But, the pathophysiological mechanisms of neuropathic pain is poorly defined. In several previous studies, [38–40] it has been suggested that neurotransmitter or channelopathy is the pathophysiology of MS pain through animal models.

There are no specific tests for MS. Instead, a diagnosis of multiple sclerosis often relies on ruling out other conditions that might produce similar signs and symptoms. Therefore, if a patient diagnosed with MS has trigeminal neuralgia, TN caused by MS can be suspected. Some studies have reported enhancements on T1-weighted images or hyperintense lesions on T2-weighted images of the cisternal portion of the nerve or its root entry zone [41, 42]. Also, plaques were found around the pons on MRI [43].

MS-related trigeminal neuralgia is treated mainly with antiepileptic medications acting on voltage-dependent sodium channels, such as carbamazepine and lamotrigine [44, 45]. Although carbamazepine is effective in treating trigeminal neuralgia, it may cause adverse effects, including reversible worsening of MS symptoms [44–46]. A lack of data makes it difficult to make an evidence-based medical treatment decision for the MS-related TN. Pain can usually be controlled with glycerol injections, radiofrequency lesioning, or radiosurgery [47–50]. However, there is a risk of side effects such as hypoesthesia/hyperesthesia, decreased corneal reflex, and transitory masticatory weakness. Some have reported on the efficacy of microvascular decompression, but this is considered to be very limited [51–53]. Noory et al. [54] suggested that demyelination along the trigeminal afferents in the intra-pontine trigeminal line is the primary cause of TN in MS. Therefore, neurovascular conflict does not play a role in the etiology of MS-related TN (Fig. 3).

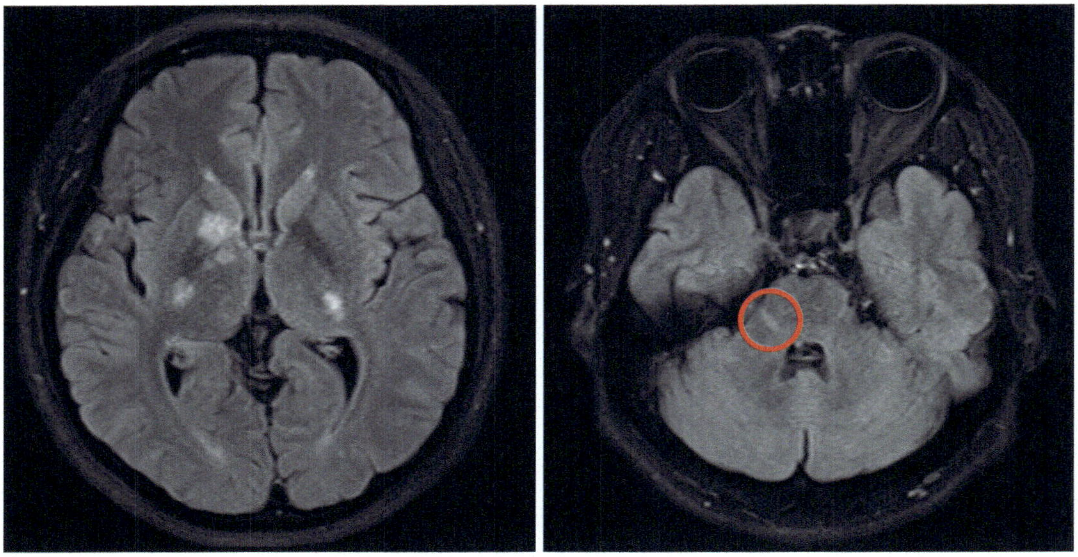

Fig. 3 A 40-year-old female patient with Rt. Facial numbness and pain, known multiple sclerosis patient. Multiple high-signal nodules were observed on brain MRI. She was treated with steroid pulse therapy. The pain was relieved after steroid treatment

4 Conclusion

Trigeminal neuralgia can be caused by various causes other than neurovascular conflict syndrome. In this case, the symptoms may be somewhat different from typical neuralgia. An MRI must be performed to confirm other causes. In the case of TN caused by a mass such as meningioma or schwannoma, if it is surgically risky, radiosurgery can be tried, but it is recommended to consider surgical treatment if possible rather than radiosurgery. In addition, it is necessary to know that MVD surgery is ineffective in patients with multiple sclerosis and trigeminal neuralgia.

References

1. Cruccu G, et al. Diagnostic accuracy of trigeminal reflex testing in trigeminal neuralgia. Neurology. 2006;66(1):139–41.
2. Maarbjerg S, et al. Trigeminal neuralgia—a prospective systematic study of clinical characteristics in 158 patients. Headache. 2014;54(10):1574–82.
3. Di Stefano G, et al. Triggering trigeminal neuralgia. Cephalalgia. 2018;38(6):1049–56.
4. Zhang YQ, et al. Surgical treatment of secondary Trigeminal neuralgia induced by cerebellopontine angle Tumors: a single-Center experience. World Neurosurg. 2020;141:e508–13.
5. Nakagawa K, et al. [Clinical and operative findings in patients with trigeminal neuralgia caused by brain tumors]. No Shinkei Geka. 2009;37(9):863–71.
6. Bly R, et al. Lateral transorbital neuroendoscopic approach to the lateral cavernous sinus. J Neurol Surg B Skull Base. 2014;75:11–7.
7. Cockerham K, et al. Surgery for orbital tumors. Part II: transorbital approaches. Neurosurg Focus. 2001;10(5):E3.
8. Dallan I, et al. Transorbital endoscopic assisted resection of a superior orbital fissure cavernous haemangioma: a technical case report. Eur Arch Otorhinolaryngol. 2015;272:3851–6.
9. Fukaya R, et al. Trigeminal schwannomas: experience with 57 cases and a review of the literature. Neurosurg Rev. 2010;34:159–71.
10. Inoue T, et al. Surgical approaches to the cavernous sinus: a microsurgical study. Neurosurgery. 1990;26:903–32.
11. Jefferson G. The trigeminal neurinomas with some remarks on malignant invasion of the gasserian ganglion. Clin Neurosurg. 1953;1:11–54.
12. Kassam A, et al. The front door to Meckel's cave: an anteromedial corridor via expanded endoscopic endonasal approach—technical considerations and clinical series. Neurosurgery. 2009;64(3 Suppl):ons71–83.
13. Dallan I, et al. Transorbital endoscopic assisted management of intraorbital lesions: lessons learned from our first 9 cases. Rhinology. 2016;54:247–53.

14. Al-Mefty O, Ayoubi S, Smith R. The petrosal approach: indications, technique, and results. In: Processes of the cranial midline. Springer; 1991. p. 166–70.
15. Cho CW, Al-Mefty O. Combined petrosal approach to petroclival meningiomas. Neurosurgery. 2002;51(3):708–18.
16. Nanda A, Javalkar V, Banerjee AD. Petroclival meningiomas: study on outcomes, complications and recurrence rates: clinical article. J Neurosurg JNS. 2011;114(5):1268–77.
17. Bir SC, et al. Management of recurrent trigeminal neuralgia associated with petroclival meningioma. J Neurological Surg Part B: Skull Base. 2016;77(01):047–53.
18. Bullitt E, Tew JM, Boyd J. Intracranial tumors in patients with facial pain. J Neurosurg. 1986;64(6):865–71.
19. Park HH, et al. Radiosurgery vs. microsurgery for newly diagnosed, small petroclival meningiomas with trigeminal neuralgia. Neurosurg Rev. 2020;43(6):1631–40.
20. Park HH, et al. Endoscopic transorbital and endonasal approach for trigeminal schwannomas: a retrospective multicenter analysis (KOSEN-005). J Neurosurg. 2020;133(2):467–76.
21. McCormick PC, Bello JA, Post KD. Trigeminal schwannoma: Surgical series of 14 cases with review of the literature. J Neurosurg. 1988;69(6): 850–60.
22. Ramina R, et al. Surgical management of trigeminal schwannomas. Neurosurg Focus. 2008;25(6):E6. discussion E6
23. Li M, et al. Trigeminal schwannoma: a single-center experience with 43 cases and review of literature. Br J Neurosurg. 2021;35(1):49–56.
24. Samii M, et al. Surgical treatment of trigeminal schwannomas. J Neurosurg. 1995;82(5):711–8.
25. Cho KR, et al. Gamma knife radiosurgery for trigeminal neuralgia secondary to benign lesions. Headache. 2016;56(5):883–9.
26. Peciu-Florianu I, et al. Trigeminal neuralgia secondary to meningiomas and vestibular schwannoma is improved after stereotactic radiosurgery: a systematic review and meta-analysis. Stereotact Funct Neurosurg. 2021;99(1):6–16.
27. Muçaj S, et al. Role of MRI in diagnosis of ruptured intracranial dermoid cyst. Acta Informatica Medica. 2017;25(2):141.
28. Akhaddar A, et al. Chronic headache and hemiparkinsonism due to a sylvian fissure dermoid cyst. Headache J head Face Pain. 2010;50(3):479–80.
29. Kocaeli, H., et al., Sylvian cistern dermoid cyst presenting with dysgeusia. 2009.
30. Tun K, et al. Dermoid tumour of the lateral wall of the cavernous sinus. J Clin Neurosci. 2008;15(7):820–3.
31. Balasundaram P, et al. Evolution of epidermoid cyst into dermoid cyst: embryological explanation and radiological-pathological correlation. Neuroradiol J. 2019;32(2):92–7.
32. Esaki T, et al. Unusual case of trigeminal neuralgia caused by remote effect of dermoid cyst in the ipsilateral cerebellar hemisphere. Clin Neurol Neurosurg. 2013;115(3):339–41.
33. Ochoa A, et al. Ruptured dermoid cyst in the Meckel's cave presenting with trigeminal neuralgia in a pediatric patient: a case report. Childs Nerv Syst. 2020;36(12):3141–6.
34. Tanabe N, et al. Dermoid cyst in meckel's cave presenting with oculomotor nerve palsy and trigeminal neuralgia:a case report. No Shinkei Geka. 2016;44(10):863–7.
35. Osterberg A, Boivie J, Thuomas KA. Central pain in multiple sclerosis—prevalence and clinical characteristics. Eur J Pain. 2005;9(5):531–42.
36. Solaro C, et al. The prevalence of pain in multiple sclerosis: a multicenter cross-sectional study. Neurology. 2004;63(5):919–21.
37. Hooge JP, Redekop WK. Trigeminal neuralgia in multiple sclerosis. Neurology. 1995;45(7):1294–6.
38. Olechowski CJ, Truong JJ, Kerr BJ. Neuropathic pain behaviours in a chronic-relapsing model of experimental autoimmune encephalomyelitis (EAE). Pain. 2009;141(1–2):156–64.
39. Aicher SA, et al. Hyperalgesia in an animal model of multiple sclerosis. Pain. 2004;110(3):560–70.
40. Thibault K, Calvino B, Pezet S. Characterisation of sensory abnormalities observed in an animal model of multiple sclerosis: a behavioural and pharmacological study. Eur J Pain. 2011;15(3):231.e1–16.
41. da Silva CJ, et al. Trigeminal involvement in multiple sclerosis: magnetic resonance imaging findings with clinical correlation in a series of patients. Mult Scler. 2005;11(3):282–5.
42. Nakashima I, et al. Linear pontine trigeminal root lesions in multiple sclerosis: clinical and magnetic resonance imaging studies in 5 cases. Arch Neurol. 2001;58(1):101–4.
43. Meaney JF, et al. Association between trigeminal neuralgia and multiple sclerosis: role of magnetic resonance imaging. J Neurol Neurosurg Psychiatry. 1995;59(3):253–9.
44. Ramsaransing G, Zwanikken C, De Keyser J. Worsening of symptoms of multiple sclerosis associated with carbamazepine. BMJ. 2000;320(7242):1113.
45. Solaro C, et al. An open-label trial of gabapentin treatment of paroxysmal symptoms in multiple sclerosis patients. Neurology. 1998;51(2):609–11.
46. Solaro C, et al. Antiepileptic medications in multiple sclerosis: adverse effects in a three-year follow-up study. Neurol Sci. 2005;25(6):307–10.
47. Berk C, Constantoyannis C, Honey CR. The treatment of trigeminal neuralgia in patients with multiple sclerosis using percutaneous radiofrequency rhizotomy. Can J Neurol Sci. 2003;30(3):220–3.
48. Kondziolka D, Lunsford LD, Bissonette DJ. Long-term results after glycerol rhizotomy for multiple sclerosis-related trigeminal neuralgia. Can J Neurol Sci. 1994;21(2):137–40.

49. Broggi G, Franzini A. Radiofrequency trigeminal rhizotomy in treatment of symptomatic non-neoplastic facial pain. J Neurosurg. 1982;57(4):483–6.
50. Huang E, et al. Gamma knife radiosurgery for treatment of trigeminal neuralgia in multiple sclerosis patients. Stereotact Funct Neurosurg. 2002;79(1):44–50.
51. Broggi G, et al. Role of microvascular decompression in trigeminal neuralgia and multiple sclerosis. Lancet. 1999;354(9193):1878–9.
52. Paulo DL, et al. Microvascular decompression for trigeminal neuralgia in patients with multiple sclerosis: predictors of treatment success. World Neurosurg. 2020;136:e165–70.
53. Montano N, et al. Microvascular decompression in patients with trigeminal neuralgia and multiple sclerosis: results and analysis of possible prognostic factors. Acta Neurol Belg. 2020;120(2):329–34.
54. Noory N, et al. Neurovascular contact plays no role in trigeminal neuralgia secondary to multiple sclerosis. Cephalalgia. 2021;41(5):593–603.

Glossopharyngeal Neuralgia Focusing on Microvascular Decompression

Jae Sung Park and Young Hwan Ahn

1 Introduction

Glossopharyngeal neuralgia (GPN) refers to an excruciating pain syndrome that is paroxysmal and located in the sensory distribution of the glossopharyngeal nerve (GN) and sensory branches of the vagus nerve (VN)—the ear, base of the tongue, tonsillar fossa, or beneath the angle of the jaw. The first symptomatic description appeared in a case report in 1910 on a patient who had been diagnosed with tic douloureux for 6 years; the authors suggested that the symptoms were attributed to a certain irritation of the ninth and twelfth cranial nerves [1]. The term GPN was first used by Harris to describe paroxysms of pain in the back of the tongue, throat, etc., in 1921 [2]. The incidence of GPN is roughly estimated as 1% of trigeminal neuralgia (TN) [3].

The GPN is categorized as classical, secondary, and idiopathic GPN [4] in the classification of the international headache society (IHS). In classical GPN, neurovascular compression on the GN root is typically identified on magnetic resonance imaging (MRI) or during MVD. An underlying disease accounting for neuralgia constitutes the diagnosis of secondary GPN, whereas idiopathic GPN refers to a condition where neither an underlying disease nor neurovascular compression is demonstrated to cause the GPN symptoms. GPN, except for secondary one, affects only adults, with seemingly a predilection for the left side and the female gender, although no meta-analysis is available to verify the predilection [5].

The propriety of the term GPN has been questioned, for the syndrome may involve the sensory tributary of the VN as well, resulting in cardiovascular episodes, such as bradycardia, asystole, or hypotension [1, 6, 7]. As we concur with Sindou and Chen, vago-glossopharyngeal neuralgia (VGPN) might be a better terminology than GPN [6]. Our intraoperative findings of 30 GPN patients demonstrated that it was more common for a vessel or vessels to compress both the GN and VN rather than to compress the GN selectively, due to their anatomical proximity [8].

Pathophysiology of GPN has been considered partially analogous to that of TN; thus, an assumption was made that treatment options for the latter could also be applied to the former. Accordingly, intracranial sectioning of the GN was performed by Singleton and Dandy in 1926 and 1927, respectively, and the concept of microvascular decompression (MVD) was first

J. S. Park
Department of Neurosurgery, Konyang University Hospital, Konyang University College of Medicine, Daejeon, South Korea

Y. H. Ahn (✉)
Department of Neurosurgery, Ajou University School of Medicine, Ajou University Hospital, Suwon, Republic of Korea

Department of Biomedical Sciences, Graduate School of Ajou University, Suwon, Republic of Korea
e-mail: yhahn@ajou.ac.kr

K. Park, K. R. Cho (eds.), *Trigeminal Neuralgia*, https://doi.org/10.1007/978-981-19-9171-4_25

employed on this disease entity by Laha and Jannetta in 1977 [9–11]. In addition, Gamma knife radiosurgery (GKRS) which had proved to be effective for treatment of TN, also started to be used for GPN since 2005 on the same theoretical basis [12]. Among available treatment options for GPN, Microvascular decompression (MVD) is the only one that can offer a long-term cure in a non-destructive fashion. In this review, we will discuss and share our experience, especially focused on the application of the transposition technique during MVD.

2 Anatomy and Pathophysiology

Understanding the surgical anatomy of the GN and pathophysiology of GPN is imperative to the establishment of treatment strategy. The GN is a mixed sensorimotor nerve which is small and lies deep within the neck, and sometimes is called "the neglected cranial nerve," as it is often unnoticed in surgical dissections [13]. The GN projections exit the lateral aspect of the pons between the inferior olive and the inferior cerebellar peduncle. The somatic sensation of the GN is derived from the posterior two-thirds of the tongue, middle ear, and pharynx, whereas the visceral sensation of it receives inputs from the carotid body. Parasympathetic fibers to the parotid gland also travel via the GN; they arise from the inferior salivatory nucleus of the pons and leave the GN as tympanic nerve, which then joins the lesser petrosal nerve. Motor fibers of the GN originate in the nucleus ambiguous of the medulla and innervate stylopharyngeal muscle [13, 14].

The VN, a part of autonomic nervous system, comprises sensory and motor fibers, and interfaces with the parasympathetic control of the heart, lung, and gastrointestinal tract. This nerve arises from the medulla oblongata and their rootlets exit lateral to olive between the olive and the inferior cerebellar peduncle [14]. The fibers from VN consist of branchial motor, visceral sensory, visceral motor, special, and general sensory fibers. The brachial motor fibers of the VN are mainly involved in phonation and swallowing, by stimulating muscles in the pharynx, larynx, and soft palate, as well as cardiac muscles. The visceral motor fibers stimulate involuntary contractions in the digestive tract, including the esophagus, stomach, and most of the intestines. The somatic sensory fibers of the VN receive sensory information from the skin behind the ear, the external part of the ear canal, and certain parts of the throat, whereas the visceral sensory ones convey the sensory input from the larynx, esophagus, lungs, trachea, heart, and most of the digestive tract. Taste near the root of the tongue travels through the special sensory fibers of the VN [14].

The GN and VN are thinner than the trigeminal nerve; the mean diameter of the former is about 1.2 ± 0.3 mm, whereas that of the latter is 2.84 mm, and it can get up to 9.7 (4.6–9.3) mm as the trigeminal ganglion in the Meckel's cave [15, 16]. The length of the GN in the cistern is estimated as 16.2 ± 1.9 mm, while that of the trigeminal nerve is 9.66 ± 1.71 mm [17, 18]. Among 5–6 rootlets of the VN, the proximal 2–3 are sensory branches while the remaining 2–3 are motor ones [19]. Given that the GN and VN are thinner and longer than the trigeminal nerve, the former might be more prone to iatrogenic insult during MVD. Also, the REZ of the glossopharyngeal-vagus complex is positioned caudal to that of the trigeminal nerve, which demands a craniotomy for GPN to be extended further toward the skull base. These anatomical features of the GN might present additional challenges for neurosurgeons when performing MVD.

A compression on the root entry zone (REZ) of the GN by a vessel or vessels has been acknowledged as the cause of GPN in the great majority of cases [6, 8, 11]. Several cases of secondary GPN have been reported: tumor in the cerebellopontine angle, infections, multiple sclerosis, Paget's disease, trauma, dental procedure, etc. [1, 7, 20]. A true idiopathic GPN where no cause was demonstrated around the GN appears to be extremely rare. Given the rarity of GPN, there are no precise data on how many percent of GPN are attributed to neurovascular compression. Our own observation demonstrated that 77 of 78 cases were caused by the compression by a vessel or two on the REZ of the GN alone or both GN and VN. There were two cases where no definite offending artery was found around the REZ during MVD, but one could not automatically conclude that they were completely idiopathic. In one of the two subjects, we speculate that the arachnoid membrane had been tethering the exceptionally tortuous posterior inferior cerebellar artery (PICA) to the REZ, yet upon the release of the arachnoid membrane, the PICA was no longer present at the REZ. The fact that the patient became symptom-free following the surgery where only wide dissection of the arachnoid membrane was performed could support our assumption. As for the other one, although there was no artery compressing the REZ, small arterioles did exist around it. During the surgery, instead of the conventional MVD, the arterioles were simply detached from the REZ of the GN, following which the patient became symptom-free, and no recurrence has been reported until now for more than 3 years. We suspect that some of idiopathic GPN could have been named so due to lack of or incomplete exploration around the GN. A thorough investigation around both the GN and VN during MVD is crucial to accomplish a cure, since a decompression on the GN only may result in remaining vagal symptoms such as swallowing difficulty or paroxysmal cough with or without GPN.

Vascular compression on the REZ in GPN, as in hemifacial spasm (HFS) or TN, may lead to microscopic disruption of the integrity of myelination, and then, in turn, ephaptic transmission in the nerve fibers [13, 21]. Although it is still undetermined whether or not the vascular compression per se could alter the structure in the nucleus related to the GN, the demyelination and consequential ephaptic conduction resulting in neural hyperexcitability appear to be the proper etiology for GPN. A relatively high success rate (higher than 90%) of MVD for GPN also advocates this theory [6, 22].

A combination of TN, hemifacial spasm (HFS), and GPN or subparts of them is referred to as hyperactive dysfunction syndrome (HDS) of cranial nerves; according to large cohort studies among HFS patients, the prevalence of HDS was reported as up to 3% [23, 24]. The only statistically proven risk factor for HDS was the advanced age that may be associated with atherosclerosis in multiple vessels [24].

3 Diagnosis

The diagnosis is basically important. If it was properly done, physicians should be able to provide its natural course, treatment options, possible complications, and prognosis, which this article seeks to address.

Diagnosis of GPN, the key to successful treatment, must be based on clinical symptoms. The symptoms are characterized by unilateral brief paroxysmal lancinating pain in the sensory distributions of the GN and sometimes vagus nerve (VN) (Table 1) [4]. The distribution of the GN is defined as the posterior part of the tongue, tonsillar fossa, pharynx, or angle of the lower jaw and/ or in the ear [8]. More than half of the patients with GPN complaint an associated radiating neuralgic pain to ipsilateral deep ear that is difficult to define the exact location by each patient. Vagal manifestations such as bradycardia, syncope, hypotension, or cardiac arrest are reported to be found approximately in 10% of GPN patients [8, 21, 25, 26]. If the term "vagal manifestation" refers to responses via visceral sensory component of the vagal nerve, we also have encountered those vagal manifestations in patients of our series: swallowing difficulty or hoarseness,

Table 1 Diagnostic criteria of glossopharyngeal neuralgia

A.	Recurring paroxysmal attacks of unilateral pain in the distribution of the glossopharyngeal nerve and fulfilling criterion B
B.	Pain has all of the following characteristics:
1.	Lasting from a few seconds to 2 min
2.	Severe intensity
3.	Electric shock-like, shooting, stabbing, or sharp in quality
4.	Precipitated by swallowing, coughing, talking, or yawning
C.	Not better accounted for by another ICHD-3 (international classification of headache disorders-third edition)

developed separately or together with the pain attack. Considering that the pain in the deep throat, one of the most common symptoms of GPN, is accounted for by both the GN and somatic sensory component of the vagal nerve, we advocate the term VGPN [27].

The GPN pain can also radiate to other areas including the eye, nose, chin, or shoulder, which mimics some symptoms of TN, GPN could be misdiagnosed as TN. Therefore, the symptoms of GPN must be differentiated from TN or other various atypical facial pain syndromes, as well as dental diseases. Differentiation between GPN and TN is not always straightforward, because parts of the distribution of the glossopharyngeal (GP) nerve may overlap with that of the mandibular branch of the trigeminal nerve; GPN can be misdiagnosed as TN, and vice versa. Therefore, an elaborate and insightful history taking is the key to the correct diagnosis; also, one must not overlook the possibility of the coexistence of both diseases. Patients' verbal complaints are often limited to the most severe symptom even when they have both TN and GPN, which can allow one of them neglected. It must be reminded that the diagnosis of one of them does not automatically rule out the other, and symptoms related to the other must be inquired as well, since some patients may need two separate MVDs. In our opinion, the pain of GPN can be more intense than that of TN, which may allow omission of diagnosis of TN. GPN and TN may share the same triggering actions including chewing, talking, or brushing teeth, but the distribution of the former must include the throat, deep ear, or deep neck, which the latter generally does not involve.

When the pain in the distribution of the GP nerve is not a typical neuralgic pain, i.e., atypical pain syndrome, MVD should not be considered, as MVD can be beneficial only for typical GPN.

The importance of accurate diagnosis cannot be over-emphasized for a successful treatment for GPN. As the first patient with GPN symptom reported in 1910, misdiagnosed as TN, we also misdiagnosed our first GPN patient who visited our clinic. The patient complained of typical pain suggesting GPN but was simply misdiagnosed as a TN, and received MVD for TN which failed to yield pain relief. When the patient was reinquired afterwards about the symptoms with much greater detail, we realized that the pain that he had described was ignored by us during the initial encounter. On a later consideration, the patient also had radiating pain to the ipsilateral deep ear as an important diagnostic clue for GPN. A second MVD was performed for GPN and it resulted in a complete cure. Lessons we learned from the diagnostic failure of the first patient are as follows: (1) possibility of GPN need always to be considered. (2) Diagnosis of GPN must be made only whenever we meet the patient with severe facial pain including TN, and vice versa, (3) both typical TN and typical GPN may be triggered by coughing, talking, chewing, or swallowing; the absence of these precipitation factors can indicate atypical GPN or atypical TN. What can separate GPN and TN is always the distribution of the pain, not the pain characteristics or precipitation factors, (4) the tongue base is where innervation by the GN overlaps with that by the trigeminal nerve. When patients' main symptom is located in the tongue base, other accompanying symptoms must be inquired; concomitant pain in the deep throat may indicate GPN, whereas that in the face may be consistent with TN, (5) coexistence of both TN and GPN should also be in consideration.

4 Treatment

GPN, at least during the early stage, tends to be responsive to medications, such as carbamazepine, oxcarbazepine, gabapentin, or pregabalin [28, 29]. When combined with cardiovascular presentation, atropine can be administered, although it does not alleviate the neuralgic pain. For those whose GPN symptoms are medically intractable, advantages and disadvantages of various surgical options could be offered: GP rhizotomy with or without partial VN rhizotomy, percutaneous radiofrequency thermocoagulation, trigeminal tractotomy, MVD, and gamma knife radiosurgery (GKRS). Among them, MVD surgery is only the therapeutic modality aiming the

GPN to be curative, all other surgical methods are more or less destructive, but are not curative.

4.1 Microvascular Decompression (MVD)

MVD is a marvelous product of modern microscope-assisted surgical techniques and anatomical research demonstrating the neurovascular relationships; since it was successfully applied to TN and HFS by Jannetta et al. in 1970, it has become the treatment of choice for both diseases [22, 30, 31]. Encouraged by the satisfactory results of MVD for TN and HFS, Jannetta et al. employed it for GPN as well in 1977 [11]. According to a review of the literature by Sindou et al. in 2014, the total relief rate was reported between 50 and 100%, yet the authors suggested that the results seemed to be largely dependent on the level of equipment, surgeons' experience, and the use of neurophysiological monitoring whether or not the procedure [6].

Decompression on the REZ of the GN and VN begins with a separation from the compression vessel, and ultimately from the pulsatile signal from it. Then, the physical separation needs to be maintained to achieve long-term cure. MVD can be a safe and efficient procedure for GPN as much as for TN or HFS with a success rate higher than 90%, in a well-equipped facility. The only statistically proven risk factor for HDS was the advanced age that may be associated with atherosclerosis in multiple vessels [24]. Surgical difficulty might be more associated with existence of perforators originating from the offending artery and the location of the perforators which make the long-term maintenance of decompressed state of the causative artery difficult.

In the author's institution, all MVDs were performed by a single surgeon (Y. A.) with the use of a CT-guided navigation system for suboccipital craniotomy (Fig. 1) [32]. Computed tomography (CT) navigation-guided craniotomy was used to expose the margin of the sigmoid sinus from its beginning to the region behind the mastoid tip and to reduce the risks of bleeding from the sigmoid sinus. Intraoperative brainstem auditory evoked potentials and sensory evoked potentials (Viasys Healthcare, Conshohocken, PA, USA) were monitored throughout the operation to check the function of the brainstem and cranial nerves.

The lateral suboccipital infra-floccular approach with a park-bench position was employed as this approach is enough to achieve a wide surgical field [33]. The extradural tissues were covered with saline-soaked gauze to avoid tissue dry-up during the surgery. A C-shaped dural incision was made and reflected over the sigmoid sinus. The arachnoid membrane was dissected carefully to allow cerebrospinal fluid (CSF) drainage and to expose the lower cranial nerves and the vessels responsible for GPN. A retractor with a 2 mm-wide tip was applied intermittently during the arachnoid dissection. A wide arachnoid dissection was carried out to avoid any retraction or injury from arachnoid. Several pieces of Teflon (Bard PTFE felt, Tempe, AZ, USA) and a Tisseel glue (Baxter Healthcare Corp., Glendale, CA, USA) were prepared as a prefilled syringe. A glue-coated Teflon sling was manually crafted just before use [15]. While a more extensive craniotomy such as a transcondylar fossa approach could be considered, such an approach known failed to overcome a limitation associated with perforating arteries [34]. Therefore, conventional method with a lateral suboccipital infra-floccular approach is appropriate for the GPN MVD as is enough to have an optimal surgical field.

Upon visualization of REZ of the GN, the decompression was carried out using one of four surgical techniques depending on the surgical finding: simple transposition of the vessel using Teflon pieces (Fig. 2), transposition of the vessel using one or two glue-coated Teflon slings (Fig. 3a, b); interposition of Teflon pieces underneath the offending vessel or vessels (Fig. 4), and cauterization of offending veins [8]. According to our previous report with 30 cases of GPN, the most commonly performed technique was simple transposition with Teflon pieces, followed by transposition using a glue-coated Teflon sling and interposition of Teflon pieces in that order (Table 2) [32, 35].

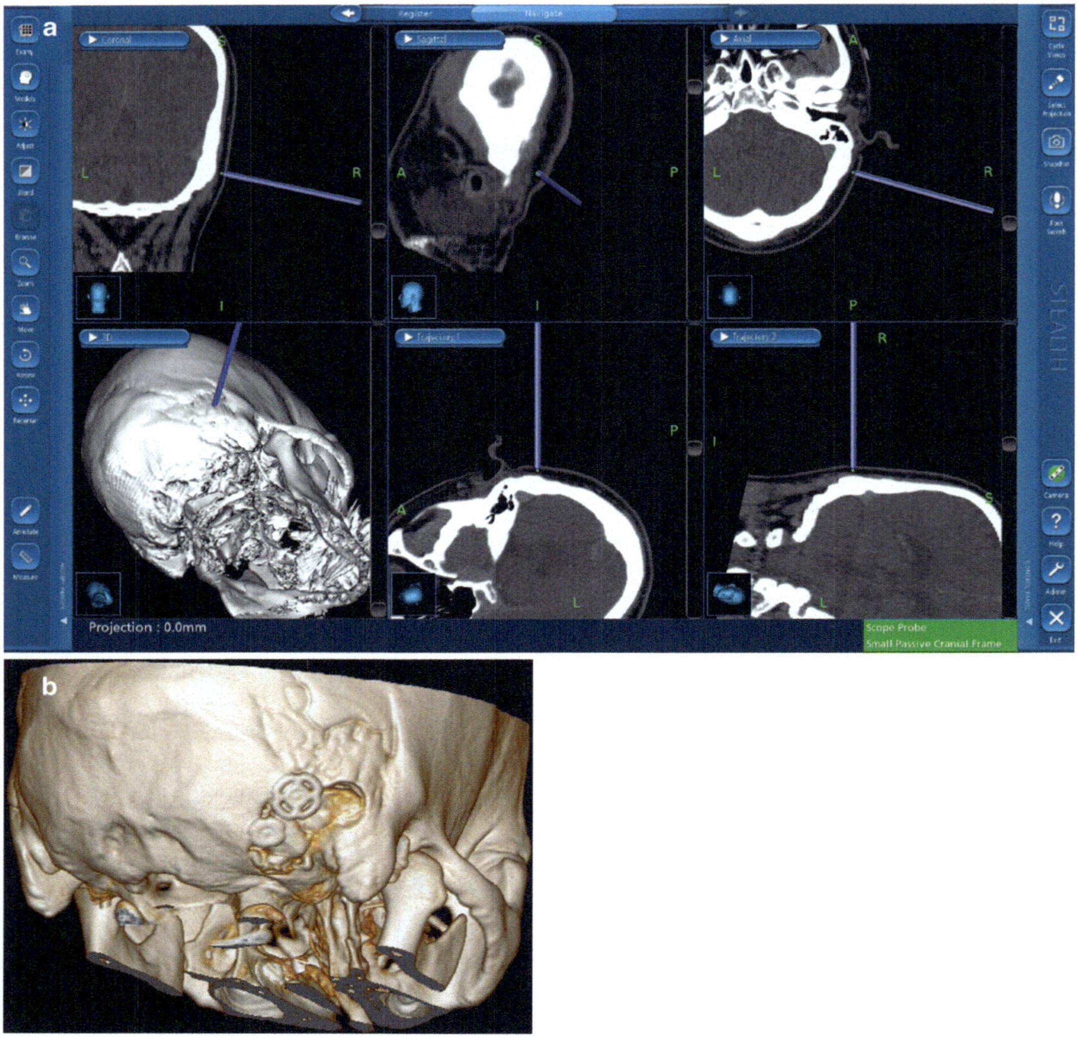

Fig. 1 (**a**) CT-guided navigation for identification of the sigmoid sinus and mastoid air cells. (**b**) Postoperative 3D CT image showing the size and shape of the suboccipital craniotomy

Cauterization of the vein was applied for one case. No additional rhizotomy was accompanied in our series.

1. *Transposition using Teflon pieces*

   When Jannetta et al. originally introduced this technique of inserting insulating materials (IM) between the offending artery and the REZ for TN, HFS, and GPN, they addressed this as "interposition" [11]. In our opinion, it can better be named "transposition" than "interposition," when the insertion of IM causes the vessel securely displaced from its original position, i.e., on the REZ. A mere interposition of IM and its insulating effect per se, with no definite change of force vector from the offending vessel, cannot explain the whole mechanism of decompression. In "transposition" technique, Teflon pieces are inserted not to become an insulation material, but to change the position and direction of the compressing vessel. Therefore, the REZ can be released not only from the physical compression by the offending vessel but also from the pulsatile

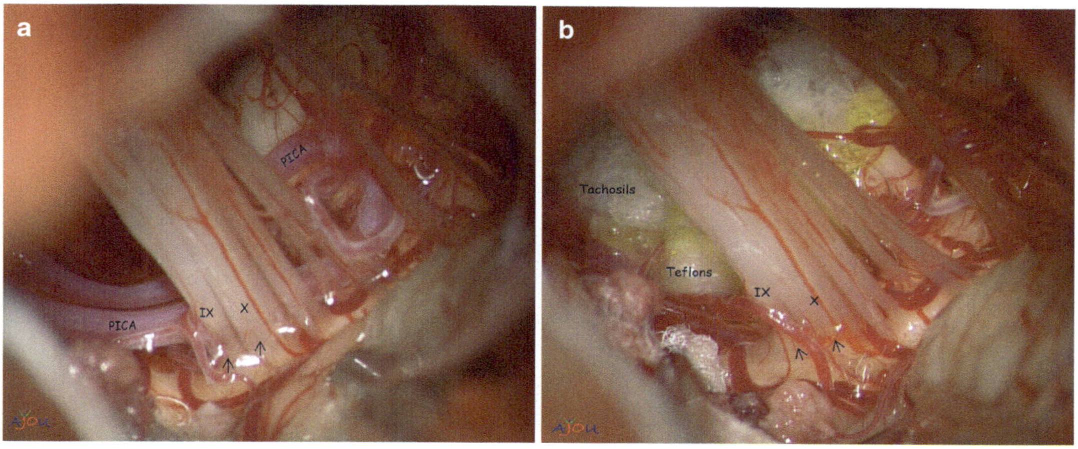

Fig. 2 Simple transposition using Teflon pieces. (**a**) PICA is compressing the REZ (arrow) of the IX nerve. (**b**) The position and trajectory of the PICA are altered by the inserted Teflon, but Teflon is not located at the REZ (arrow) as an insulation material. Since Teflon was not used as an insulation material, we define this technique "transposition". *IX* the glossopharyngeal nerve, *X* the vagus nerve, *PICA* posterior inferior cerebellar artery

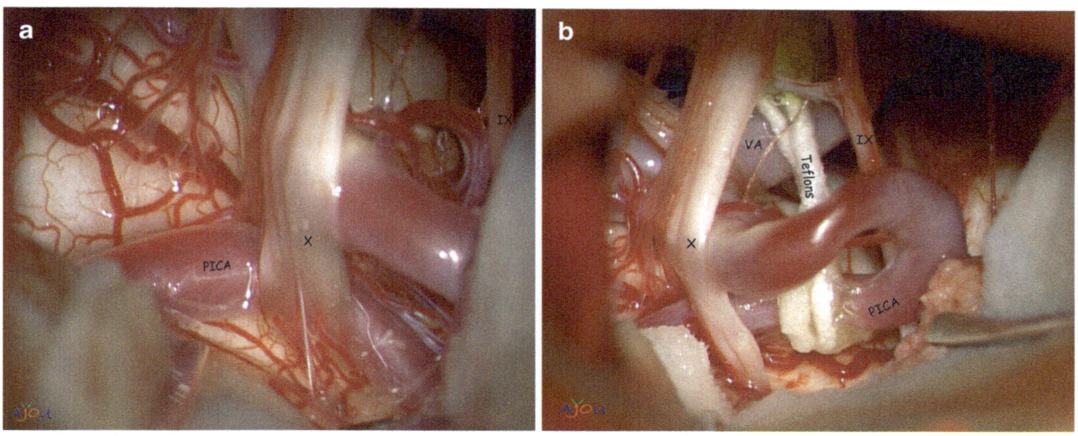

Fig. 3 Transposition using a Teflon sling. (**a**) Very tortuous PICA is compressing the REZ of the IX and X nerves. (**b**) A fibrin glue coated sling is lifting up PICA to change its position and trajectory off the REZ. We define this technique 'transposition using a Teflon sling'. *IX* the glossopharyngeal nerve, *X* the vagus nerve, *PICA* posterior inferior cerebellar artery

force from it, because the force vector can be redirected off the REZ. The concept "off the REZ" epitomizes the superiority of the transposition technique over others, because it indicates complete release from compression not only by the offending vessel but also by Teflon pieces [32]. We propose that the term interposition can better be used for occasions where the interposed Teflon pieces merely insulate the REZ, changing neither position nor force vector of the vessel. In our series, transposition using Teflon pieces and fibrin glue was always attempted with a few exceptions.

2. *Transposition using a fibrin glue-coated Teflon sling*

   Once transposition using Teflon pieces was successfully performed, some "transposed" arteries needed to be further secured to an immovable part in the surgery field: the petrosal dura in our series [35]. Since a recurrence

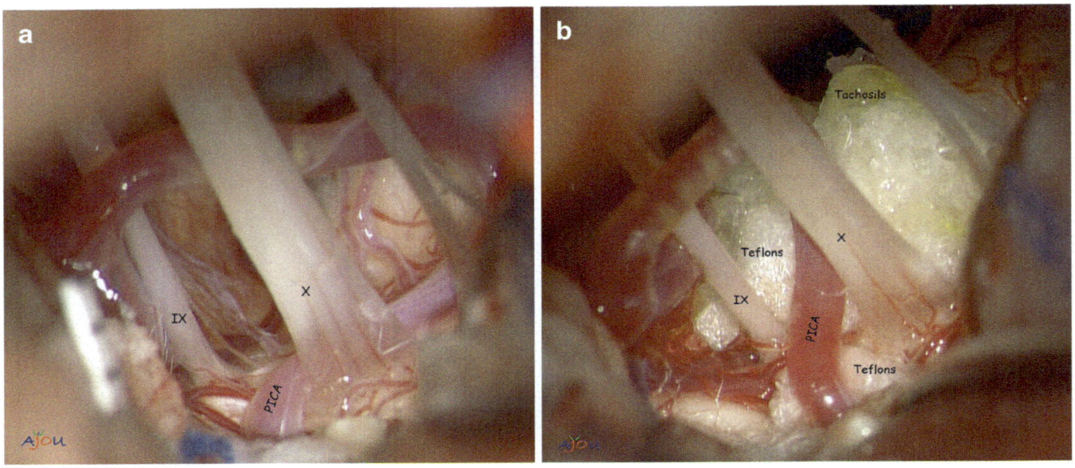

Fig. 4 Interposition of insulating material (IM). (**a**) PICA compressing the IX nerve. While PICA being maneuvered, it appears unfeasible to transpose PICA to another position, owing to several perforators tethering PICA to the brain stem. (**b**) Teflon pieces are inserted between the REZ and the vessel as an IM. *IX* the glossopharyngeal nerve, *X* the vagus nerve, *PICA* posterior inferior cerebellar artery

Table 2 Surgical techniques used for microvascular decompression

Decompression technique	Number of patients
Transposition using Teflon pieces	15 (50%)
Transposition using a glue-coated Teflon sling	9 (30%)
Interposition of insulating materials (IM)	5 (16.7%)
Cauterization of veins	1 (3.3%)
Total	30

can take place when the transposed artery is no longer "transposed," we applied this maneuver to sustain the transposition. For this procedure, a fibrin glue-coated Teflon sling was hand-crafted by the surgeon, using small pieces of glue-coated Teflon (Fig. 5). Several Teflon threads were manually twisted and combined with help of fibrin glue until it formed an elongated strand. The length and thickness of the strand, i.e., the sling, were modified in accordance with each individual's anatomical feature. One should be reminded that the sling never has to be thicker than necessary, for an excessively thick sling may complicate the procedure. The sling was positioned to encircle the offending artery, and then the ends of it were fixated to the petrosal dura or on the top of the brain stem using fibrin glue or fibrin glue plus TachoSil® pieces. When fibrin glue and Tachosil pieces were expected to be insufficient to secure the sling to the constant part of the brain, additional fixating procedures including one or two stitches to the petrosal dura were carried out (Figs. 2, 3, 4, and 5).

3. *Interposition of IM*

   The true interposition was performed only when the offending vessel failed to be manipulated enough to be transposed off the REZ [8, 35]. In five of 78 cases in our series, short perforating arteries from the offending artery were tightly tethering it to the REZ, which precluded the application of transposition; hence, the interposition. Unlike the "transposition" technique, interposition of IM solely contributed to decompression of the REZ without alteration of the position or course of the vessel.

4. *Cauterization of vein*

   On rare occasions, a thorough investigation around the REZ of GN and VN failed to locate a compressing artery, although several engorged veins appeared to compress the REZ. Considering that venous compression as the sole cause of TN is not unheard of, the

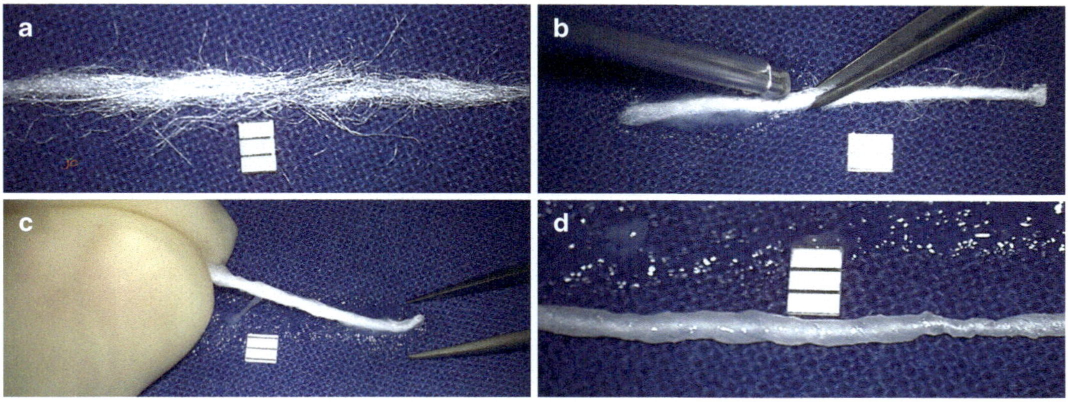

Fig. 5 Manually crafted glue-coated Teflon. (**a**) Dry pieces of Teflon fiber (the scale of the measuring key is 1 mm). (**b**) Fibrin glue being sprayed on the Teflon strands. (**c**) Twisting of the fibrin glue-coated Teflon strands to form a sling. (**d**) Lint free and sleek fibrin glue-coated Teflon sling, kept in normal saline until used

same etiology can contribute to GPN [36]. In the case of our series, as the veins were profusely anastomosed with other collateral ones, the engorged portion of the vein on the REZ was cauterized and divided, using the lowest possible power setting of the bipolar coagulator. The patient became symptom-free after the cauterization of the vein.

Since no cohort-based statistics are available on the success rate of transposition procedure-based MVD for GPN, we present our own results. A total of 78 typical GPN patients underwent MVD in our institute for the past two decades, and all had a follow-up of at least 6 months. The Barrow neurological institute pain intensity score (BNI) was used for the evaluation of the pain. Seventy six (97.4%) of 78 patients became pain-free (BNI grade 1) or with only occasional pain (BNI grade 2) after MVD. There were 49 GPN patients with a longer follow-up (more than 5 years); 48 (97.9%) of them became BNI 1 or 2 in 1 year after MVD. On a chronological analysis, eight of those 49 patients had stated that their pain belonged to BNI grade 3 after MVD, but 7 of them became BNI grade 1 or 2 in 1 year. One individual has remained in BNI grade 3 who needs intermittent medications, despite her general satisfaction with the result. While there were three patients who experienced transient complications, such as dysphagia, dysphonia, and decreased hearing ability, neither mortality nor permanent complication occurred in our series. Also, no VN-related complication took place.

Considering that the success rate of MVD for TN (80–85%) reported by cohort studies is somewhat lower than that for HFS (90%), we cautiously speculate that MVD might be more beneficial to GPN than to TN [37–39]. The relatively high success rate of MVD for GPN might be attributed to the anatomical simplicity of the ninth and tenth cranial nerves, and no bony structure to encompass it except for the jugular foramen. In such sense, it is probably more likely for a successful MVD to provide a long-term cure for GPN than for TN. However, revision surgeries for GPN should be avoided at all costs, given its anatomical features. Compared to the trigeminal nerve, the GN and VN are much thinner and a hypothetical injury to them may cause irreversible, sometimes life-threatening consequences. Therefore, we suggest that the "transposition" technique should always be aimed for, as the mere "interposition" cannot guarantee a long-term cure. Regardless of the kind of surgical technique, perforating arteries must not be jeopardized, and maneuvering the vessels should be limited to the minimum in order to prevent vasospasm.

Although some case reports advocate selective glossopharyngeal rhizotomy (GNR) in addition to MVD for GPN, we believe that it should not be considered as a standard treatment [40].

Selective GNR alone or with an additional rhizotomy of the sensory branches of the VN may partially alleviate the pain, but complications following them are not negligible: irritative cough, foreign body sensation in the throat, hoarseness, dysphagia, etc [41]. A review article with 454 MVD and 157 GNR cases reported that permanent complications after GNR (19.1%) was three times greater than those after MVD (5.1%) [42]. Another research regarding selective GNR with or without partial VN rhizotomy in 103 patients with a follow-up of 2.3 years reported that the pain relief and immediate complications did not significantly differ between the two groups, while the long-term complications after GNR with partial VN rhizotomy (35.8%) were much more frequent than those after GNR without VN rhizotomy (3.8%) [43]. The authors concluded that GNR, especially without VN rhizotomy, can be a safe and effective treatment option for GPN, yet we cannot concur with their conclusion, given a relatively short follow-up (2.3 years) and the high rate of long-term complications after GNR with partial VN rhizotomy. In our opinion, there is no need to add an adjuvant rhizotomy during MVD for GPN. We believe that MVD alone is the treatment of choice for GPN, in that it is non-destructive and can afford the cure.

5 Conclusion

GPN is one of the neurovascular compression syndromes alongside HFS and TN; also, its treatment strategy has been established, largely based on that of the other two more common diseases. The GN is unique in that it shares nerve projections with the VN and it travels with great proximity to the jugular vein and internal carotid artery. Symptoms of GPN must be carefully evaluated and differentiated from other pain syndromes, especially TN, and the optimal treatment plan should be offered after thorough consideration of each patient's radiological features around the GN, medical status, and preference. Medication can initially be prescribed, and yet when it fails to alleviate the pain, MVD should be considered as the primary choice of treatment. In addition, we advocate the use of the transposition technique during an MVD, because it employs "off the REZ" policy, which can fundamentally prevent a recurrence. For those who are not eligible for a craniotomy, GKRS can be a reasonable alternative.

Disclosure The Majority of contents in this article are based on our recent publication in JKNS (Journal of Korean Neurosurgical Society). However, all the figures that are used for this chapter are original and not bound to copyright restrictions.

No grants pertinent to the paper exist.

Authors state that they have no personal or institutional financial interest in drugs, materials, or devices described in their submission.

References

1. White JC, Sweet WH. Pain and the neurosurgeon: a forty-year experience. CC Thomas; 1969.
2. Harris W. Persistent pain in lesions of the peripheral and central nervous system. Br Med J. 1921;2(3178):896.
3. Sarlani E, Grace EG, Balciunas BA, Schwartz AH. Trigeminal neuralgia in a patient with multiple sclerosis and chronic inflammatory demyelinating polyneuropathy. J Am Dent Assoc. 2005;136(4):469–76.
4. Arnold M. Headache classification committee of the international headache society (IHS) the international classification of headache disorders. Cephalalgia. 2018;38(1):1–211.
5. Rozen TD. Trigeminal neuralgia and glossopharyngeal neuralgia. Neurol Clin. 2004;22(1):185–206.
6. Chen J, Sindou M. Vago-glossopharyngeal neuralgia: a literature review of neurosurgical experience. Acta Neurochir. 2015;157(2):311–21.
7. Rushton JG, Stevens JC, Miller RH. Glossopharyngeal (vagoglossopharyngeal) neuralgia a study of 217 cases. Arch Neurol. 1981;38(4):201–5.
8. Kim MK, Park JS, Ahn YH. Microvascular decompression for glossopharyngeal neuralgia: clinical analyses of 30 cases. J Korean Neurosurg Soc. 2017;60(6):738.
9. Singleton AO. Glossopharyngeal neuralgia and its surgical relief. Ann Surg. 1926;83(3):338.
10. Dandy WE. Glossopharyngeal neuralgia (tic douloureux): its diagnosis and treatment. Arch Surg. 1927;15(2):198–214.
11. Laha RK, Jannetta PJ. Glossopharyngeal neuralgia. J Neurosurg. 1977;47(3):316–20.
12. Stieber VW, Bourland JD, Ellis TL. Glossopharyngeal neuralgia treated with gamma knife surgery: treatment outcome and failure analysis: case report. J Neurosurg. 2005;102(Spl_Suppl):155–7.

13. Pearce J. Glossopharyngeal neuralgia. Eur Neurol. 2006;55(1):49–52.
14. Tubbs RS, Shoja MM, Loukas M. Anatomy of the glossopharyngeal nerve. In: Nerves and Nerve Injuries, vol. 1. Elsevier; 2015. p. 371–83.
15. Wang C, Kundaria S, Fernandez-Miranda J, Duvvuri U. A description of the anatomy of the glossopharyngeal nerve as encountered in transoral surgery. Laryngoscope. 2016;126(9):2010–5.
16. Ajayi N, Lazarus L, Satyapal K. Trigeminal cave and ganglion: an anatomical review. Int J Morphol. 2013;31(4):1444–8.
17. Kakizawa Y, Seguchi T, Kodama K, et al. Anatomical study of the trigeminal and facial cranial nerves with the aid of 3.0-tesla magnetic resonance imaging. J Neurosurg. 2008;108(3):483–90.
18. Wang M, Chae R, Shehata J, et al. Comparative analysis of surgical exposure and freedom between the subtonsillar, endoscope-assisted subtonsillar, and far-lateral approaches to the lower clivus: a cadaveric study. J Clin Neurosci. 2020;72:412–9.
19. Peris-Celda M, Oushy S, Perry A, et al. Nervus intermedius and the surgical management of geniculate neuralgia. J Neurosurg. 2018;131(2):343–51.
20. Koratkar H, Parashar V, Koratkar S. A review of neuropathic pain conditions affecting teeth. Gen Dent. 2010;58(5):436–41. quiz 442
21. Blumenfeld A, Nikolskaya G. Glossopharyngeal neuralgia. Curr Pain Headache Rep. 2013;17(7):343.
22. Patel A, Kassam A, Horowitz M, Chang Y-F. Microvascular decompression in the management of glossopharyngeal neuralgia: analysis of 217 cases. Neurosurgery. 2002;50(4):705–11.
23. Manzoni G, Torelli P. Epidemiology of typical and atypical craniofacial neuralgias. Neurol Sci. 2005;26(2):s65–7.
24. Yang K-H, Na J-H, Kong D-S, Park K. Combined hyperactive dysfunction syndrome of the cranial nerves. J Korean Neurosurg Soc. 2009;46(4):351.
25. Kong Y, Heyman A, Entman ML, Mcintosh HD. Glossopharyngeal neuralgia associated with bradycardia, syncope, and seizures. Circulation. 1964;30(1):109–13.
26. Barbash GI, Keren G, Korczyn AD, et al. Mechanisms of syncope in glossopharyngeal neuralgia. Electroencephalogr Clin Neurophysiol. 1986;63(3):231–5.
27. Sibilla L, Agarwal N. Cranial Nerve IX: glossopharyngeal. In: Neuroimaging: anatomy meets function. Springer; 2018. p. 207–10.
28. Fromm GH. Clinical pharmacology of drugs used to treat head and face pain. Neurol Clin. 1990;8(1):143–51.
29. Moretti R, Torre P, Antonello R, Bava A, Cazzato G. Gabapentin treatment of glossopharyngeal neuralgia: a follow-up of four years of a single case. Eur J Pain. 2002;6(5):403–7.
30. Hardy DG, Rhoton AL. Microsurgical relationships of the superior cerebellar artery and the trigeminal nerve. J Neurosurg. 1978;49(5):669–78.
31. Janetta P. Microsurgical exploration and decompression of the facial nerve in hemifacial spasm. Curr Top Surg Res. 1970;2:217–20.
32. Park JS, Ahn YH. Glossopharyngeal Neuralgia. J Korean Neurosurg Soc. 2022;66(1):12–23.
33. Sampson JH, Grossi PM, Asaoka K, Fukushima T. Microvascular decompression for glossopharyngeal neuralgia: long-term effectiveness and complication avoidance. Neurosurgery. 2004;54(4):884–90.
34. Kawashima M, Matsushima T, Inoue T, Mineta T, Masuoka J, Hirakawa N. Microvascular decompression for glossopharyngeal neuralgia through the transcondylar fossa (supracondylar transjugular tubercle) approach. *Operative*. Neurosurgery. 2010;66(suppl_2):ons275–80.
35. Lee SH, Park JS, Ahn YH. Bioglue-coated teflon sling technique in microvascular decompression for hemifacial spasm involving the vertebral artery. J Korean Neurosurg Soc. 2016;59(5):505.
36. Matsushima T, Huynh-Le P, Miyazono M. Trigeminal neuralgia caused by venous compression. Neurosurgery. 2004;55(2):334–9.
37. Linskey ME, Ratanatharathorn V, Peñagaricano J. A prospective cohort study of microvascular decompression and gamma knife surgery in patients with trigeminal neuralgia. J Neurosurg. 2008;109(Supplement):160–72.
38. Breeze R, Ignelzi RJ. Microvascular decompression for trigeminal neuralgia: results with special reference to the late recurrence rate. J Neurosurg. 1982;57(4):487–90.
39. Park JS, Lee S, Park S-K, Lee J-A, Park K. Facial motor evoked potential with paired transcranial magnetic stimulation: prognostic value following microvascular decompression for hemifacial spasm. J Neurosurg. 2018;131(6):1780–7.
40. Ozenci M, Karaoguz R, Conkbayir C, Altin T, Kanpolat Y. Glossopharyngeal neuralgia with cardiac syncope treated by glossopharyngeal rhizotomy and microvascular decompression. Europace. 2003;5(2):149–52.
41. Bohm E, Strang R. Glossopharyngeal neuralgia. Brain. 1962;85(2):371–88.
42. Rey-Dios R, Cohen-Gadol AA. Current neurosurgical management of glossopharyngeal neuralgia and technical nuances for microvascular decompression surgery. Neurosurg Focus. 2013;34(3):E8.
43. Ma Y, Li Y-f, Wang Q-c, Wang B, Huang H-t. Neurosurgical treatment of glossopharyngeal neuralgia: analysis of 103 cases. J Neurosurg. 2016;124(4):1088–92.

Otalgia and Geniculate Neuralgia

Chang-Hee Kim

1 Introduction

Otalgia is an ear pain and is common affecting people of all ages with almost a 100% lifetime prevalence [1, 2]. Otalgia can be broken down into two categories of primary (otogenic) otalgia and secondary otalgia regarding its causes. Primary otalgia arises as a consequence of otologic diseases, and secondary otalgia arises from pathologic processes in structures other than the ear. Otalgia can be referred to as a primary otalgia when the etiology of otalgia is limited within the affected ear and the cause of otalgia can be identified by otoendoscopic examination. Primary otalgia can be caused by otitis externa, acute or chronic otitis media, impacted cerumen, mastoiditis, folliculitis, myringitis, and neoplasm [3]. Primary otalgia is far more common in children than in adults, and secondary otalgia is more common in adults [1–3]. When the pathoetiology of otalgia cannot be identified through physical examination and otoendoscopy, the cause of secondary otalgia should be investigated. Sensory innervation of the ear is provided by a complex neural network as a result of complex embryogenic development. Because the ear shares this complex neural network with other organs, numerous sources of secondary otalgia can be possible. Cranial nerves (CNs) V (trigeminal), VII (facial), IX (glossopharyngeal), X (vagus), and branches from the cervical plexus (C1, C2, and C3) all innervate the middle ear, external auditory canal, auricle and peri-auricular tissues, and irritation of any portion of CNs V, VII, IX, X or C1, 2, and 3 may cause otalgia. The auricle is innervated by CNs V, VII, X, C2, and C3, the external auditory canal is innervated by CNs V, VII, and X, the tympanic membrane is innervated by CNs VII, IX, and X, and the middle ear is innervated by CNs V, VII, and IX. The location of nerve irritation can be remote from the ear, and, for example, otalgia may be the sole manifestation of myocardial ischemia because the CN X innervates both the ear and heart [4–6]. Furthermore, although most secondary otalgia is caused by the problems of the neck, cervical spine, and temporomandibular joints, more ominous causes of otalgia such as occult malignancy should be taken into consideration.

Specific nerves which are related to otalgia are as follows. The CN V is composed of the ophthalmic (V1), maxillary (V2), and mandibular (V3) branches. The CN V provides sensory innervation for the temporomandibular joint, teeth, palate, sinuses, and face. Dental and temporomandibular joint disorders are the most common causes of secondary otalgia. The CN VII innervates the taste of the anterior two-thirds of the tongue and provides sensory innervation of facial

C.-H. Kim (✉)
Department of Otorhinolaryngology-Head and Neck Surgery, Konkuk University Medical Center, Konkuk University School of Medicine,
Seoul, Republic of Korea
e-mail: changhee.kim@kuh.ac.kr

K. Park, K. R. Cho (eds.), *Trigeminal Neuralgia*, https://doi.org/10.1007/978-981-19-9171-4_26

deep soft tissue. The CN IX innervates the posterior one-third of the tongue, carotid body, and oropharynx. The CN X innervates the sinuses, thyroid gland, pharynx, and larynx. It also innervates distant organs such as the lung, heart, and parts of the gastrointestinal tract. The branches of the cervical plexus innervate the back of the head, sternocleidomastoid muscle, and cervical paraspinal muscles.

2 Etiology and Differential Diagnosis

The etiology of otalgia is classified into primary versus secondary or referred causes. For the differential diagnosis between primary and secondary otalgia, it is imperative that a complete history and comprehensive physical examination be conducted. Primary otalgia is generally attributed to infectious, mechanical, neoplastic, and inflammatory causes, and secondary otalgia is best classified based on organ systems. Dental and temporomandibular joint problems are included in more proximal causes of the head and neck area, and cardiac, gastrointestinal, and lung pathology are included in distant etiologies of secondary otalgia. The characteristics of pain may be of help to differentiate the etiology of otalgia. Primary otalgia associated with infection tends to be continuous, and wax and wane in intensity according to the degree of the infection control. Infection is unlikely to produce pain that lasts for a few minutes and then resolves spontaneously. Intermittent episodes of abrupt pain are more likely to be related to musculoskeletal conditions. Otalgia associated with the temporomandibular joint or other myofascial disorders shows the characteristics of this pattern. Other associated otologic symptoms such as hearing loss, otorrhea, tinnitus, aural fullness, and vertigo may point to primary otalgia. Recent history of trismus, sore throat, odynophagia, reflux symptoms, hoarseness, pain in paranasal sinus area, or dental caries may point to secondary otalgia. Careful inspection of the auricle, postauricular area, external auditory canal, and tympanic membrane should be performed. Besides, a full examination of the nasal cavity, oral cavity, neck, larynx, and pharynx should be carried out. Although the causes of otalgia are able to be identified by the history and physical examination in most cases, cross-sectional imaging studies may be needed when the cause of otalgia is not identified after an appropriate history and physical examination. Temporal bone CT is the first-line imaging technique for assessing etiologies arising from the ear and temporal bone. For the evaluation of the lesions in the larynx, pharynx, and other neck regions, contrast-enhanced neck CT is the first-line choice, although neck MRI may be superior to CT for soft tissue assessment. Especially, identification of the cause of secondary otalgia is sometimes more challenging, because of the complex interplay of multiple upper cervical, lower cranial, and peripheral nerves providing sensory information to and from the ear.

3 Primary Otalgia

3.1 Causes of the Middle Ear

The common cause of primary otalgia is infection. Especially in children, acute otitis media ranks as the number one cause of primary otalgia. Because the middle ear mucosa takes up part of the upper respiratory tract, acute otitis media follows acute upper respiratory tract infection. In adults, chronic otitis media is the most common primary otalgia, although chronic ear infections are rarely painful.

Acute otitis media can be diagnosed when middle ear effusion is present, accompanying signs and symptoms of acute inflammation. Acute otitis media is exclusively more common in children and is usually concurrent with acute upper respiratory tract infection. The common bacterial organisms causing acute otitis media are Streptococcus pneumoniae, Haemophilus influenzae, and Moraxella catarrhalis. The otalgia associated with acute otitis media usually begins as a mild dull pain, accompanying aural fullness in the affected ear. The intensity of pain becomes severe as the inflammation gets worse. The severity of pain improves if treatment is successful, spontaneous resolution begins, or the inflamed middle ear effusion is discharged through the ruptured tympanic membrane. At its worst, the pain of acute otitis media is described as severe, pulsating pain deep in the ear. Although the intensity of otalgia in acute otitis media may be very severe, the ear is not tender, which may provide an important clue to distinguish middle ear disease from disorders of the external auditory canal. Because it is known that spontaneous resolution of disease occurs in about 80% of acute otitis media, a day or two of observation may be allowed before the administration of systemic antibiotics. It has to be noted that adequate pain control should be implemented even before the start of antibiotics. Bullous myringitis, which shows bullae on the tympanic membrane, is commonly accompanied by acute otitis media and is usually caused by an acute bacterial infection. Bullous myringitis is extremely painful and the pain is significantly relieved by puncturing the bullae.

Although acute mastoiditis is a contemporarily rare disease since the widespread use of systemic antibiotics, acute mastoiditis may cause severe otalgia [7]. The mastoid cavity is usually inflamed in chronic otitis media, and acute mastoiditis develops from acute otitis media. Acute mastoiditis may be manifested as otalgia, postauricular pain, and high fever. Because acute mastoiditis can occur despite previous systemic antibiotics for acute otitis media, the possibility of mastoiditis should be suspected when acute otitis media does not respond to the proper treatment of 7 days or more. Outward protrusion of the auricle and postauricular erythema may be present, and, if progressed to develop subperiosteal abscess, postauricular induration and fluctuation may occur. Missed diagnosis of acute mastoiditis can result in intriguing complications such as facial paralysis, and labyrinthitis. Intracranial complications such as extradural abscess, meningitis, cerebellar abscess, sigmoid sinus thrombophlebitis, and otogenic hydrocephalus may be devastating. It is noteworthy that external otitis, when the inflammation extends to the postauricular tissues, can manifest clinical findings similar to acute mastoiditis. Bony erosion of the mastoid air cells with coalescence of air cells into a single cavity is observed on temporal bone CT. A CT scan will show bony destruction of the mastoid air cells with the coalescence of air cells into a single cavity. Intravenous antibiotic therapy should be started as early as possible based on the result of the culture. When there is any evidence of intracranial progression or severe bony erosion, surgical treatment such as mastoidectomy with myringotomy is required.

Acute barotrauma is caused by flight, hyperbaric oxygen therapy, or scuba diving, and may lead to severe otalgia [5, 8–12]. Rapid development of negative pressure in the middle ear space results in hemotympanum and can cause acute retraction of the tympanic membrane, resulting in perforation of the tympanic membrane. Intratympanic membrane bleeding can also develop due to the rupture of capillaries within the tympanic membrane [13]. Acute barotrauma may involve the paranasal sinuses, which may lead to secondary otalgia.

3.2 Causes of the External Auditory Canal

The impacted cerumen in the external auditory canal may cause severe, dull otalgia. In progressed cases, impacted cerumen implements pressure effect on the bony external auditory canal, causing thinning of skin and bony erosion. Attempting to remove impacted cerumen may cause severe pain due to trauma to the external auditory canal skin [14, 15].

Acute otitis externa is an inflammation of the external auditory canal and is usually caused by a bacterial infection, following the breakdown of protective barrier of the skin and cerumen [16–18]. The skin of the external auditory canal is weakly acidic in a normal condition, which provides an important protective environment. However, alkalinization of the external auditory canal may predispose bacterial infection. External otitis, traditionally, has been referred to as "swimmer's ear," because the infection occurs more frequently in conjunction with elevated humidity and temperature. Predisposing factors for external otitis media include canal obstruction by hearing aids, impacted cerumen or the use of an ear plug, chronic seborrheic dermatitis, and trauma from scratching. Clinical symptoms include otalgia, itching, aural fullness, and hearing loss. Otoendoscopic examination shows that the external auditory canal is erythematous and wet. In more severe cases, the edematous skin may completely obstruct the canal, resulting in nonvisualization of the tympanic membrane. Moreover, cellulitis may extend to the soft tissues of the pre- or postauricular area. Traction of the auricle and touching the tragus may cause intense pain, which helps differential diagnosis between acute external otitis and acute otitis media. The infection is typically polymicrobial, and pseudomonas aeruginosa is the most common cause of infection, followed by staphylococcus aureus, and other gram-negative bacilli. Although fungal infection is common in chronic otitis externa, fungal involvement is uncommon in acute infection. Treatment begins with thorough cleansing of debris and exudates, and the infection is generally well-controlled by topical therapy in early, uncomplicated cases. Topical ear drops deliver a very high concentration of the antimicrobial to the infected external auditory canal skin, and proper administration of ear drops is important to ensure adequate delivery of antibiotics [16, 19, 20]. The addition of a steroid to topical ear drops may help in the elimination of pain. Inadequate delivery of topical ear drops is the most common cause of failure of medical therapy. If the skin of the external auditory canal is swollen due to the progression of infection enough to obstruct the canal, the antibiotic-soaked wicks should be placed to ensure that the topical antibiotics reach the tissues. Oral analgesia can be administered for pain control, and oral antibiotics can be administered if cellulitis extends to the surrounding soft tissues of the face or postauricular area. Early use of systemic antibiotics is guaranteed in patients with uncontrolled diabetes or immune-compromised patients [16, 20, 21]. Furthermore, special attention should be paid when the otalgia persists despite treatment, especially in the elderly, patients with diabetes mellitus, or immunocompromised patients. In this case, the possibility of necrotizing external otitis must be ruled out. Necrotizing external otitis, also called malignant external otitis, represents extension of the infection into the underlying bone and may be a potentially fatal condition. Symptoms include persistent, deep-seated otalgia and headache for more than 1 week, persistent purulent otorrhea with granulation tissue in the external auditory canal, and/or the development of lower cranial nerve palsy, most commonly facial nerve palsy. Early therapeutic intervention is imperative because progression to death can be rapid [22–30].

Otalgia may be elicited in tumorous lesions in the external auditory canal. Benign tumors such as neuroma and ceruminoma rarely produce severe otalgia, and malignant squamous cell carcinoma of the external auditory canal may be painless at early stage. Deep-seated otalgia associated with granulation tissue in the external auditory canal should raise the suspicion of squamous cell carcinoma. The list of differential diagnosis includes cholesteatoma of the external auditory canal and keratosis obturans. A contrast-enhanced temporal bone CT is performed to establish the extent of temporal bone involvement and help rule out the possibility of other benign neoplasms [31–33].

3.3 Causes of the Auricle

Acute perichondritis refers to acute inflammation of the auricular perichondrium, which may be caused by extension of infections from the external auditory canal, trauma to the auricle, or piercing in the auricle. Acute perichondritis typically presents with severe pain and itching. The affected area is erythematous and edematous and may progress to involve adjacent soft tissues. Cultures of the exudates in the infected area are necessary, and Pseudomonas aeruginosa is the most common pathogen, followed by Staphylococcus aureus. Initial management includes use of topical and oral antibiotics, and, if progressed despite therapy, the skin in the affected region will begin to desquamate and the underlying cartilage can begin to weep, consequently resulting in the deformity of the auricular cartilage. If the infection becomes chronic, with continued weeping despite medical management, surgical debridement of affected cartilage is indicated [34, 35].

Relapsing polychondritis is characterized by recurrent episodes of inflammation of the perichondrium and cartilage, which eventually progress to fibrosis. It is known as one of the autoimmune diseases. Other organs may be involved in this autoimmune process, and the diagnosis of relapsing polychondritis should be considered when three or more of below-mentioned symptoms; (1) inflammation of the cartilage in both ears, (2) inflammation of the cartilage in the nose, (3) inflammation of the cartilage in the airway, (4) arthritis in five or more joints at the same time, (5) hearing or balance problems (vertigo, hearing loss, tinnitus), and (6) eye inflammation (conjunctivitis, episcleritis, scleritis, and/or uveitis). The auricle is the most commonly involved organ, and otalgia may be the only complaint. The auricle is erythematous, swollen, and tender at the early stage, and then deformed at the progressed stage [36].

4 Secondary Otalgia

Secondary otalgia is also called as "referred otalgia," and is suspected when the physical examination of the ear is normal despite of otalgia. It is important to note that the intensity of pain does not directly correspond to the severity of its underlying cause. Generally, pain is caused by heat, chemical, and mechanical stimuli, which are sensed by primary afferent nociceptors in the skin, muscles, and viscera. Because secondary pain is subjective and difficult to measure objectively, the mechanism of secondary otalgia is incompletely understood. Thus, we can perceive subjective pain without activity in primary afferent nociceptors, and there can be activity in primary afferent nociceptors without subjective pain. Moreover, afferent nociceptors from deep structures are not easy to localize and may be misinterpreted as originating from a site distant from the actual site of stimulation. Proposed hypotheses for the elusive phenomenon of secondary or referred pain are as follows; (1) A single nociceptor afferent may synapse on multiple second-order neurons, which are latent under normal conditions. When prolonged and repetitive nociceptive stimulation is implicated, previously latent second-order neurons become activated, allowing information from the unrelated site to be conveyed to higher centers of the brain [37]. (2) Sympathetic nerves may elicit referred pain by sensitizing nociceptors or restricting blood flow [38]. (3) Referred pain may be caused by the central sensitization theory, in which previously subthreshold synaptic inputs are recruited and stimulated to generate an action potential output [39, 40]. (4) A single second-order neuron receives nociceptive input from multiple primary nociceptor afferents from separate regions, but the brain cannot accurately distinguish which site the stimulus originated from thus it misinterprets and incorrectly localizes the sensation [41].

4.1 Causes of Head and Neck Problems

It has been reported that the problems of temporomandibular joint are the most common cause of secondary otalgia, and temporomandibular joint-related disorders take up about 25% of all causes of secondary otalgia [42]. Musculoskeletal disorders around the joint or the muscles of mastication may cause temporomandibular joint problems. Due to the anatomical proximity, approximately 65% of patients with temporomandibular joint disorders complain of otalgia [43]. Spasms of the mastication muscles such as temporalis, masseter, internal and external pterygoid muscles, dental problems such as bruxism, jaw clenching during sleep, and malocclusion may elicit temporomandibular joint-related secondary otalgia. Previous history of mandibulomaxillary trauma and emotional stress may predispose this type of secondary otalgia. Pain can be elicited from intrinsic joint disease, which is manifested as the mobile condyle when the mouth is opened and closed, dislocation of the disc, and clicking with mouth opening. Synovitis or osteoarthritis of the temporomandibular joint can also cause otalgia. The intensity of pain may vary and may show diurnal variation according to the cause of otalgia. If nocturnal bruxism or nocturnal jaw clenching is the cause, pain is often most severe in the morning on awakening and improves during the course of the day. Temporomandibular joint may be tender to palpation and be accompanied by other otologic symptoms such as aural fullness, tinnitus, and dizziness [44]. Spasm of the mastication muscles may occur with intrinsic temporomandibular joint disorders. Myofascial pain of the temporomandibular joint is another common cause of secondary otalgia and characterized by dull pain during mastication. The location of pain can be retro-auricular or deep in the ear. When the temporalis muscle is the cause of secondary otalgia, recurrent temporal headache is commonly accompanied. When the pterygoid muscles are suspected as the cause of secondary otalgia, intraoral palpation should be performed to evaluate for spasm. To treat temporomandibular disorders causing secondary otalgia, resting the temporomandibular joint is crucial. To rest temporomandibular joint and muscles, patients are instructed to eat a soft diet, avoid chewing gum, and apply heat around the joint. Nonsteroidal anti-inflammatory drugs relieve the symptom in most cases, though refractory cases sometimes require low-dose tricyclic antidepressants or short-term use of systemic steroids. Because the therapeutic efficacy of oral splints is still controversial, the use of oral splints is only recommended as short-term therapy. Surgery is limitedly indicated when a structural defect in the temporomandibular joint is identified by imaging or arthroscopy.

Myofascial pain syndrome can be a cause of secondary otalgia, in which muscles develop trigger points, tight bands, or shortening [45]. Mastication muscles are the most commonly involved in cases with secondary otalgia, and the lateral cervical, posterior cervical, and shoulder muscles are often involved in association with degenerative cervical spine disease. The prevalence of cervical myofascial pain syndrome is reported to be 3.6–7.0% of the population [45]. Besides otalgia, which is often described as deep ear pain, otologic symptoms such as aural fullness are common accompanying symptoms. The interval and intensity of pain expression are variable. A history of neck pain is present in the majority of patients with cervically related myofascial pain syndrome. The diagnosis of myofascial pain syndrome can be made when muscle pathology is identified and findings of degenerative upper cervical spine disease on radiographic imaging are present [42]. Physical examination focuses on careful inspection of the mastication, cervical, and shoulder muscles. Trigger points can be identified by palpation of affected muscles. Nonsteroidal anti-inflammatory drugs may relieve the symptoms. Physical therapy including ice or heat massage, myofascial release, and range-of-motion exercises may be helpful, and trigger point injection with local anesthetic can be performed in severe cases. Various inflammatory conditions in the cervical area may cause secondary otalgia. Acute lymphadenopathy and thyroiditis can produce secondary otalgia. Inflammation of the carotid sheath can also cause ear pain as well as dysphagia, odynophagia, and local carotid tenderness. Inflammation in the larynx, pharynx due to laryngopharyngeal reflux may elicit referred pain to one or both ears.

The maxillary branch of CN V innervates the maxillary and ethmoid sinuses, and problems in these paranasal sinuses may produce secondary otalgia. Acute rhinosinusitis can elicit dull, aching otalgia which fluctuates in severity. Nasal obstruction, mucopurulent rhinorrhea, anosmia, and postnasal drip are frequent symptoms. Pain and tenderness of the upper molars or maxillary area are common. Systemic symptoms such as fever and malaise are also common. Nasal endoscopic examination demonstrates hyperemic, engorged nasal mucosa, nasal obstruction, and mucopurulent nasal discharge. For the treatment of acute rhinosinusitis, systemic antibiotics, decongestants, nasal saline sprays, or irrigations are used. Because dental and periodontal structures are innervated by CN V, dental problems are common causes of secondary otalgia. Dental caries, impacted wisdom teeth, poorly fitted dentures, and peri-apical abscesses are common causes of secondary otalgia [46]. Therefore, a history of dental disease should be thoroughly sought, and the dentition should be carefully inspected. Gingiva may be swollen, erythematous, and tender. If tooth decay extends through dentine into the tooth pulp, pain is often poorly localized and commonly radiates to the cheek and ear, causing secondary otalgia [45]. Oral ulcers, such as aphthous ulcers, may also elicit otalgia, especially when they are located in the posterior tongue or peri-tonsillar area.

4.2 Causes of Aerodigestive Tract Problems

The CN IX innervates the pharynx and the larynx, and disorders in the pharynx or larynx are common causes of secondary otalgia. It has to be noted that the referred otalgia is often more intense that the pain at the primary site of pathology. Disorders in the posterior or lateral oropharynx such as ulcers, acute upper respiratory infection, and benign or malignant tumors can elicit ear pain. Eagle's syndrome, which is calcification of the styloid ligament leading to elongation of the styloid process, is uncommon cause of secondary otalgia. In this case, an elongated styloid process can be palpated manually in the tonsillar fossa. Acute pharyngitis and acute tonsillitis can often generate secondary otalgia, which is exacerbated during swallowing. Acute epiglottitis, which is characterized by severe odynophagia, hoarseness, dyspnea, and fever, may cause severe ear pain. Arytenoid arthritis may also elicit hoarseness and secondary otalgia. It is noteworthy that otalgia may be the only or most prominent symptom of a neoplasm in the pharynx or larynx. Unexplained otalgia, especially in an adult, requires a thorough evaluation of the entire pharynx and the larynx, to identify neoplasm. Malignancy should be suspected especially when weight loss, odynophagia, dysphagia, or hoarseness are associated symptoms.

5 Geniculate Neuralgia or Nervus Intermedius Neuralgia

Because branches of CN VII directly innervate parts of the ear, ear pain may develop in idiopathic acute facial nerve palsy (Bell's palsy). Geniculate neuralgia or nervus intermedius neuralgia is an uncommon condition and is characterized by severe shock-like pain deep in the ear [47, 48]. Geniculate neuralgia is related to disorders of nervus intermedius and generally assumed to be caused by microvascular compression or varicella zoster infection [49]. The name nervus intermedius originated from its intermediate position between the facial nerve and superior portion of the vestibular nerves. Three types of fibers are included in the nervus intermedius: (1) Somatic sensory afferents from the external auditory canal, tympanic membrane, retro-auricular skin, and soft palate. (2) Special sensory (taste) from the anterior two-thirds of the tongue, floor of the mouth, and palate. (3) Parasympathetic efferents to the lacrimal, sublingual, submandibular, and nasopalatine glands. Neuronal cell bodies of the gustatory and sensory fibers are located in the geniculate ganglion. Resection of the nervus intermedius resulted in a decrease in the cutaneous sensitivity around the cavum concha, part of the external auditory canal, tympanic membrane, anterior nasopharynx, and the area behind the ear over that mastoid process [50]. The International Headache Society defines geniculate neuralgia as intermittent episodes of pain located deep in the ear that last for seconds or minutes and describes the posterior wall of the auditory canal may be a trigger zone [51]. Problems in taste, salivation, and/or lacrimation may be accompanyingsymptoms. Definitive diagnosis of geniculate neuralgia is difficult in most cases, because sensory innervation of the external auditory canal is made by not only CN VII but also CNs III, IX, and X. Clinically, the "deep ear pain" in geniculate neuralgia is indistinguishable to that in trigeminal neuralgia or glossopharyngeal neuralgia. Peris-Celda et al. reported that 64% of patients with geniculate neuralgia presented with complex symptoms exhibiting features consistent with geniculate neuralgia and at least one additional cranial neuralgia [49]. Treatment for geniculate neuralgia generally begins with medical management by carbamazepine, gabapentin, opioid, baclofen, lamotrigine, oxcarbazepine, or nonsteroidal anti-inflammatory drugs. If medical therapy fails, two surgical options may be considered; microvascular decompression or sectioning of the nervus intermedius. When neurovascular cross-compression of nervus intermedius is encountered, the anterior inferior cerebellar artery is often the offending vessel [48]. Successful sectioning of the nervus intermedius was first reported for the treatment of geniculate neuralgia in 1909 [52], and, however, the efficacy of exploratory surgery with sectioning of nervus intermedius for long-term relief of geniculate neuralgia remains unconvincing [53–55].

6 Summary

Otalgia is a common symptom, and the causes can be either otologic or non-otologic. To identify diverse causes of otalgia, a comprehensive history taking and physical examination are important. Furthermore, complex innervation by CNs V, VII, IX, and X in this area should be well understood for the differential diagnosis between primary and secondary otalgia.

References

1. Harrison E, Cronin M. Otalgia. Aust Fam Physician. 2016;45(7):493–7.
2. Olsen KD. The many causes of otalgia. Infection, trauma, cancer. Postgrad Med. 1986;80(6):50–2., 55–56, 61–53. https://doi.org/10.1080/00325481.1986.11699588.
3. Neilan RE, Roland PS. Otalgia. Med Clin North Am. 2010;94(5):961–71. https://doi.org/10.1016/j.mcna.2010.05.004.
4. Yanagisawa K, Kveton JF. Referred otalgia. Am J Otolaryngol. 1992;13(6):323–7. https://doi.org/10.1016/0196-0709(92)90072-2.
5. Mirza S, Richardson H. Otic barotrauma from air travel. J Laryngol Otol. 2005;119(5):366–70. https://doi.org/10.1258/0022215053945723.
6. Ely JW, Hansen MR, Clark EC. Diagnosis of ear pain. Am Fam Physician. 2008;77(5):621–8.
7. Garcia C, Salgueiro AB, Luís C, Correia P, Brito MJ. Acute mastoiditis in children: middle ear cultures may help in reducing use of broad spectrum antibiotics. Int J Pediatr Otorhinolaryngol. 2017;92:32–7. https://doi.org/10.1016/j.ijporl.2016.11.002.
8. Al-Khudari S, Loochtan M, Yaremchuk K. Roller coaster-induced barotrauma. Laryngoscope. 2011;121(3):501–2. https://doi.org/10.1002/lary.21424.
9. Blanshard J, Toma A, Bryson P, Williamson P. Middle ear barotrauma in patients undergoing hyperbaric oxygen therapy. Clin Otolaryngol Allied Sci. 1996;21(5):400–3. https://doi.org/10.1046/j.1365-2273.1996.00813.x.
10. Carmichael ML, Boyev KP. Middle ear barotrauma causing transient facial nerve paralysis after scuba diving. Diving Hyperb Med. 2016;46(4):260–1.
11. Jansen S, Meyer MF, Boor M, Felsch M, Kluenter HD, Pracht ED, Hüttenbrink KB, Beutner D, Grosheva M. Prevalence of barotrauma in recreational scuba divers after repetitive saltwater dives. Otol Neurotol. 2016;37(9):1325–31. https://doi.org/10.1097/mao.0000000000001158.
12. Wang MC, Liu CY, Shiao AS, Wang T. Ear problems in swimmers. J Chin Med Assoc: JCMA. 2005;68(8):347–52. https://doi.org/10.1016/s1726-4901(09)70174-1.
13. Kim CH, Shin JE. Hemorrhage within the tympanic membrane without perforation. J Otolaryngol Head Neck Surg. 2018;47(1):66. https://doi.org/10.1186/s40463-018-0300-0.
14. Gabriel OT. Cerumen impaction: challenges and management profile in a rural health facility. Niger J med Assoc. 2015;56(6):390–3. https://doi.org/10.4103/0300-1652.171620.
15. Soy FK, Ozbay C, Kulduk E, Dundar R, Yazıcı H, Sakarya EU. A new approach for cerumenolytic treatment in children: in vivo and in vitro study. Int J Pediatr Otorhinolaryngol. 2015;79(7):1096–100. https://doi.org/10.1016/j.ijporl.2015.04.039.
16. Rosenfeld RM, Schwartz SR, Cannon CR, Roland PS, Simon GR, Kumar KA, Huang WW, Haskell HW, Robertson PJ. Clinical practice guideline: acute otitis externa. Otolaryngol Head Neck Surg. 2014;150(1 Suppl):S1–s24. https://doi.org/10.1177/0194599813517083.
17. Price J. Otitis externa in children. J R Coll Gen Pract. 1976;26(169):610–5.
18. Sarrell EM, Mandelberg A, Cohen HA. Efficacy of naturopathic extracts in the management of ear pain associated with acute otitis media. Arch Pediatr Adolesc Med. 2001;155(7):796–9. https://doi.org/10.1001/archpedi.155.7.796.
19. Rosenfeld JA, Clarity G. Acute otitis media in children. Prim Care. 1996;23(4):677–86. https://doi.org/10.1016/s0095-4543(05)70356-0.
20. Rosenfeld RM, Shin JJ, Schwartz SR, Coggins R, Gagnon L, Hackell JM, Hoelting D, Hunter LL,

Kummer AW, Payne SC, Poe DS, Veling M, Vila PM, Walsh SA, Corrigan MD. Clinical practice guideline: otitis media with effusion (update). Otolaryngol Head Neck Surg. 2016;154(1 Suppl):S1–s41. https://doi.org/10.1177/0194599815623467.
21. Roland PS, Belcher BP, Bettis R, Makabale RL, Conroy PJ, Wall GM, Dupre S, Potts S, Hogg G, Weber K. A single topical agent is clinically equivalent to the combination of topical and oral antibiotic treatment for otitis externa. Am J Otolaryngol. 2008;29(4):255–61. https://doi.org/10.1016/j.amjoto.2007.09.002.
22. Babiatzki A, Sadé J. Malignant external otitis. J Laryngol Otol. 1987;101(3):205–10. https://doi.org/10.1017/s0022215100101549.
23. Barrow HN, Levenson MJ. Necrotizing 'malignant' external otitis caused by Staphylococcus epidermidis. Arch Otolaryngol Head Neck Surg. 1992;118(1):94–6. https://doi.org/10.1001/archotol.1992.01880010098023.
24. Di Lullo AM, Russo C, Piroli P, Petti A, Capriglione P, Cantone E, Motta G, Iengo M, Elefante A, Cavaliere M. Malignant otitis external: our experience and literature review. Am J Med Case Rep. 2020;21:e925060. https://doi.org/10.12659/ajcr.925060.
25. Ferlito S, Maniaci A, Di Luca M, Grillo C, Mannelli L, Salvatore M, La Mantia I, Spinato G, Cocuzza S. From uncommon infection to multi-cranial palsy: malignant external otitis insights. Dose Response. 2020;18(4):1559325820963910. https://doi.org/10.1177/1559325820963910.
26. Karaman E, Yilmaz M, Ibrahimov M, Haciyev Y, Enver O. Malignant otitis externa. J Craniofac Surg. 2012;23(6):1748–51. https://doi.org/10.1097/SCS.0b013e31825e4d9a.
27. Rubin J, Yu VL. Malignant external otitis: insights into pathogenesis, clinical manifestations, diagnosis, and therapy. Am J Med. 1988;85(3):391–8. https://doi.org/10.1016/0002-9343(88)90592-x.
28. Rubin J, Yu VL, Stool SE. Malignant external otitis in children. J Pediatr. 1988;113(6):965–70. https://doi.org/10.1016/s0022-3476(88)80564-x.
29. Shimizu T, Ishinaga H, Seno S, Majima Y. Malignant external otitis: treatment with prolonged usage of antibiotics and Burow's solution. Auris Nasus Larynx. 2005;32(4):403–6. https://doi.org/10.1016/j.anl.2005.05.010.
30. Yu LH, Shu CH, Tu TY, Shiao AS, Lien CF. Malignant otitis externa. Chinese Med J Free China Ed. 1999;62(6):362–8.
31. Al-Shihabi BA. Carcinoma of temporal bone presenting as malignant otitis externa. J Laryngol Otol. 1992;106(10):908–10. https://doi.org/10.1017/s0022215100121255.
32. Chee G, Mok P, Sim R. Squamous cell carcinoma of the temporal bone: diagnosis, treatment and prognosis. Singap Med J. 2000;41(9):441–6.
33. Leong SC, Youssef A, Lesser TH. Squamous cell carcinoma of the temporal bone: outcomes of radical surgery and postoperative radiotherapy. Laryngoscope. 2013;123(10):2442–8. https://doi.org/10.1002/lary.24063.
34. Bress E, Cohn JE. Perichondritis: inspect the lobule. Int J Emerg Med. 2020;13(1):51. https://doi.org/10.1186/s12245-020-00310-z.
35. Savastano M, Ferraro SM, Marioni G. Perichondritis with or without external otitis and intradermal injection: a new therapeutic approach. J Otolaryngol Head Neck Surg. 2009;38(5):568–72.
36. Borgia F, Giuffrida R, Guarneri F, Cannavò SP. Relapsing polychondritis: an updated review. Biomedicine. 2018;6(3):84. https://doi.org/10.3390/biomedicines6030084.
37. Murray GM. (2009) referred pain, allodynia and hyperalgesia. J Am Dent Assoc. 1939;140(9):1122–4. https://doi.org/10.14219/jada.archive.2009.0339.
38. Procacci P, Zoppi M, Maresca M, Sereni E. [Analgesic action of tetracosactide in chronic pain syndromes]. Clin Ter. 1981;98(6):643–6.
39. Pace MC, Passavanti MB, De Nardis L, Bosco F, Sansone P, Pota V, Barbarisi M, Palagiano A, Iannotti FA, Panza E, Aurilio C. Nociceptor plasticity: a closer look. J Cell Physiol. 2018;233(4):2824–38. https://doi.org/10.1002/jcp.25993.
40. Woolf CJ. Central sensitization: implications for the diagnosis and treatment of pain. Pain. 2011;152(3 Suppl):S2–s15. https://doi.org/10.1016/j.pain.2010.09.030.
41. Foreman RD, Schmidt RF, Willis WD. Effects of mechanical and chemical stimulation of fine muscle afferents upon primate spinothalamic tract cells. J Physiol. 1979;286:215–31. https://doi.org/10.1113/jphysiol.1979.sp012615.
42. Jaber JJ, Leonetti JP, Lawrason AE, Feustel PJ. Cervical spine causes for referred otalgia. Otolaryngol Head Neck Surg. 2008;138(4):479–85. https://doi.org/10.1016/j.otohns.2007.12.043.
43. Charlett SD, Coatesworth AP. Referred otalgia: a structured approach to diagnosis and treatment. Int J Clin Pract. 2007;61(6):1015–21. https://doi.org/10.1111/j.1742-1241.2006.00932.x.
44. Cooper BC, Cooper DL. Recognizing otolaryngologic symptoms in patients with temporomandibular disorders. Cranio J Craniomandib Pract. 1993;11(4):260–7. https://doi.org/10.1080/08869634.1993.11677977.
45. Teachey WS. Otolaryngic myofascial pain syndromes. Curr Pain Headache Rep. 2004;8(6):457–62. https://doi.org/10.1007/s11916-004-0067-z.
46. Kreisberg MK, Turner J. Dental causes of referred otalgia. Ear Nose Throat J. 1987;66(10):398–408.
47. Nanda A, Khan IS. Nervus intermedius and geniculate neuralgia. World Neurosurg. 2013;79(5–6):651–2. https://doi.org/10.1016/j.wneu.2012.05.002.
48. Ouaknine GE, Robert F, Molina-Negro P, Hardy J. Geniculate neuralgia and audio-vestibular disturbances due to compression of the intermediate and eighth nerves by the postero-inferior cerebellar artery. Surg Neurol. 1980;13(2):147–50.
49. Peris-Celda M, Oushy S, Perry A, Graffeo CS, Carlstrom LP, Zimmerman RS, Meyer FB, Pollock

BE, Link MJ. Nervus intermedius and the surgical management of geniculate neuralgia. J Neurosurg. 2018;131(2):343–51. https://doi.org/10.3171/2018.3.Jns172920.
50. Rowed DW. Chronic cluster headache managed by nervus intermedius section. Headache. 1990;30(7):401–6. https://doi.org/10.1111/j.1526-4610.1990.hed3007401.x.
51. Headache Classification Committee of the International Headache Society. Classification and diagnostic criteria for headache disorders, cranial neuralgias and facial pain. Cephalalgia. 1988;8(Suppl 7):1–96.
52. Clark L, Taylor A. Ture tic douloureux of the sensory filaments of the facial nerve. I. Clinical report of a case in which cure was effected by physiological extirpation of the geniculate ganglion: Report of surgical treatment JAMA. J Am Med Assoc. 1909;53:2144–6.
53. Rupa V, Saunders RL, Weider DJ. Geniculate neuralgia: the surgical management of primary otalgia. J Neurosurg. 1991;75(4):505–11. https://doi.org/10.3171/jns.1991.75.4.0505.
54. Pulec JL. Geniculate neuralgia: long-term results of surgical treatment. Ear Nose Throat J. 2002;81(1):30–3.
55. Sakas DE, Panourias IG, Stranjalis G, Stefanatou MP, Maratheftis N, Bontozoglou N. Paroxysmal otalgia due to compression of the intermediate nerve: a distinct syndrome of neurovascular conflict confirmed by neuroimaging. Case report. J Neurosurg. 2007;107(6):1228–30. https://doi.org/10.3171/jns-07/12/1228.

The manufacturer's authorised representative in the EU is Springer
Nature Customer Service Centre GmbH, Europaplatz 3, 69115 Heidelberg,
Germany. If you have any concerns regarding our products, please
contact ProductSafety@springernature.com

Printed and bound by CPI Group (UK) Ltd, Croydon, CR0 4YY
30/09/2026
02225240-0018